Amsler's Grid

The chart on the opposite page is patterned after the grid devised by Professor Marc Amsler. It can provide for the rapid detection of small irregularities in the central 20° of the field of vision. The chart is composed of a grid of lines containing a central white fixation spot. The squares on the grid are 5 mm in size and subtend a visual angle of 1° at 30 cm viewing distance.

The chart is to be viewed in modest light monocularly at a distance of 28-30 cm utilizing the correct refraction for this distance. Viewing should be accomplished without previous ophthalmoscopy and without instillation of any drugs affecting pupillary size or accommodation.

A series of questions should be asked while the patient is viewing the central white spot.

1) Is the center spot visible? The absence of the spot may indicate the presence of a central scotoma.

2) While viewing the center white spot can you see all four sides? The inability to perceive these areas may indicate the presence of an arcuate scotoma of glaucoma encroaching upon the central area or a centrocecal scotoma.

3) Do you see the entire grid intact? Are there any defects? If an area of the grid is not visible, then a paracentral scotoma is present.

4) Are the horizontal and vertical lines straight and parallel? If not, then metamorphopsia is present. The parallel lines may "bend" inwards giving rise to micropsia or "bend" outwards giving rise to macropsia.

5) Do you see any blur or distortion in the grid? Any movement? A color aberration? These changes may be present prior to the appearance of a definite scotoma.

PDR® -for all of your drug information needs.

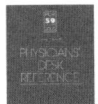
2005 Physicians' Desk Reference®
Physicians have turned to the PDR for the latest word on prescription drugs for 59 years. Today, PDR is still considered the standard prescription drug reference and can be found in virtually every physician's office, hospital and pharmacy in the United States. You can search the more than 4,000 drugs by using one of many indices and look at more than 2,100 full-color photos of drugs cross-referenced to the label information.

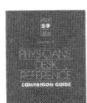
2005 PDR® Companion Guide
This unique 1,900-page all-in-one clinical companion to the PDR ensures safe, appropriate drug selection with eight critical checkpoint indices including *Indications, Side Effects, Interactions,* and much more.

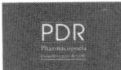
PDR® Pharmacopoeia Pocket Dosing Guide – Fifth Edition 2005
This pocket dosing guide brings important dispensing information to the practitioner's fingertips. Organized in tabular format, this small, 300-page quick reference is easy to navigate and gives important FDA-approved dosing information, black box warning summaries and much more, whenever it is needed. At the point of care, rely on PDR Pharmacopoeia for quick dosing information.

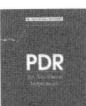
PDR® for Nutritional Supplements – 1st Edition
The definitive information source for more than 300 nutritional supplements. This unique, comprehensive, unbiased source of solid, evidence-based information about nutritional supplements provides practitioners with more than 700 pages of the most current and reliable information available.

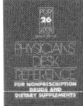
2005 PDR® for Nonprescription Drugs and Dietary Supplements
This acknowledged authority offers full FDA-approved descriptions of the most commonly used OTC medicines in four separate indices within more than 400 pages. Plus, it includes a section on supplements, vitamins and herbal remedies.

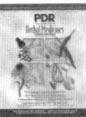
PDR® for Herbal Medicines – 3rd Edition
The third edition goes far beyond the original source, adding a new section on Nutritional Supplements and new information aimed at greatly enhancing patient management by medical practitioners. All monographs have been updated to include recent scientific findings on efficacy, safety and potential interactions; clinical trials (including abstracts); case reports; and meta-analysis results. This new information has resulted in greatly expanded Effects, Contraindications, Precautions and Adverse Reactions, and Dosage sections of each monograph.

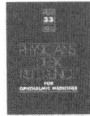
2005 PDR® for Ophthalmic Medicines
The definitive reference for the eye-care professional offers 230 pages of detailed information on drugs and equipment used in the fields of ophthalmology and optometry. With five full indices and information on specialized instruments, lenses and much more, this guide is the most comprehensive of its kind.

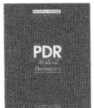
PDR® Medical Dictionary – 2nd Edition
The second edition reflects the thorough revision performed by 44 medical consultants as well as a team of skilled editors and lexicographers. This fully updated edition, with more than 2,100 pages, includes 1,000 images, numerous tables, an innovative Genus Finder to help you find the genus of organisms, and much more!

PDR® Drug Guide for Mental Health Professionals – 2nd Edition
The *PDR® Drug Guide for Mental Health Professionals* was created to help you understand the beneficial effects—and the dangerous side effects—of today's potent psychotherapeutic medications. Over 75 common psychotropic drugs are profiled by brand name. All this vital information is presented in an easy-to-read format, written in nontechnical language, and drawn from the FDA-approved PDR database.

PDR® Monthly Prescribing Guide™
This portable monthly digest provides healthcare professionals with the most up-to-date prescribing information for over 2,000 commonly prescribed medications. Each monograph includes clear and concise prescribing details, cross-referenced to the annual PDR.

Complete Your 2005 PDR® Library NOW! Enclose payment and save shipping costs.

Code		Item	Price	$
260000	_____ copies	**2005 Physicians' Desk Reference®**	$92.95 ea.	$_____
260018	_____ copies	**2005 PDR® Companion Guide**	$71.95 ea.	$_____
260059	_____ copies	**PDR® Pharmacopoeia Pocket Dosing Guide***	$8.95 ea.	$_____
260133	_____ copies	**PDR® for Nutritional Supplements, 1st EDITION!**	$59.95 ea.	$_____
260026	_____ copies	**2005 PDR® for Nonprescription Drugs and Dietary Supplements**	$59.95 ea.	$_____
260125	_____ copies	**PDR® for Herbal Medicines, 3rd EDITION!**	$59.95 ea.	$_____
260034	_____ copies	**2005 PDR® for Ophthalmic Medicines**	$67.95 ea.	$_____
260158	_____ copies	**PDR® Medical Dictionary, 2nd EDITION!**	$49.95 ea.	$_____
260117	_____ copies	**PDR® Drug Guide for Mental Health Professionals 2nd EDITION!**	$39.95 ea.	$_____
	_____ copies	**PDR® Monthly Prescribing Guide™ (yearly subscription)**	$49.00 ea.	$_____
		Shipping & Handling (Add $9.95 S&H per book if paying later*)		$_____
		Sales Tax (FL, IA, & NJ)		$_____
		Total Amount of Order		$_____

(*Shipping and handling is $1.95 for PDR Pharmacopoeia)

Mail this order form to: **PDR**, P.O. Box 10336, Des Moines, IA 50336-0689
e-mail: PDR.customerservice@thomson.com

**For Faster Service—FAX YOUR ORDER (515) 284-6714
or CALL TOLL-FREE (888) 859-8053**
Do not mail a confirmation order in addition to this fax.
Valid for 2005 editions only, prices and shipping & handling higher outside U.S.

PLEASE INDICATE METHOD OF PAYMENT:
Payment Enclosed (shipping & handling FREE)
☐ Check payable to PDR
☐ VISA ☐ MasterCard
☐ Discover ☐ American Express

Account No. _____
Exp. Date _____
Telephone No. _____
Signature _____
Name _____
Address _____
City _____
State/Zip _____

☐ **Bill me later** (Add $9.95 per book for shipping and handling*)

SAVE TIME AND MONEY EVERY YEAR AS A STANDING ORDER SUBSCRIBER
☐ Check here to enter your standing order for future editions of publications ordered. They will be shipped to you automatically, after advance notice. As a standing order subscriber, you are **guaranteed** our lowest price offer, earliest delivery and FREE shipping and handling.

KEY 773101

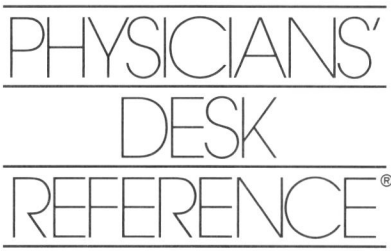

FOR OPHTHALMIC MEDICINES

Editorial Consultants and Contributors

Douglas J. Rhee, MD, Assistant Surgeon, Glaucoma Service, Wills Eye Hospital; Assistant Professor of Ophthalmology; and Assistant Professor of Pathology, Anatomy, and Cell Biology, Jefferson Medical College of Thomas Jefferson University, Philadelphia, PA
Christopher J. Rapuano, MD, Attending Surgeon, Cornea Service, Wills Eye Hospital; and Professor of Ophthalmology; Jefferson Medical College of Thomas Jefferson University, Philadelphia, PA
Theresa L. Belzer, RPh, Pharmacy Manager, Jefferson Hospital for Neuroscience and Wills Eye Hospital, Philadelphia, PA
F.W. Fraunfelder, MD, Director, National Registry of Drug-Induced Ocular Side Effects; and Assistant Professor of Ophthalmology, Casey Eye Institute, Oregon Health & Science University, Portland, OR

Executive Vice President, PDR: David Duplay

Vice President, Sales and Marketing: Dikran N. Barsamian
Senior Director, Pharmaceutical Sales: Anthony Sorce
Account Managers: Kevin McGlynn, Eileen Sullivan
Director of Trade Sales: Bill Gaffney
Senior Director, Brand and Product Management: Valerie E. Berger
Director, Brand and Product Management: Carmen Mazzatta
Finance Director: Mark S. Ritchin
Senior Director, Publishing Sales and Marketing: Michael Bennett
Associate Director of Marketing: Jennifer M. Fronzaglia
Senior Marketing Manager: Kim Marich
Direct Mail Manager: Lorraine M. Loening
Manager of Marketing Analysis: Dina A. Maeder
Promotion Manager: Linda Levine
Vice President, Regulatory Affairs: Mukesh Mehta, RPh
Vice President, PDR Services: Brian Holland
Director of Operations: Rob Klein
Director of PDR Content: Jeffrey D. Schaefer
Clinical Content Operations Manager: Thomas Fleming, PharmD
Manager, Editorial Services: Bette LaGow
Senior Pharmacy Manager: Tammy Chernin, RPh

Drug Information Specialists: Min Ko, PharmD; Sheila Talatala, PharmD; Greg Tallis, RPh
Project Editor: Harris Fleming
Senior Editor: Lori Murray
Production Editor: Gwynned L. Kelly
PDR Production Manager: Joseph F. Rizzo
Manager, Production Purchasing: Thomas Westburgh
Production Specialist: Christina Klinger
Senior Production Coordinator: Gianna Caradonna
Production Coordinator: Yasmin Hernández
Senior Index Editors: Noel Deloughery, Shannon Reilly
Format Editor: Michelle S. Guzman
Production Associate: Joan K. Akerlind
Production Design Supervisor: Adeline Rich
Senior Electronic Publishing Designer: Livio Udina
Electronic Publishing Designers: Bryan C. Dix, Rosalia Sberna
Digital Imaging Manager: Christopher Husted
Digital Imaging Coordinator: Michael Labruyere
Director of Client Services: Stephanie Struble

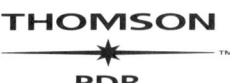

Copyright © 2004 and published by Thomson PDR at Montvale, NJ 07645-1742. All rights reserved. None of the content of this publication may be reproduced, stored in a retrieval system, resold, redistributed, or transmitted in any form or by any means (electronic, mechanical, photocopying, recording, or otherwise) without the prior written permission of the publisher. PHYSICIANS' DESK REFERENCE®, PDR®, Pocket PDR®, PDR Family Guide to Prescription Drugs®, PDR Family Guide to Women's Health and Prescription Drugs®, and PDR Family Guide to Nutrition and Health® are registered trademarks used herein under license. PDR® for Ophthalmic Medicines, PDR® for Nonprescription Drugs and Dietary Supplements, PDR® Companion Guide, PDR® Pharmacopoeia, PDR® for Herbal Medicines, PDR® for Nutritional Supplements, PDR® Medical Dictionary, PDR® Nurse's Drug Handbook™, PDR® Nurse's Dictionary, PDR® Family Guide Encyclopedia of Medical Care, PDR® Family Guide to Natural Medicines and Healing Therapies, PDR® Family Guide to Common Ailments, PDR® Family Guide to Over-the-Counter Drugs, PDR® Family Guide to Nutritional Supplements, and PDR® Electronic Library are trademarks used herein under license.

Officers of Thomson Healthcare, Inc.: *President and Chief Executive Officer:* Richard Noble; *Chief Financial Officer:* Paul Hilger; *Executive Vice President, Clinical Trials:* Tom Kelly; *Executive Vice President, Medical Education:* Jeff MacDonald; *Executive Vice President, Clinical Solutions:* Jeff Reihl; *Executive Vice President, PDR:* David Duplay; *Senior Vice President, Business Development:* Robert Christopher; *Vice President, Human Resources:* Pamela M. Bilash; *President, Physician's World:* Marty Cearnal

ISBN: 1-56363-502-X

FOREWORD TO THE THIRTY-THIRD EDITION

Thomson PDR is pleased to provide eyecare professionals with the nation's most authoritative guide to ophthalmic pharmaceuticals. Completely revised for 2005, the *PDR® for Ophthalmic Medicines* includes complete, FDA-approved guidelines for hundreds of leading eyecare products, as well as information on of newly released medications. In addition, the book's opening sections feature useful tables summarizing the major pharmaceutical alternatives currently available in ophthalmology, as well as a brief guide to suture materials and information on vision standards and low vision. There are also lens comparison and conversion tables and a directory of soft contact lenses manufacturers. Four detailed indices help you locate products by manufacturer, trade name, product category, and active ingredient; and a full-color product identification section features photos of many leading ophthalmic medications.

The special reference sections near the beginning of *PDR for Ophthalmic Medicines* have been prepared with the assistance of Douglas J. Rhee, MD, Christopher J. Rapuano, MD, and Theresa L. Belzer, RPh, of Wills Eye Hospital in Philadelphia. Our thanks also go to F.W. Fraunfelder, MD, of Oregon Health & Science University in Portland, who edited the section on ocular toxicology. The opinions expressed in these sections are those of the authors and are not necessarily endorsed by the publisher.

Essential Prescribing Aids from PDR

For complicated cases and special patient problems, there is of course no substitute for the in-depth data contained in *Physicians' Desk Reference*. But on other occasions, you may find that the *PDR® Monthly Prescribing Guide™* provides a practical alternative. Distilled from the pages of *PDR*, this 350-page digest-sized reference presents the key facts on more than 1,000 drugs, including the form, strength, and route; therapeutic class; approved indications; dosage; contraindications; warnings; precautions; pregnancy rating; drug interactions; and adverse reactions. Each entry alerts you to the significant precautions you need to take, spells out the most common or dangerous adverse effects, summarizes the recommended adult and pediatric dosages, and supplies you with the *PDR* page number to turn to for further prescribing information.

Issued monthly, the guide is continuously updated with the latest FDA-approved revisions to existing product information, augmented with detailed descriptions of recently approved medications. In addition, you'll receive bulletins about major new pharmaceutical developments, an overview of important new agents nearing approval, an update on the latest news on herbal and nutritional supplements, and a handy reminder of upcoming medical meetings. In fact, in one neat package you'll find just about everything you need to make a routine prescribing decision—secure in the knowledge that you're acting on the latest FDA-approved data. To order your personal subscription to this important new monthly publication, simply call 800-232-7379.

If you prefer to keep information such as this on a handheld device like a Palm or Pocket PC, another of our other reference guides may be just what you're looking for. Called **mobilePDR®**, this easy-to-use software allows you to instantly retrieve the basic facts you need on any drug, lets you run automatic interaction checks on multidrug regimens, and even alerts you to significant events such as product recalls, new product introductions, and new dosing and indication approvals. Covering a total of 1,600 drugs, this portable electronic reference is updated daily based on the latest FDA-approved package inserts. mobilePDR is available for downloading at www.PDR.net. It works with both the Palm and Pocket PC operating systems, and it's free to U.S.–based MDs, DOs, NPs, and PAs in full-time patient practice as well as to medical students and residents.

PDR and its major companion volumes are also found in the *PDR® Electronic Library* on CD-ROM, now used in over 100,000 practices. This Windows-compatible disc provides users with a complete database of *PDR* prescribing information, electronically searchable for instant retrieval. A standard subscription includes *PDR's* sophisticated search software and an extensive file of chemical structures, illustrations, and full-color product photographs. Optional enhancements include the complete contents of *The Merck Manual Seventeenth Edition, Stedman's Medical Dictionary,* and *Stedman's Spellchecker.* For anyone who wants to run a fast double check on a proposed prescription, there's also the *PDR® Drug Interactions and Side Effects System* — sophisticated software capable of automatically screening a 20-drug regimen for conflicts, then proposing alternatives for any problematic medication. This unique decision-making tool now comes free with the *PDR Electronic Library.*

For more information on these or any other members of the growing family of *PDR* products, please call, toll-free, 800-232-7379 or fax 201-722-2680.

About This Book

Physicians' Desk Reference for Ophthalmic Medicines is made possible through the courtesy of the manufacturers whose products appear in it. The information on each pharmaceutical product described in the book has been prepared by the manufacturer and edited and approved by the manufacturer's medical department, medical director, or medical counsel.

Under the federal Food, Drug & Cosmetics (FD&C) Act, a drug approved for marketing may be labeled, promoted, and advertised by the manufacturer for only those uses for which the drug's safety and effectiveness have been established. The Code of Federal Regulations 201.100(d)(1) pertaining to labeling for prescription products requires that in the text of *Physicians' Desk Reference for Ophthalmic Medicines,* "indications, effects, dosages, routes, methods, and frequency and duration of administration and any relevant warnings, hazards, contraindications, side effects, and precautions" must be in the "*same language and emphasis*" as the approved labeling for the products. FDA regards the words *same language and emphasis* as requiring VERBATIM use of the approved labeling information. Furthermore, information in the approved labeling that is emphasized by the use of capitals, boldface, or italics, or that is placed in a box, must be given the same emphasis in *Physicians' Desk Reference for Ophthalmic Medicines.*

The FDA has also recognized that the FD&C Act does not, however, limit the manner in which a physician may use an approved drug. Once a product has been approved for marketing, a physician may prescribe it for uses or in treatment regimens or patient populations that are not included in approved labeling. The FDA also observes that accepted medical practice often includes drug use that is not reflected in approved drug labeling. For products that do not have official package circulars, the publisher has emphasized the necessity of describing such products comprehensively, so that physicians have access to all information essential for intelligent and informed decision making. Particularly in the case of over-the-counter dietary supplements, it should be remembered that this information has not been evaluated by the FDA, and that such products are not intended to diagnose, treat, cure, or prevent any disease.

The function of the publisher is the compilation, organization, and distribution of this information. In organizing and presenting the material in *Physicians' Desk Reference for Ophthalmic Medicines,* the publisher does not warrant or guarantee any of the products described, or perform any independent analysis in connection with any of the product information contained herein. *Physicians' Desk Reference for Ophthalmic Medicines* does not assume, and expressly disclaims, any obligation to obtain and include any information other than that provided to it by the manufacturer. It should be understood that by making this material available the publisher is not advocating the use of any product described herein, nor is the publisher responsible for misuse of a product due to typographical error. Additional information on any product may be obtained from the manufacturer.

CONTENTS

Section 1. Indices — Page I
1. Manufacturers' Index I
2. Product Name Index III
3. Product Category Index V
4. Active Ingredients Index VII

Section 2. Pharmaceuticals in Ophthalmology — Page 1
1. Mydriatics and Cycloplegics 2
2. Antimicrobial Therapy 2
3. Ocular Anti-Inflammatory Agents 8
4. Anesthetic Agents 10
5. Agents for Treatment of Glaucoma 11
6. Medications for Dry Eye 14
7. Ocular Decongestants 15
8. Ophthalmic Irrigating Solutions 16
9. Hyperosmolar Agents 16
10. Diagnostic Agents 16
11. Viscoelastic Materials Used in Ophthalmology 17
12. Off-Label Drug Applications in Ophthalmology 18
13. Ocular Toxicology 19

Section 3. Suture Materials — Page 23

Section 4. Ophthalmic Lenses — Page 25
1. Comparison and Conversion Tables 25
2. Soft Contact Lenses Manufacturer Directory 28

Section 5. Vision Standards and Low-Vision Aids — Page 30
1. Vision Standards 30
2. Low-Vision Aids 32

Section 6. Product Identification Guide — Page 101

Section 7. Product Information on Pharmaceuticals and Equipment — Page 201

Section 8. Intraocular Product Information — Page 297

Amsler's Grid .... Inside Front Cover

SECTION 1
INDICES

This section offers four ways to locate the product information you need:

1. Manufacturers' Index: Gives the location of each participating manufacturer's product information. If two page numbers appear, the first refers to photographs in the Product Identification Guide, the second to product information. Also listed are the addresses and telephone numbers of the company's headquarters and regional offices.

2. Product Name Index: Lists page numbers of product information alphabetically by brand name. A diamond symbol to the left of a name indicates that a photograph of the item appears in the Product Identification Guide. For these products, the first page number refers to the photograph, the second to an entry in one of the Product Information Sections. All pharmaceuticals, equipment, and intraocular products are included.

3. Product Category Index: Lists products alphabetically by type or category, such as "Anti-Infectives" or "Hypertonic Agents." All pharmaceuticals, equipment, and intraocular products are included.

4. Active Ingredients Index: Groups products alphabetically by generic name or material, such as "Atropine Sulfate" or "Dexamethasone." Under each heading, all fully described products are listed first, followed by those with only partial descriptions. Equipment is not included.

PART I/MANUFACTURERS' INDEX

ALCON LABORATORIES, INC.   201
and its Affiliates
Corporate Headquarters
6201 South Freeway
Fort Worth, TX 76134
Direct Inquiries to:
Pharmaceutical/Consumer Products:
(800) 451-3937
(Therapeutic Drugs/Lens Care)
Surgical: (800) 862-5266
(Instrumentation/Surgical Meds)

ALLERGAN   103, 215
2525 Dupont Drive
P.O. Box 19534
Irvine, CA 92623-9534
For Medical Information, Contact:
Outside CA: (800) 433-8871
CA: (714) 246-4500
Sales and Ordering:
Outside CA: (800) 377-7790
CA: (714) 246-4500

BAUSCH & LOMB INCORPORATED   244
Surgical Division
180 East Via Verde
San Dimas, CA 91773
Direct Inquiries to:
Customer Service
(800) 338-2020

BAUSCH & LOMB INCORPORATED   104, 244
8500 Hidden River Parkway
Tampa, FL 33637
Direct Inquiries to:
Customer Service Department:
(800) 323-0000
(813) 975-7700

DURAMED PHARMACEUTICALS, INC.   257
Subsidiary of Barr Pharmaceuticals, Inc.
2 Quaker Road
Pomona, NY 10970
Direct Inquires to:
(877) 405-0369

FALCON PHARMACEUTICALS LTD.   258
6201 South Freeway
Fort Worth, TX 76134
Direct Inquiries to:
Falcon Pharmaceuticals, Ltd.
(800) 343-2133

KING PHARMACEUTICALS, INC.   104, 261
501 Fifth Street
Bristol, TN 37620
Direct Inquiries to:
(800) 776-3637
(423) 989-8786

MERCK & CO., INC.   104, 264
P.O. Box 4
West Point, PA 19486-0004
For Product and Service Information, and Adverse Experience Reports, call the Merck National Service Center, 8:00 AM to 7:00 PM (ET), Monday through Friday:
(800) NSC-MERCK
(800) 672-6372
FAX: (800) MERCK-68
FAX: (800) 637-2568
24-Hour Emergency Product Information for Healthcare Professionals, Call:
(800) NSC-MERCK
(800) 672-6372
For Product Orders and Direct Account Inquiries Only, call the Order Management Center, 8:00 AM to 7:00 PM (ET), Monday through Friday:
(800) MERCK RX
(800) 637-2579

MONARCH PHARMACEUTICALS
(See KING PHARMACEUTICALS, INC)

NOVARTIS OPHTHALMICS, INC.   105, 281
One Health Plaza
East Hanover, NJ 07936
Direct Inquiries to:
Customer Service
(888) 669-6682
www.novartisophthalmics.com

PFIZER CONSUMER HEALTHCARE   105, 286
Pfizer Inc
182 Tabor Road
Morris Plains, NJ 07950
Direct Inquiries to:
Consumer Affairs
(800) 223-0182

PFIZER CONSUMER HEALTHCARE— *cont.*
For Consumer Product Information Call:
(800) 223-0182
www.prodhelp.com

PHARMACIA & UPJOHN   **106, 289**
A Pfizer Company
235 East 42nd Street
New York, NY 10017
For Medical Information Contact:
24 hours a day, 7 days a week:
(800) 438-1985

SANTEN INC.
(See VISTAKON PHARMACEUTICALS, LLC.)

VISTAKON PHARMACEUTICALS, LLC   **106, 290**
7500 Centurion Parkway
Jacksonville, FL 32256
Direct Inquires to:
(866) 427-6815

WYETH PHARMACEUTICALS   **295**
Division of Wyeth
P.O. Box 8299
Philadelphia, PA 19101
For Product Information Contact:
(800) 934-5556
For Product Quality Contact:
(800) 999-9384
For Professional Services Contact:
(800) 395-9938
For Customer Service and Ordering Information Contact:
Pharmaceuticals: (800) 666-7248
Vaccines: (800) 572-8221
For Patient Assistance Program Contact:
(800) 568-9938
For All Other Inquiries:
(610) 688-4400
www.wyeth.com

PART II/PRODUCT NAME INDEX

A

Acular LS Ophthalmic Solution
(Allergan) 216
◆ Acular Ophthalmic Solution
(Allergan) 103, 215
◆ Acular PF Ophthalmic
Solution (Allergan) 103, 217
◆ Alamast Ophthalmic Solution
(Vistakon) 106, 290
Albalon Ophthalmic Solution
(Allergan) 218
◆ Alphagan P Ophthalmic
Solution (Allergan) 103, 218
◆ Alrex Ophthalmic Suspension
0.2% (Bausch & Lomb) 104, 246
Amvisc (Bausch & Lomb) *298*
Amvisc Plus (Bausch & Lomb) 297
Atropine Sulfate Ophthalmic
Ointment USP, 1% (Bausch &
Lomb) *244*
Atropine Sulfate Ophthalmic
Solution USP, 1% (Bausch &
Lomb) *244*
Azopt Ophthalmic Suspension
(Alcon) 201

B

Bacitracin Zinc & Polymyxin B
Sulfate Ophthalmic Ointment,
USP (Bausch & Lomb) *244*
Betadine 5% Ophthalmic Solution
(Alcon) 202
Betagan Liquifilm (Allergan) 219
Betagan Liquifilm with C CAP
Compliance Cap (Allergan) 219
◆ Betimol Ophthalmic Solution
(Vistakon) 106, 291
Betoptic S Ophthalmic Suspension
(Alcon) 203
Bion Tears Lubricant Eye Drops
(Alcon) 204
Bleph-10 Ophthalmic Solution 10%
(Allergan) 221
◆ Blephamide Ophthalmic
Suspension (Allergan) 103, 222
◆ Blephamide Sterile
Ophthalmic Ointment
(Allergan) 103, 223
◆ Brimonidine Tartrate
Ophthalmic Solution 0.2%
(Bausch & Lomb) 104, 247
BSS (15 mL, 30 mL, 250 mL, &
500 mL) Sterile Irrigating
Solution (Alcon) *204*
BSS Plus (Alcon) *204*

C

Carteolol Hydrochloride Ophthalmic
Solution USP, 1% (Bausch &
Lomb) 248
Ciloxan Ophthalmic Ointment
(Alcon) 204
Ciloxan Ophthalmic Solution (Alcon) .. 206
◆ Cortisporin Ophthalmic
Suspension Sterile (King) 104, 261
◆ Cosopt Sterile Ophthalmic
Solution (Merck) 104, 264
◆ Crolom Cromolyn Sodium
Sterile Ophthalmic
Solution USP 4% (Bausch
& Lomb) 104, 249
Cyclopentolate Hydrochloride
Ophthalmic Solution USP, 1%
(Bausch & Lomb) *244*

D

◆ Daranide Tablets (Merck) 104, 267
Dexamethasone Sodium Phosphate
Ophthalmic Solution USP, 0.1%
(Bausch & Lomb) *244*

Diamox Sequels Sustained-Release
Capsules (Duramed) 257
Dipivefrin Hydrochloride Ophthalmic
Solution USP, 0.1% (Bausch &
Lomb) *244*

E

Elestat Ophthalmic Solution
(Allergan) 225
Epifrin Sterile Ophthalmic Solution
(Allergan) 226
Erythromycin Ophthalmic Ointment
USP, 0.5% (Bausch & Lomb) *244*

F

Fluorescein Sodium & Benoxinate
HCl Ophthalmic Solution USP,
0.25%/0.4% (Bausch & Lomb) *244*
Fluorescite Injection (Alcon) 207
◆ Fluor-I-Strip A.T. Ophthalmic
Strips 1 mg (Bausch &
Lomb) 104, 251
◆ Fluor-I-Strip Ophthalmic Strips
9 mg (Bausch & Lomb) 104, 251
Fluorometholone Ophthalmic
Suspension USP, 0.1% (Bausch
& Lomb) *244*
Flurbiprofen Sodium Ophthalmic
Solution USP, 0.03% (Bausch &
Lomb) *244*
◆ FML Ophthalmic Ointment
(Allergan) 103, 228
FML Ophthalmic Suspension
(Allergan) 227
FML Forte Ophthalmic Suspension
(Allergan) 226
FML-S Liquifilm Sterile Ophthalmic
Suspension (Allergan) 229

G

Genoptic Sterile Ophthalmic
Solution (Allergan) 230
Gentamicin Sulfate Ophthalmic
Solution USP, 0.3% (Bausch &
Lomb) *244*
◆ GenTeal Lubricant Eye Drops
(Novartis Ophthalmics) 105, 282
◆ GenTeal Lubricant Gel
(Novartis Ophthalmics) 105, 282
◆ GenTeal Mild Lubricant Eye
Drops (Novartis
Ophthalmics) 105, 282

H

HMS Sterile Ophthalmic Suspension
(Allergan) 231
HypoTears Lubricant Eye Drops
(Novartis Ophthalmics) *281*
HypoTears PF Lubricant Eye Drops
(Novartis Ophthalmics) *281*

L

◆ Lacrisert Sterile Ophthalmic
Insert (Merck) 105, 268
Levobunolol Hydrochloride
Ophthalmic Solution USP,
0.25%/0.5% (Bausch & Lomb) *244*
Livostin Ophthalmic Suspension
(Novartis Ophthalmics) *281*
◆ Lotemax Ophthalmic
Suspension 0.5% (Bausch
& Lomb) 104, 251
◆ Lumigan Ophthalmic Solution
(Allergan) 103, 232

M

Metipranolol Ophthalmic Solution
0.3% (Bausch & Lomb) *244*
Millennium Microsurgical System
(Bausch & Lomb) *298*

Miochol-E Intraocular Solution
(Novartis Ophthalmics) *281*
Miochol-E System Pak (Novartis
Ophthalmics) *281*
◆ Muro 128 Ophthalmic
Ointment (Bausch & Lomb) .. 104, 253
◆ Muro 128 Ophthalmic
Solution 2% and 5%
(Bausch & Lomb) 104, 252
Murocel Ophthalmic Solution USP,
1% (Bausch & Lomb) *244*
Murocoll 2 Ophthalmic Solution
(Bausch & Lomb) *244*

N

Naphazoline Hydrochloride
Ophthalmic Solution USP, 0.1%
(Bausch & Lomb) *244*
Naphcon-A Eye Drops (Alcon) 208
Natacyn Antifungal Ophthalmic
Suspension (Alcon) 208
Neomycin and Polymyxin B Sulfates
and Bacitracin Zinc Ophthalmic
Ointment, USP (Bausch & Lomb) .. *244*
Neomycin and Polymyxin B
Sulfates, Bacitracin Zinc and
Hydrocortisone Ophthalmic
Ointment, USP (Bausch & Lomb) .. *244*
Neomycin and Polymyxin B Sulfates
and Dexamethasone Ophthalmic
Ointment, USP (Bausch & Lomb) .. *244*
Neomycin and Polymyxin B Sulfates
and Dexamethasone Ophthalmic
Suspension, USP (Bausch &
Lomb) *244*
Neomycin and Polymyxin B Sulfates
and Gramicidin Ophthalmic
Solution, USP (Bausch & Lomb) ... *244*
Neosporin Ophthalmic Solution
Sterile (King) 262

O

Ocucoat (Bausch & Lomb) *298*
Ocufen Ophthalmic Solution
(Allergan) 233
◆ Ocuvite Lutein Vitamin and
Mineral Supplement
(Bausch & Lomb) 104, 254
◆ Ocuvite PreserVision Vitamin
and Mineral Supplement
(Bausch & Lomb) 104, 254
◆ Ocuvite Vitamin and Mineral
Supplement (Bausch &
Lomb) 104, 253
◆ Ocuvite Extra Vitamin and
Mineral Supplement
(Bausch & Lomb) 104, 253
Ofloxacin Ophthalmic Solution 0.3%
(Bausch & Lomb) 254
Ophetic Ophthalmic Solution
(Allergan) 234
◆ OptiPranolol Metipranolol
Ophthalmic Solution 0.3%
(Bausch & Lomb) 104, 254

P

Patanol Ophthalmic Solution (Alcon) .. 208
Phenylephrine Hydrochloride
Ophthalmic Solution USP, 2.5%
(Bausch & Lomb) *244*
Phospholine Iodide for Ophthalmic
Solution (Wyeth) 295
Pilocarpine Hydrochloride
Ophthalmic Solution USP, 0.5%,
1%, 2%, 3%, 4%, 6% (Bausch &
Lomb) *244*
Polymyxin B Sulfate and
Trimethoprim Sulfate
Ophthalmic Solution USP
(Bausch & Lomb) *244*
Poly-Pred Liquifilm Ophthalmic
Suspension (Allergan) 234

◆ Shown in Product Identification Guide

Italic Page Number Indicates Brief Listing

Polytrim Ophthalmic Solution
(Allergan) 235
◆ Pred Forte Ophthalmic
Suspension (Allergan) 103, 236
Pred Mild Sterile Ophthalmic
Suspension (Allergan) 239
Pred-G Ophthalmic Suspension
(Allergan) 236
Pred-G Sterile Ophthalmic Ointment
(Allergan) 238
Prednisolone Sodium Phosphate
Ophthalmic Solution USP, 1%
(Bausch & Lomb) *244*
Proparacaine Hydrochloride
Ophthalmic Solution USP, 0.5%
(Bausch & Lomb) *244*
Propine Ophthalmic Solution
(Allergan) 239

Q

◆ Quixin Ophthalmic Solution
(Vistakon) 106, 293

R

◆ Refresh Celluvisc Lubricant
Eye Drops (Allergan).......... 103, 240
◆ Refresh Endura Lubricant Eye
Drops (Allergan)............... 103, 240
◆ Refresh Liquigel (Allergan) 103, 241
◆ Refresh P.M. Lubricant Eye
Ointment (Allergan)........... 103, 241
◆ Refresh Plus Lubricant Eye
Drops (Allergan)............... 103, 241
◆ Refresh Tears Lubricant Eye
Drops (Allergan)............... 103, 242
◆ Restasis Ophthalmic Emulsion
(Allergan) 103, 242
◆ Rēv-Eyes Ophthalmic
Eyedrops 0.5% (Bausch &
Lomb) 104, 256

S

Sulfacetamide Sodium and
Prednisolone Sodium Phosphate
Ophthalmic Solution 10%/
0.23% (Bausch & Lomb) *244*
Sulfacetamide Sodium Ophthalmic
Solution USP, 10% (Bausch &
Lomb)................................ *244*
Systane Lubricant Eye Drops
(Alcon).............................. 209

T

Tears Naturale Forte Lubricant Eye
Drops (Alcon)....................... 209
Tears Naturale Free Lubricant Eye
Drops (Alcon)....................... 209
Tetracaine Hydrochloride
Ophthalmic Solution USP, 0.5%
(Bausch & Lomb) *244*
Timolol GFS (Falcon) 258
Timolol Maleate Ophthalmic
Solution USP, 0.25% and 0.5%
(Bausch & Lomb) *244*
◆ Timoptic in Ocudose (Merck) 105, 273
◆ Timoptic Sterile Ophthalmic
Solution (Merck) 105, 269
◆ Timoptic-XE Sterile
Ophthalmic Gel Forming
Solution (Merck).............. 105, 275
TobraDex Ophthalmic Ointment
(Alcon).............................. 211
TobraDex Ophthalmic Suspension
(Alcon).............................. 210
Tobramycin Ophthalmic Solution
USP, 0.3% (Bausch & Lomb) *244*
Travatan Ophthalmic Solution
(Alcon).............................. 212
Tropicamide Ophthalmic Solution
USP, 0.5% and 1% (Bausch &
Lomb)................................ *244*
◆ Trusopt Sterile Ophthalmic
Solution (Merck) 105, 279

V

Vasocon-A Eye Drops (Novartis
Ophthalmics)....................... *281*
Vigamox Ophthalmic Solution
(Alcon)................................ 213
◆ Visine Original Eye Drops
(Pfizer Consumer)............. 105, 288
◆ Visine A.C. Seasonal Itching
and Redness Relief Drops
(Pfizer Consumer)............. 105, 287
◆ Advanced Relief Visine Eye
Drops (Pfizer Consumer)...... 105, 286
◆ Visine For Contacts
Rewetting Drops (Pfizer
Consumer) 106, 287
◆ Visine L.R. Long Lasting Eye
Drops (Pfizer Consumer)...... 105, 288
◆ Visine Tears Eye Drops (Pfizer
Consumer) 106, 288
◆ Visine Tears Preservative Free
Eye Drops (Pfizer
Consumer) 106, 288
◆ Visine-A Eye Allergy Relief
Eye Drops (Pfizer
Consumer) 106, 287
◆ Visudyne for Injection
(Novartis Ophthalmics)....... 105, 282
Visudyne Patient Treatment Kit
(Novartis Ophthalmics)............ *281*
Voltaren Ophthalmic Sterile
Ophthalmic Solution 0.1%
(Novartis Ophthalmics) 285

X

◆ Xalatan Ophthalmic Solution
(Pharmacia & Upjohn) 106, 289

Z

◆ Zaditor Ophthalmic Solution
(Novartis Ophthalmics)....... 105, 286
◆ Zymar Ophthalmic Solution
(Allergan) 103, 243

PART III/PRODUCT CATEGORY INDEX

A

ADRENERGIC AGONISTS
(see under:
SYMPATHOMIMETICS & COMBINATIONS)

ANESTHETICS
Ophthetic Ophthalmic Solution
  (Allergan)............................**234**

ANTIBIOTICS
(see under:
ANTI-INFECTIVES
  ANTIBIOTICS & COMBINATIONS)

ANTIGLAUCOMA AGENTS
(see under:
BETA ADRENERGIC BLOCKING AGENTS
CARBONIC ANHYDRASE INHIBITORS
MIOTICS
PROSTAGLANDINS
SYMPATHOMIMETICS & COMBINATIONS)

ANTIHISTAMINE & MAST CELL STABILIZER COMBINATIONS
Elestat Ophthalmic Solution
  (Allergan)............................**225**
Patanol Ophthalmic Solution (Alcon)...**208**
Zaditor Ophthalmic Solution
  (Novartis Ophthalmics).......**105, 286**

ANTIHISTAMINES & COMBINATIONS
Visine-A Eye Allergy Relief Eye
  Drops (Pfizer Consumer)......**106, 287**

ANTI-INFECTIVES

ANTIBIOTICS & COMBINATIONS
Betadine 5% Ophthalmic Solution
  (Alcon)..............................**202**
Cortisporin Ophthalmic
  Suspension Sterile (King)....**104, 261**
Genoptic Sterile Ophthalmic
  Solution (Allergan)..................**230**
Neosporin Ophthalmic Solution
  Sterile (King)........................**262**
Poly-Pred Liquifilm Ophthalmic
  Suspension (Allergan)..............**234**
Polytrim Ophthalmic Solution
  (Allergan)............................**235**
Pred-G Ophthalmic Suspension
  (Allergan)............................**236**
Pred-G Sterile Ophthalmic Ointment
  (Allergan)............................**238**
TobraDex Ophthalmic Ointment
  (Alcon)..............................**211**
TobraDex Ophthalmic Suspension
  (Alcon)..............................**210**

ANTIFUNGALS
Natacyn Antifungal Ophthalmic
  Suspension (Alcon) **208**

QUINOLONES
Ciloxan Ophthalmic Ointment (Alcon)..**204**
Ciloxan Ophthalmic Solution (Alcon)...**206**
Ofloxacin Ophthalmic Solution 0.3%
  (Bausch & Lomb) **254**
Quixin Ophthalmic Solution
  (Vistakon)....................**106, 293**
Vigamox Ophthalmic Solution
  (Alcon)..............................**213**
Zymar Ophthalmic Solution
  (Allergan)....................**103, 243**

SULFONAMIDES & COMBINATIONS
Bleph-10 Ophthalmic Solution 10%
  (Allergan)............................**221**
Blephamide Ophthalmic
  Suspension (Allergan)........**103, 222**
Blephamide Sterile Ophthalmic
  Ointment (Allergan)..........**103, 223**
FML-S Liquifilm Sterile Ophthalmic
  Suspension (Allergan).............**229**

ANTI-INFLAMMATORY AGENTS
NONSTEROIDAL ANTI-INFLAMMATORY DRUGS (NSAIDS)
Acular LS Ophthalmic Solution
  (Allergan)............................**216**
Acular Ophthalmic Solution
  (Allergan)....................**103, 215**
Acular PF Ophthalmic Solution
  (Allergan)....................**103, 217**
Ocufen Ophthalmic Solution
  (Allergan)............................**233**
Voltaren Ophthalmic Sterile
  Ophthalmic Solution 0.1%
  (Novartis Ophthalmics)............**285**

STEROIDAL ANTI-INFLAMMATORY AGENTS & COMBINATIONS
Alrex Ophthalmic Suspension
  0.2% (Bausch & Lomb).......**104, 246**
Blephamide Ophthalmic
  Suspension (Allergan)........**103, 222**
Blephamide Sterile Ophthalmic
  Ointment (Allergan)..........**103, 223**
Cortisporin Ophthalmic
  Suspension Sterile (King)....**104, 261**
FML Ophthalmic Ointment
  (Allergan)....................**103, 228**
FML Ophthalmic Suspension
  (Allergan)............................**227**
FML Forte Ophthalmic Suspension
  (Allergan)............................**226**
FML-S Liquifilm Sterile Ophthalmic
  Suspension (Allergan).............**229**
HMS Sterile Ophthalmic Suspension
  (Allergan)............................**231**
Lotemax Ophthalmic
  Suspension 0.5% (Bausch
  & Lomb)......................**104, 251**
Poly-Pred Liquifilm Ophthalmic
  Suspension (Allergan).............**234**
Pred Forte Ophthalmic
  Suspension (Allergan)........**103, 236**
Pred Mild Sterile Ophthalmic
  Suspension (Allergan).............**239**
Pred-G Ophthalmic Suspension
  (Allergan)............................**236**
Pred-G Sterile Ophthalmic Ointment
  (Allergan)............................**238**
TobraDex Ophthalmic Ointment
  (Alcon)..............................**211**
TobraDex Ophthalmic Suspension
  (Alcon)..............................**210**

ARTIFICIAL TEARS/LUBRICANTS & COMBINATIONS
Bion Tears Lubricant Eye Drops
  (Alcon)..............................**204**
GenTeal Lubricant Eye Drops
  (Novartis Ophthalmics).......**105, 282**
GenTeal Lubricant Gel
  (Novartis Ophthalmics).......**105, 282**
GenTeal Mild Lubricant Eye
  Drops (Novartis
  Ophthalmics)................**105, 282**
GenTeal PF Lubricant Eye
  Drops (Novartis
  Ophthalmics)................**105, 282**
Lacrisert Sterile Ophthalmic
  Insert (Merck)................**105, 268**
Refresh Celluvisc Lubricant
  Eye Drops (Allergan).........**103, 240**
Refresh Endura Lubricant Eye
  Drops (Allergan)..............**103, 240**
Refresh Liquigel (Allergan) **103, 241**
Refresh P.M. Lubricant Eye
  Ointment (Allergan)..........**103, 241**
Refresh Plus Lubricant Eye
  Drops (Allergan)..............**103, 241**
Refresh Tears Lubricant Eye
  Drops (Allergan)..............**103, 242**
Restasis Ophthalmic Emulsion
  (Allergan)....................**103, 242**
Systane Lubricant Eye Drops (Alcon)..**209**
Tears Naturale Forte Lubricant Eye
  Drops (Alcon).......................**209**

Tears Naturale Free Lubricant Eye
  Drops (Alcon).......................**209**
Advanced Relief Visine Eye
  Drops (Pfizer Consumer)......**105, 286**
Visine For Contacts Rewetting
  Drops (Pfizer Consumer)......**106, 287**
Visine Tears Eye Drops (Pfizer
  Consumer) **106, 288**
Visine Tears Preservative Free
  Eye Drops (Pfizer
  Consumer) **106, 288**

B

BETA ADRENERGIC BLOCKING AGENTS
Betagan Liquifilm (Allergan) **219**
Betagan Liquifilm with C CAP
  Compliance Cap (Allergan) **219**
Betimol Ophthalmic Solution
  (Vistakon)....................**106, 291**
Betoptic S Ophthalmic Suspension
  (Alcon)..............................**203**
Carteolol Hydrochloride Ophthalmic
  Solution USP, 1% (Bausch &
  Lomb)..............................**248**
Cosopt Sterile Ophthalmic
  Solution (Merck) **104, 264**
OptiPranolol Metipranolol
  Ophthalmic Solution 0.3%
  (Bausch & Lomb) **104, 254**
Timolol GFS (Falcon)....................**258**
Timoptic in Ocudose (Merck).....**105, 273**
Timoptic Sterile Ophthalmic
  Solution (Merck) **105, 269**
Timoptic-XE Sterile Ophthalmic
  Gel Forming Solution
  (Merck).......................**105, 275**

BETA ADRENERGIC BLOCKING AGENT & CARBONIC ANHYDRASE INHIBITOR COMBINATIONS
Cosopt Sterile Ophthalmic
  Solution (Merck) **104, 264**

C

CARBONIC ANHYDRASE INHIBITORS
Azopt Ophthalmic Suspension
  (Alcon)..............................**201**
Cosopt Sterile Ophthalmic
  Solution (Merck) **104, 264**
Daranide Tablets (Merck).........**104, 267**
Diamox Sequels Sustained-Release
  Capsules (Duramed)................**257**
Trusopt Sterile Ophthalmic
  Solution (Merck) **105, 279**

CORNEAL DEHYDRATING AGENTS
(see under:
HYPERTONIC AGENTS)

D

DECONGESTANTS
(see under:
SYMPATHOMIMETICS & COMBINATIONS)

DIAGNOSTIC AIDS
Fluorescite Injection (Alcon) **207**
Fluor-I-Strip A.T. Ophthalmic
  Strips 1 mg (Bausch &
  Lomb) **104, 251**
Fluor-I-Strip Ophthalmic Strips
  9 mg (Bausch & Lomb).......**104, 251**

Italic Page Number **Indicates Instrumentation and Equipment**

G

GLAUCOMA, AGENTS FOR
(see under:
BETA ADRENERGIC BLOCKING AGENTS
CARBONIC ANHYDRASE INHIBITORS
HYPERTONIC AGENTS
MIOTICS
PROSTAGLANDINS
SYMPATHOMIMETICS & COMBINATIONS)

H

HYPERTONIC AGENTS
Muro 128 Ophthalmic
   Ointment (Bausch & Lomb) .. **104, 253**
Muro 128 Ophthalmic Solution
   2% and 5% (Bausch &
   Lomb) **104, 252**

L

LUBRICANTS
(see under:
ARTIFICIAL TEARS/LUBRICANTS & COMBINATIONS)

M

MAST CELL STABILIZERS
Alamast Ophthalmic Solution
   (Vistakon) **106, 290**
Crolom Cromolyn Sodium
   Sterile Ophthalmic Solution
   USP 4% (Bausch & Lomb).... **104, 249**

MIOTICS
ALPHA ADRENERGIC BLOCKING AGENTS
Rēv-Eyes Ophthalmic Eyedrops
   0.5% (Bausch & Lomb) **104, 256**

P

PROSTAGLANDINS
Lumigan Ophthalmic Solution
   (Allergan) **103, 232**
Travatan Ophthalmic Solution
   (Alcon) **212**
Xalatan Ophthalmic Solution
   (Pharmacia & Upjohn) **106, 289**

S

SURGICAL AIDS
(see also under:
VISCOELASTIC AGENTS
ANESTHETICS)
Ocufen Ophthalmic Solution
   (Allergan) **233**

SYMPATHOMIMETICS & COMBINATIONS
Albalon Ophthalmic Solution
   (Allergan) **218**
Alphagan P Ophthalmic
   Solution (Allergan) **103, 218**
Brimonidine Tartrate
   Ophthalmic Solution 0.2%
   (Bausch & Lomb) **104, 247**
Epifrin Sterile Ophthalmic Solution
   (Allergan) **226**
Naphcon-A Eye Drops (Alcon)........... **208**
Propine Ophthalmic Solution
   (Allergan) **239**
Visine Original Eye Drops
   (Pfizer Consumer) **105, 288**
Visine A.C. Seasonal Itching
   and Redness Relief Drops
   (Pfizer Consumer) **105, 287**
Advanced Relief Visine Eye
   Drops (Pfizer Consumer) **105, 286**
Visine L.R. Long Lasting Eye
   Drops (Pfizer Consumer) **105, 288**
Visine-A Eye Allergy Relief Eye
   Drops (Pfizer Consumer) **106, 287**

V

VASOCONSTRICTORS
(see under:
SYMPATHOMIMETICS & COMBINATIONS)

VISCOELASTIC AGENTS
Amvisc Plus (Bausch & Lomb) **297**
Ocucoat (Bausch & Lomb) **298**

VITAMINS & COMBINATIONS
Ocuvite Lutein Vitamin and
   Mineral Supplement
   (Bausch & Lomb) **104, 254**
Ocuvite PreserVision Vitamin
   and Mineral Supplement
   (Bausch & Lomb) **104, 254**
Ocuvite Vitamin and Mineral
   Supplement (Bausch &
   Lomb) **104, 253**
Ocuvite Extra Vitamin and
   Mineral Supplement
   (Bausch & Lomb) **104, 253**

PART IV/ACTIVE INGREDIENTS INDEX

A

ACETAZOLAMIDE
Diamox Sequels Sustained-Release
Capsules (Duramed) **257**

ACETYLCHOLINE CHLORIDE
Miochol-E Intraocular Solution
(Novartis Ophthalmics) *281*
Miochol-E System Pak (Novartis
Ophthalmics) *281*

ANTAZOLINE PHOSPHATE
Vasocon-A Eye Drops (Novartis
Ophthalmics) *281*

ATROPINE SULFATE
Atropine Sulfate Ophthalmic
Ointment USP, 1% (Bausch &
Lomb) *244*
Atropine Sulfate Ophthalmic
Solution USP, 1% (Bausch &
Lomb) *244*

B

BACITRACIN ZINC
Bacitracin Zinc & Polymyxin B
Sulfate Ophthalmic Ointment,
USP (Bausch & Lomb) *244*
Neomycin and Polymyxin B Sulfates
and Bacitracin Zinc Ophthalmic
Ointment, USP (Bausch & Lomb) ... *244*
Neomycin and Polymyxin B Sulfates,
Bacitracin Zinc and
Hydrocortisone Ophthalmic
Ointment, USP (Bausch & Lomb) ... *244*

BALANCED SALT SOLUTION
BSS (15 mL, 30 mL, 250 mL, &
500 mL) Sterile Irrigating
Solution (Alcon) *204*
BSS Plus (Alcon) *204*

BENOXINATE HYDROCHLORIDE
Fluorescein Sodium & Benoxinate
HCl Ophthalmic Solution USP,
0.25%/0.4% (Bausch & Lomb) *244*

BETAXOLOL HYDROCHLORIDE
Betoptic S Ophthalmic Suspension
(Alcon) **203**

BIMATOPROST
Lumigan Ophthalmic Solution
(Allergan) **103, 232**

BRIMONIDINE TARTRATE
Alphagan P Ophthalmic
Solution (Allergan) **103, 218**
Brimonidine Tartrate
Ophthalmic Solution 0.2%
(Bausch & Lomb) **104, 247**

BRINZOLAMIDE
Azopt Ophthalmic Suspension
(Alcon) **201**

C

CARBOXYMETHYLCELLULOSE SODIUM
Refresh Celluvisc Lubricant
Eye Drops (Allergan) **103, 240**
Refresh Liquigel (Allergan) **103, 241**
Refresh Plus Lubricant Eye
Drops (Allergan) **103, 241**
Refresh Tears Lubricant Eye
Drops (Allergan) **103, 242**

CARTEOLOL HYDROCHLORIDE
Carteolol Hydrochloride Ophthalmic
Solution USP, 1% (Bausch &
Lomb) **248**

CIPROFLOXACIN HYDROCHLORIDE
Ciloxan Ophthalmic Ointment (Alcon) .. **204**
Ciloxan Ophthalmic Solution (Alcon) ... **206**

CORTISOL
(*see under:* **HYDROCORTISONE**)

CROMOLYN SODIUM
Crolom Cromolyn Sodium
Sterile Ophthalmic Solution
USP 4% (Bausch & Lomb) **104, 249**

CYCLOPENTOLATE HYDROCHLORIDE
Cyclopentolate Hydrochloride
Ophthalmic Solution USP, 1%
(Bausch & Lomb) *244*

CYCLOSPORINE
Restasis Ophthalmic Emulsion
(Allergan) **103, 242**

D

DAPIPRAZOLE HYDROCHLORIDE
Rēv-Eyes Ophthalmic Eyedrops
0.5% (Bausch & Lomb) **104, 256**

DEXAMETHASONE
TobraDex Ophthalmic Ointment
(Alcon) **211**
TobraDex Ophthalmic Suspension
(Alcon) **210**
Neomycin and Polymyxin B Sulfates
and Dexamethasone Ophthalmic
Ointment, USP (Bausch & Lomb) ... *244*
Neomycin and Polymyxin B Sulfates
and Dexamethasone Ophthalmic
Suspension, USP (Bausch &
Lomb) *244*

DEXAMETHASONE SODIUM PHOSPHATE
Dexamethasone Sodium Phosphate
Ophthalmic Solution USP, 0.1%
(Bausch & Lomb) *244*

DEXTRAN 70
Bion Tears Lubricant Eye Drops
(Alcon) **204**
Tears Naturale Forte Lubricant Eye
Drops (Alcon) **209**
Tears Naturale Free Lubricant Eye
Drops (Alcon) **209**
Advanced Relief Visine Eye
Drops (Pfizer Consumer) **105, 286**

DICHLORPHENAMIDE
Daranide Tablets (Merck) **104, 267**

DICLOFENAC SODIUM
Voltaren Ophthalmic Sterile
Ophthalmic Solution 0.1%
(Novartis Ophthalmics) **285**

DIPIVEFRIN HYDROCHLORIDE
Propine Ophthalmic Solution
(Allergan) **239**
Dipivefrin Hydrochloride Ophthalmic
Solution USP, 0.1% (Bausch &
Lomb) *244*

DORZOLAMIDE HYDROCHLORIDE
Cosopt Sterile Ophthalmic
Solution (Merck) **104, 264**
Trusopt Sterile Ophthalmic
Solution (Merck) **105, 279**

E

ECHOTHIOPHATE IODIDE
Phospholine Iodide for Ophthalmic
Solution (Wyeth) *295*

EPINASTINE HYDROCHLORIDE
Elestat Ophthalmic Solution
(Allergan) **225**

EPINEPHRINE
Epifrin Sterile Ophthalmic Solution
(Allergan) **226**

ERYTHROMYCIN
Erythromycin Ophthalmic Ointment
USP, 0.5% (Bausch & Lomb) *244*

F

FLUORESCEIN SODIUM
Fluorescite Injection (Alcon) **207**
Fluor-I-Strip A.T. Ophthalmic
Strips 1 mg (Bausch &
Lomb) **104, 251**
Fluor-I-Strip Ophthalmic Strips
9 mg (Bausch & Lomb) **104, 251**
Fluorescein Sodium & Benoxinate
HCl Ophthalmic Solution USP,
0.25%/0.4% (Bausch & Lomb) *244*

FLUOROMETHOLONE
FML Ophthalmic Ointment
(Allergan) **103, 228**
FML Ophthalmic Suspension
(Allergan) **227**
FML Forte Ophthalmic Suspension
(Allergan) **226**
FML-S Liquifilm Sterile Ophthalmic
Suspension (Allergan) **229**
Fluorometholone Ophthalmic
Suspension USP, 0.1% (Bausch
& Lomb) *244*

FLURBIPROFEN SODIUM
Ocufen Ophthalmic Solution
(Allergan) **233**
Flurbiprofen Sodium Ophthalmic
Solution USP, 0.03% (Bausch &
Lomb) *244*

G

GATIFLOXACIN
Zymar Ophthalmic Solution
(Allergan) **103, 243**

GENTAMICIN SULFATE
Genoptic Sterile Ophthalmic
Solution (Allergan) **230**
Pred-G Ophthalmic Suspension
(Allergan) **236**
Pred-G Sterile Ophthalmic Ointment
(Allergan) **238**
Gentamicin Sulfate Ophthalmic
Solution USP, 0.3% (Bausch &
Lomb) *244*

GLYCERIN
Refresh Endura Lubricant Eye
Drops (Allergan) **103, 240**
Tears Naturale Forte Lubricant Eye
Drops (Alcon) **209**
Visine For Contacts Rewetting
Drops (Pfizer Consumer) **106, 287**
Visine Tears Eye Drops (Pfizer
Consumer) **106, 288**
Visine Tears Preservative Free
Eye Drops (Pfizer
Consumer) **106, 288**

Italic Page Number **Indicates Brief Listing**

GRAMICIDIN
Neosporin Ophthalmic Solution Sterile (King) 262
Neomycin and Polymyxin B Sulfates and Gramicidin Ophthalmic Solution, USP (Bausch & Lomb) 244

H

HYDROCORTISONE
Cortisporin Ophthalmic Suspension Sterile (King) **104, 261**
Neomycin and Polymyxin B Sulfates, Bacitracin Zinc and Hydrocortisone Ophthalmic Ointment, USP (Bausch & Lomb) ... 244

HYDROXYPROPYL CELLULOSE
Lacrisert Sterile Ophthalmic Insert (Merck) **105, 268**

HYDROXYPROPYL METHYLCELLULOSE
Ocucoat (Bausch & Lomb) 298
Visine For Contacts Rewetting Drops (Pfizer Consumer) **106, 287**

HYOSCINE HYDROBROMIDE
(see under: SCOPOLAMINE HYDROBROMIDE)

HYPROMELLOSE
Bion Tears Lubricant Eye Drops (Alcon) 204
GenTeal Lubricant Eye Drops (Novartis Ophthalmics) **105, 282**
GenTeal Lubricant Gel (Novartis Ophthalmics) **105, 282**
GenTeal Mild Lubricant Eye Drops (Novartis Ophthalmics) **105, 282**
GenTeal PF Lubricant Eye Drops (Novartis Ophthalmics) **105, 282**
Tears Naturale Forte Lubricant Eye Drops (Alcon) 209
Tears Naturale Free Lubricant Eye Drops (Alcon) 209
Visine Tears Eye Drops (Pfizer Consumer) **106, 288**
Visine Tears Preservative Free Eye Drops (Pfizer Consumer) **106, 288**

K

KETOROLAC TROMETHAMINE
Acular LS Ophthalmic Solution (Allergan) 216
Acular Ophthalmic Solution (Allergan) **103, 215**
Acular PF Ophthalmic Solution (Allergan) **103, 217**

KETOTIFEN FUMARATE
Zaditor Ophthalmic Solution (Novartis Ophthalmics) **105, 286**

L

LATANOPROST
Xalatan Ophthalmic Solution (Pharmacia & Upjohn) **106, 289**

LEVOBUNOLOL HYDROCHLORIDE
Betagan Liquifilm (Allergan) 219
Betagan Liquifilm with C CAP Compliance Cap (Allergan) 219
Levobunolol Hydrochloride Ophthalmic Solution USP, 0.25%/0.5% (Bausch & Lomb) 244

LEVOCABASTINE HYDROCHLORIDE
Livostin Ophthalmic Suspension (Novartis Ophthalmics) 281

LEVOFLOXACIN
Quixin Ophthalmic Solution (Vistakon) **106, 293**

LOTEPREDNOL ETABONATE
Alrex Ophthalmic Suspension 0.2% (Bausch & Lomb) **104, 246**
Lotemax Ophthalmic Suspension 0.5% (Bausch & Lomb) **104, 251**

M

MEDRYSONE
HMS Sterile Ophthalmic Suspension (Allergan) 231

METHYLCELLULOSE
Murocel Ophthalmic Solution USP, 1% (Bausch & Lomb) 244

METIPRANOLOL
OptiPranolol Metipranolol Ophthalmic Solution 0.3% (Bausch & Lomb) **104, 254**
Metipranolol Ophthalmic Solution 0.3% (Bausch & Lomb) 244

MINERAL OIL
Refresh P.M. Lubricant Eye Ointment (Allergan) **103, 241**

MOXIFLOXACIN HYDROCHLORIDE
Vigamox Ophthalmic Solution (Alcon) .. 213

MULTIMINERALS
(see under: VITAMINS WITH MINERALS)

MULTIVITAMINS WITH MINERALS
(see under: VITAMINS WITH MINERALS)

N

NAPHAZOLINE HYDROCHLORIDE
Albalon Ophthalmic Solution (Allergan) 218
Naphcon-A Eye Drops (Alcon) 208
Visine-A Eye Allergy Relief Eye Drops (Pfizer Consumer) **106, 287**
Naphazoline Hydrochloride Ophthalmic Solution USP, 0.1% (Bausch & Lomb) 244
Vasocon-A Eye Drops (Novartis Ophthalmics) 281

NATAMYCIN
Natacyn Antifungal Ophthalmic Suspension (Alcon) 208

NEOMYCIN SULFATE
Cortisporin Ophthalmic Suspension Sterile (King) **104, 261**
Neosporin Ophthalmic Solution Sterile (King) 262
Poly-Pred Liquifilm Ophthalmic Suspension (Allergan) 234
Neomycin and Polymyxin B Sulfates and Bacitracin Zinc Ophthalmic Ointment, USP (Bausch & Lomb) ... 244
Neomycin and Polymyxin B Sulfates, Bacitracin Zinc and Hydrocortisone Ophthalmic Ointment, USP (Bausch & Lomb) ... 244
Neomycin and Polymyxin B Sulfates and Dexamethasone Ophthalmic Ointment, USP (Bausch & Lomb) ... 244
Neomycin and Polymyxin B Sulfates and Dexamethasone Ophthalmic Suspension, USP (Bausch & Lomb) 244
Neomycin and Polymyxin B Sulfates and Gramicidin Ophthalmic Solution, USP (Bausch & Lomb) 244

O

OFLOXACIN
Ofloxacin Ophthalmic Solution 0.3% (Bausch & Lomb) 254

OLOPATADINE HYDROCHLORIDE
Patanol Ophthalmic Solution (Alcon) .. **208**

OXYMETAZOLINE HYDROCHLORIDE
Visine L.R. Long Lasting Eye Drops (Pfizer Consumer) **105, 288**

P

PEMIROLAST POTASSIUM
Alamast Ophthalmic Solution (Vistakon) **106, 290**

PETROLATUM, WHITE
Refresh P.M. Lubricant Eye Ointment (Allergan) **103, 241**

PHENIRAMINE MALEATE
Naphcon-A Eye Drops (Alcon) 208
Visine-A Eye Allergy Relief Eye Drops (Pfizer Consumer) **106, 287**

PHENYLEPHRINE HYDROCHLORIDE
Murocoll 2 Ophthalmic Solution (Bausch & Lomb) 244
Phenylephrine Hydrochloride Ophthalmic Solution USP, 2.5% (Bausch & Lomb) 244

PILOCARPINE HYDROCHLORIDE
Pilocarpine Hydrochloride Ophthalmic Solution USP, 0.5%, 1%, 2%, 3%, 4%, 6% (Bausch & Lomb) 244

POLYETHYLENE GLYCOL
Systane Lubricant Eye Drops (Alcon) ... 209
Advanced Relief Visine Eye Drops (Pfizer Consumer) **105, 286**
Visine Tears Eye Drops (Pfizer Consumer) **106, 288**
Visine Tears Preservative Free Eye Drops (Pfizer Consumer) **106, 288**

POLYMYXIN B SULFATE
Cortisporin Ophthalmic Suspension Sterile (King) **104, 261**
Neosporin Ophthalmic Solution Sterile (King) 262
Poly-Pred Liquifilm Ophthalmic Suspension (Allergan) 234
Polytrim Ophthalmic Solution (Allergan) 235
Bacitracin Zinc & Polymyxin B Sulfate Ophthalmic Ointment, USP (Bausch & Lomb) 244
Neomycin and Polymyxin B Sulfates and Bacitracin Zinc Ophthalmic Ointment, USP (Bausch & Lomb) ... 244
Neomycin and Polymyxin B Sulfates, Bacitracin Zinc and Hydrocortisone Ophthalmic Ointment, USP (Bausch & Lomb) ... 244
Neomycin and Polymyxin B Sulfates and Dexamethasone Ophthalmic Ointment, USP (Bausch & Lomb) ... 244

Italic Page Number **Indicates Brief Listing**

ACTIVE INGREDIENTS INDEX

Neomycin and Polymyxin B Sulfates and Dexamethasone Ophthalmic Suspension, USP (Bausch & Lomb).................................*244*
Neomycin and Polymyxin B Sulfates and Gramicidin Ophthalmic Solution, USP (Bausch & Lomb)....*244*
Polymyxin B Sulfate and Trimethoprim Sulfate Ophthalmic Solution USP (Bausch & Lomb) *244*

POLYSORBATE 80
Refresh Endura Lubricant Eye Drops (Allergan)...............**103, 240**

POLYVINYLPYRROLIDONE
(*see under:* **POVIDONE**)

POVIDONE
Advanced Relief Visine Eye Drops (Pfizer Consumer)......**105, 286**

POVIDONE IODINE
Betadine 5% Ophthalmic Solution (Alcon)..................................**202**

PREDNISOLONE ACETATE
Blephamide Ophthalmic Suspension (Allergan) **103, 222**
Blephamide Sterile Ophthalmic Ointment (Allergan) **103, 223**
Poly-Pred Liquifilm Ophthalmic Suspension (Allergan) **234**
Pred Forte Ophthalmic Suspension (Allergan) **103, 236**
Pred Mild Sterile Ophthalmic Suspension (Allergan) **239**
Pred-G Ophthalmic Suspension (Allergan)..............................**236**
Pred-G Sterile Ophthalmic Ointment (Allergan)..............................**238**

PREDNISOLONE SODIUM PHOSPHATE
Prednisolone Sodium Phosphate Ophthalmic Solution USP, 1% (Bausch & Lomb) *244*
Sulfacetamide Sodium and Prednisolone Sodium Phosphate Ophthalmic Solution 10%/0.23% (Bausch & Lomb) *244*

PROPARACAINE HYDROCHLORIDE
Ophthetic Ophthalmic Solution (Allergan)..............................**234**
Proparacaine Hydrochloride Ophthalmic Solution USP, 0.5% (Bausch & Lomb) *244*

PROPYLENE GLYCOL
Systane Lubricant Eye Drops (Alcon)...**209**

S

SCOPOLAMINE HYDROBROMIDE
Murocoll 2 Ophthalmic Solution (Bausch & Lomb) *244*

SODIUM CHLORIDE
Muro 128 Ophthalmic Ointment (Bausch & Lomb)...**104, 253**
Muro 128 Ophthalmic Solution 2% and 5% (Bausch & Lomb)..........................**104, 252**

SODIUM HYALURONATE
Amvisc Plus (Bausch & Lomb)..........**297**
Amvisc (Bausch & Lomb) **298**

SULFACETAMIDE SODIUM
Bleph-10 Ophthalmic Solution 10% (Allergan) **221**
Blephamide Ophthalmic Suspension (Allergan) **103, 222**
Blephamide Sterile Ophthalmic Ointment (Allergan) **103, 223**
FML-S Liquifilm Sterile Ophthalmic Suspension (Allergan) **229**
Sulfacetamide Sodium and Prednisolone Sodium Phosphate Ophthalmic Solution 10%/0.23% (Bausch & Lomb) *244*
Sulfacetamide Sodium Ophthalmic Solution USP, 10% (Bausch & Lomb)..................................*244*

T

TETRACAINE HYDROCHLORIDE
Tetracaine Hydrochloride Ophthalmic Solution USP, 0.5% (Bausch & Lomb)..................................*244*

TETRAHYDROZOLINE HYDROCHLORIDE
Visine Original Eye Drops (Pfizer Consumer) **105, 288**
Visine A.C. Seasonal Itching and Redness Relief Drops (Pfizer Consumer) **105, 287**
Advanced Relief Visine Eye Drops (Pfizer Consumer)......**105, 286**

TIMOLOL HEMIHYDRATE
Betimol Ophthalmic Solution (Vistakon) **106, 291**

TIMOLOL MALEATE
Cosopt Sterile Ophthalmic Solution (Merck) **104, 264**
Timolol GFS (Falcon) **258**
Timoptic in Ocudose (Merck) **105, 273**
Timoptic Sterile Ophthalmic Solution (Merck) **105, 269**
Timoptic-XE Sterile Ophthalmic Gel Forming Solution (Merck) **105, 275**
Timolol Maleate Ophthalmic Solution USP, 0.25% and 0.5% (Bausch & Lomb)..................................*244*

TOBRAMYCIN
TobraDex Ophthalmic Ointment (Alcon)..............................**211**
TobraDex Ophthalmic Suspension (Alcon)..............................**210**
Tobramycin Ophthalmic Solution USP, 0.3% (Bausch & Lomb) *244*

TRAVOPROST
Travatan Ophthalmic Solution (Alcon)..**212**

TRIFLUOROTHYMIDINE
(*see under:* **TRIFLURIDINE**)

TRIMETHOPRIM SULFATE
Polytrim Ophthalmic Solution (Allergan) **235**
Polymyxin B Sulfate and Trimethoprim Sulfate Ophthalmic Solution USP (Bausch & Lomb) *244*

TROPICAMIDE
Tropicamide Ophthalmic Solution USP, 0.5% and 1% (Bausch & Lomb)..................................*244*

V

VERTEPORFIN
Visudyne for Injection (Novartis Ophthalmics)...................**105, 282**
Visudyne Patient Treatment Kit (Novartis Ophthalmics) *281*

VITAMINS WITH MINERALS
Ocuvite Lutein Vitamin and Mineral Supplement (Bausch & Lomb) **104, 254**
Ocuvite PreserVision Vitamin and Mineral Supplement (Bausch & Lomb) **104, 254**
Ocuvite Vitamin and Mineral Supplement (Bausch & Lomb)..........................**104, 253**
Ocuvite Extra Vitamin and Mineral Supplement (Bausch & Lomb) **104, 253**

W

WHITE PETROLATUM
(*see under:* **PETROLATUM, WHITE**)

Z

ZINC SULFATE
Visine A.C. Seasonal Itching and Redness Relief Drops (Pfizer Consumer) **105, 287**

Italic Page Number **Indicates Brief Listing**

SECTION 2
PHARMACEUTICALS IN OPHTHALMOLOGY

Douglas J. Rhee, MD, Christopher J. Rapuano, MD, and Theresa L. Belzer, RPh, (Wills Eye Hospital, Philadelphia, PA), with a section on ocular toxicology by F.W. Fraunfelder, MD (Casey Eye Institute, Portland, OR)

We are pleased to present this updated overview of pharmaceutical options in ophthalmology. This edition of the *PDR for Ophthalmic Medicines* marks the introduction of epinastine HCl (Elestat), a mast-cell inhibitor and histamine (H_1 and H_2) antagonist indicated for the prevention of itching associated with allergic conjunctivitis (see **Table 11**). Another development during the past year is the availability of the antibacterial agent levofloxacin as a 1.5% ophthalmic solution (Iquix), which is highlighted in **Table 2**. Additionally, we've included revised information on antimicrobial therapy, drug-induced ocular side effects, and off-label drug uses.

In all, this section offers 29 reference tables presenting therapeutic alternatives in all major categories of ophthalmic treatment, as well as a survey of recently identified adverse drug reactions encountered in ophthalmology. The material is divided into 13 parts as follows:

1. Mydriatics and Cycloplegics
2. Antimicrobial Therapy
3. Ocular Anti-inflammatory Agents
4. Anesthetic Agents
5. Agents for Treatment of Glaucoma
6. Medications for Dry Eye
7. Ocular Decongestants
8. Ophthalmic Irrigating Solutions
9. Hyperosmolar Agents
10. Diagnostic Agents
11. Viscoelastic Materials Used in Ophthalmology
12. Off-Label Drug Applications in Ophthalmology
13. Ocular Toxicology

There are a large number of excellent references related to pharmacology and treatment regimens in ophthalmology. Listed below are some of the ones we regard as particularly useful.

GENERAL REFERENCES

American Medical Association. *Drug Evaluations Annual.* Milwaukee, Wis: AMA Department of Drugs, Division of Toxicology.

Fraunfelder FT, Fraunfelder FW. *Drug-Induced Ocular Side Effects*, ed 5. Woburn, Mass: Butterworth-Heinemann; 2001.

Fraunfelder FT, Roy FH. *Current Ocular Therapy*, ed 5. Philadelphia, Pa: WB Saunders; 1999.

Kunimoto DY, Kanitkar KD, Makar M, et al. *The Wills Eye Manual, Fourth Edition, for PDA* (Palm OS, Windows CE, and Pocket PC). Philadelphia, PA: Lippincott Williams & Wilkins; 2004.

Rhee D, Deramo V. The Wills Eye Hospital Drug Guide, ed 2. Philadelphia, Pa: Lippincott Williams & Wilkins; 2001.

Tasman W, Jaeger EA. *Duane's Clinical Ophthalmology on CD-ROM, 2004 Edition*. Philadelphia, PA: Lippincott Williams & Wilkins; 2004.

Vaughan D, Asbury T, Riordan-Eva P. *General Ophthalmology*, ed 15. Norwalk, Conn: Appleton & Lange; 1999.

1. MYDRIATICS AND CYCLOPLEGICS

The autonomic drugs that produce mydriasis (pupillary dilation) and cycloplegia (paralysis of accommodation) are among the most frequently used topical medications in ophthalmic practice. The most commonly used mydriatic is the direct-acting adrenergic agent phenylephrine hydrochloride, usually in a 2.5% concentration. Phenylephrine is used alone or, more commonly, in combination with a cycloplegic agent for refraction or pupillary dilation. The 2.5% concentration is favored for most cases. There is a possibility of severe adverse systemic effects from the use of the 10% solution.

Anticholinergic agents have both cycloplegic and mydriatic activity. They are usually used for refraction, pupillary dilation, and relief of inflammation.

It is important to remember that the effect of these medications depends on many factors, including age, race, and eye color. For example, the mydriatics and cycloplegics tend to be less effective in dark-eyed individuals than in those with blue-eyes.

The drug dapiprazole hydrochloride (Rēv-Eyes) can be used to reverse the effects of phenylephrine and, to a lesser extent, tropicamide. Activity against phenylephrine is excellent: 88% reversal at the end of 1 hour. Against tropicamide, results are significantly lower: 38% at the end of 2 hours. It therefore remains important, when using both drugs, to instruct the patient to use sunglasses and avoid driving or operating dangerous machinery.

TABLE 1

MYDRIATICS AND CYCLOPLEGICS

GENERIC NAME	TRADE NAMES	CONCENTRATION	ONSET/DURATION OF ACTION
Phenylephrine hydrochloride	AK-Dilate Mydfrin Neo-Synephrine Available generically	Soln, 2.5%, 10% Soln, 2.5% Soln, 2.5%, 10% Soln, 2.5%, 10%	30–60 min/3–5 h
Atropine sulfate	Atropine-Care Atrosulf-1 Isopto Atropine Available generically	Soln, 1% Soln, 1% Soln, 1% Soln, 1% Ointment, 1%	45–120 min/7–14 days
Cyclopentolate hydrochloride	AK-Pentolate Cyclogyl Cylate Available generically	Soln, 1% Soln, 0.5%, 1%, 2% Soln, 1% Soln, 1%	30–60 min/6–24 h
Homatropine hydrobromide	Isopto Homatropine Available generically	Soln, 2%, 5% Soln, 2%, 5%	30–60 min/3 days
Scopolamine hydrobromide	Isopto Hyoscine	Soln, 0.25%	30–60 min/4–7 days
Tropicamide	Mydriacyl Opticyl Available generically	Soln, 0.5%, 1% Soln, 0.5%, 1% Soln, 0.5%, 1%	20–40 min/4–6 h

2. ANTIMICROBIAL THERAPY

Antibiotics are routinely used in ophthalmology for both treatment and prophylaxis. They are used prophylactically in the management of foreign bodies and corneal abrasions and in preoperative and postoperative care, administered as an ophthalmic solution, ointment, or subconjunctival injection (see **Table 2**).

Many ophthalmic institutions have been using a solution of 5% povidone-iodine (Betadine) preoperatively to "sterilize" the eye, lids, and brow. Another development is the use of collagen shields (usually 12-hour) soaked in antibiotic, with or without steroid, in place of a patch and/or subconjunctival injection after surgery. While more expensive, the shields do have the advantage of being more comfortable for the patient and are less likely to cause tissue degeneration.

Also in the literature is another prophylactic measure: the addition of antibiotics to the irrigating solution. This technique is being used in several hospitals and high-volume surgicenters throughout the country. The maximum nontoxic concentrations of antibiotics are listed in **Table 3**. For prophylaxis, however, clinicians advise using half these amounts. Note that concentrations are given in micrograms per milliliter.

Whether treating an external or intraocular infection, slides for gram and Giemsa stain and aerobic and anaerobic cultures should be secured prior to initiating therapy if the severity or site of infection dictates the necessity of culturing. When fungal, acanthamoebal, or atypical mycobacterial involvement is a possibility, additional stains to consider are: methenamine silver, acridine orange, and calcofluor white. You can also consider using Lowenstein-Jensen culture medium. When an active or suspected superficial ocular infection is accompanied by inflammation, a variety of combination agents may be considered (see **Table 4**).

Corneal ulcers and intraocular infections require vigorous management. Most physicians and hospitals have protocols for their treatment. One such protocol for treating endophthalmitis, modified from Mandelbaum and Forster, is given in **Table 5**. Serious ocular infections are usually treated by the topical, subconjunctival, and intraocular routes of administration (see **Table 6**). Corneal ulcers are usually treated with one or more of the topical solutions listed in **Table 6**, usually given every $1/2$ to 1 hour, in alternating doses if more than one solution is used. In severe cases, such as impending or actual perforation and scleral extension, medication is given by the topical, subconjunctival, oral, and/or intravenous route.

Fungal keratitis (keratomycosis) is relatively uncommon, but should be suspected in patients who have previously received topical steroids and/or antibiotics, and in patients whose corneal ulcer does not respond to antibiotics. Corneal scraping often permits correct clinical diagnosis. Natamycin 5% ophthalmic suspension (Natacyn) is recognized as one of the most potent broad-spectrum antifungal agents available for use in the eye. Amphotericin B 0.15% ophthalmic solution, which is extemporaneously prepared, is another commonly used antifungal agent.

Endogenous fungal endophthalmitis can be seen in intravenous drug users and patients with compromised immune systems. For these infections, amphotericin B has been used subconjunctivally, intravenously, and, where indicated, intravitreally. Prior to intravitreal use, a small portion of the vitreous abscess should be aspirated for microbiologic study. In addition to amphotericin B, flucytosine has also been used to treat fungal endophthalmitis. For more on treatment of fungal infections, see **Table 7**.

There has been an increase, within the last decade, in the incidence of Acanthamoeba keratitis. This has been linked, in many cases, to use of contaminated solutions for soft contact lenses — especially homemade saline solutions. Current therapy includes the concurrent use of polyhexamethylene biguanide compounded with Baquacil (PHMB), Neosporin, and chlorhexidine digluconate (CHX) (found in Boston Rewetting Drops).

In bacterial endophthalmitis, the use of intraocular and periocular antimicrobial therapy has significantly improved the final visual outcome. A diagnosis of bacterial endophthalmitis should be strongly suspected in a patient who is postoperative or posttraumatic, or when the intraocular inflammation is out of proportion to the situation. Ocular pain is often present before obvious inflammation. Preoperative and postoperative antibiotics may decrease the incidence of postoperative endophthalmitis.

Once endophthalmitis is suspected, prompt intervention is required. Samples of the aqueous and vitreous humors must be promptly secured and treatment quickly initiated with antimicrobials appropriate to the suspected organism(s). Fungal or anaerobic organisms should be considered in cases where inflammation occurs several weeks or more after surgery or in cases of trauma or immunosuppression.

Once the aqueous and vitreous humors have been cultured, antimicrobial agents should be directly injected into the vitreous. To prevent retinal toxicity, medications should be injected slowly into the anterior vitreous cavity, with particular caution after vitrectomy. Vitrectomy and intravitreal antibiotics should always be considered when treating endophthalmitis.

In a study by Pavan and Brinser, the use of intravenous antibiotics was found to make no difference in final visual acuity or media clarity. The authors concluded that "omission of systemic antibiotic treatment can reduce toxic effects, costs, and length of hospital stay."

REFERENCES

Anonymous. Results of endophthalmitis vitrectomy study. *Arch Ophthalmol.* 1995;113:1479.

Axelrod AJ, Peyman GA. Intravitreal amphotericin B treatment of experimental fungal endophthalmitis. *Am J Ophthalmol.* 1973;76:584.

Barza M. Antibacterial agents in the treatment of ocular infections. *Infect Dis Clin North Am.* 1989;3:533-551.

Baum JL. Antibiotic use in ophthalmology. In: Tasman W, Jaeger EA, eds. *Duane's Clinical Ophthalmology.* Vol. 4. Philadelphia, Pa: JB Lippincott; 1989:chap 26.

Ellis P. *Ocular Therapeutics and Pharmacology.* 7th ed. St. Louis, Mo: CV Mosby; 1985.

Forster RK. Endophthalmitis. In: Tasman W, Jaeger EA, eds. *Duane's Clinical Ophthalmology.* Vol. 4. Philadelphia, Pa: JB Lippincott; 1989:chap 24.

Gardner S. Treatment of bacterial endophthalmitis. *Ocular Therapeutics and Management.* 1991;2(1):3-4.

Lamberts DW, Potter DE, eds. *Clinical Ocular Pharmacology.* Boston, Mass: Little, Brown; 1987.

Lemp MA, Blackman HJ, Koffler BH. Therapy for bacterial and fungal infections. *Int Ophthalmol Clin.* 1980;20(3):135-145.

Pavan PR, Brinser JH. Exogenous bacterial endophthalmitis treated without systemic antibiotics. *Am J Ophthalmol.* 1987;104:121.

Peyman GA. Antibiotic administration in the treatment of bacterial endophthalmitis. II. Intravitreal injections. *Surv Ophthalmol.* 1977;21:332,339-346.

Tabbara KF, Hyndiuk RA, eds. *Infections of the Eye.* Boston, Mass: Little, Brown; 1986.

TABLE 2

COMMERCIALLY AVAILABLE OPHTHALMIC ANTIBACTERIAL AGENTS

GENERIC NAME	TRADE NAME	CONCENTRATION OPHTHALMIC SOLUTION	OPHTHALMIC OINTMENT
INDIVIDUAL AGENTS			
Bacitracin	Available generically	Not available	500 units/g
Ciprofloxacin hydrochloride	Ciloxan	0.3%	0.3%
Erythromycin	Available generically	Not available	0.5%
Gatifloxacin	Zymar	0.3%	Not available
Gentamicin sulfate	Garamycin	0.3%	0.3%
	Genoptic	0.3%	0.3%
	Gentacidin	0.3%	Not available
	Gentak	0.3%	0.3%
	Available generically	0.3%	0.3%
Levofloxacin	Iquix	1.5%	Not available
	Quixin	0.5%	Not available
Moxifloxacin	Vigamox	0.5%	Not available
Ofloxacin	Ocuflox	0.3%	Not available
Sulfacetamide sodium	AK-Sulf	Not available	10%
	Bleph-10	10%	Not available
	Sulf-10 (15-mL bottle or preservative-free dropperettes)	10%	Not available
	Available generically	10%	10%
Tobramycin sulfate	AK-Tob	0.3%	Not available
	Tobrex	0.3%	0.3%
	Tobrasol	0.3%	Not available
	Available generically	0.3%	Not available
MIXTURES			
Polymyxin B/Bacitracin Zinc	AK-Poly-Bac	Not available	10,000 units - 500 units/g
	Polysporin		
	Polycin-B		
	Available generically		
Polymyxin B/Neomycin/Bacitracin	Neosporin	Not available	10,000 units - 3.5 mg - 400 units/g
	Available generically		
Polymyxin B/Neomycin/Gramicidin	Neosporin	10,000 units - 1.75 mg - 0.025 mg/mL	Not available
	Available generically		
Polymyxin B/Trimethoprim	Polytrim	10,000 units - 1 mg/mL	Not available
	Available generically		

TABLE 3

ANTIBIOTICS IN INFUSION FLUID

AGENT	MAXIMUM NONTOXIC DOSE (mcg/mL)	AGENT	MAXIMUM NONTOXIC DOSE (mcg/mL)
Amikacin	10	Oxacillin	10
Ceftazidime	40	Tobramycin	10
Clindamycin	9	Vancomycin*	30
Gentamicin	8		
Imipenem	16		

*Usage discouraged by CDC because of increased resistant organisms.
Adapted from Peyman GA, Daun M. Prophylaxis of endophthalmitis. *Ophthalmic Surg.* 1994;25:673.

TABLE 4

COMBINATION OCULAR ANTI-INFLAMMATORY AND ANTIBIOTIC AGENTS

GENERIC NAME	TRADE NAME	PREPARATION & CONCENTRATION
Dexamethasone - Neomycin - Polymyxin B	AK-Trol Dexasporin Maxitrol Poly-Dex Available generically	Suspension, 0.1% - 3.5 mg/mL - 10,000 units/mL
	Maxitrol Poly-Dex Dexacine Available generically	Ointment, 0.1% - 3.5 mg/g - 10,000 units/g
Dexamethasone - Tobramycin	Tobradex Tobradex	Suspension, 0.1% - 0.3% Ointment, 0.1% - 0.3%
Fluorometholone - Sulfacetamide	FML-S	Suspension, 0.1% - 10%
Gentamicin - Prednisolone acetate	Pred-G Pred-G	Suspension, 0.3% - 1.0% Ointment, 0.3% - 0.6%
Hydrocortisone - Neomycin - Polymyxin B	Cortisporin Available generically	Suspension, 1% - 3.5 mg/mL - 10,000 units/mL
Hydrocortisone - Neomycin - Polymyxin B - Bacitracin	AK Spore HC Cortisporin Available generically	Ointment, 1% - 3.5 mg/g - 10,000 units/g - 400 units/g
Prednisolone acetate - Neomycin - Polymyxin B	Poly-Pred	Suspension, 0.5% - 0.35% - 10,000 units/mL
Prednisolone acetate - Sulfacetamide	Blephamide Blephamide S. O. P.	Suspension, 0.2% - 10% Ointment, 0.2% - 10%
Prednisolone sodium phosphate - Sulfacetamide	Vasocidin Available generically	Solution, 0.25% - 10% Solution, 0.25% - 10%

TABLE 5
REGIMEN FOR ENDOPHTHALMITIS

1. Diagnostic anterior chamber and vitreous aspiration; diagnostic vitrectomy when liquid vitreous fails to aspirate or in cases of suspected fungal endophthalmitis.

2. Initial therapy (in operating room after diagnostic technique).
   A. Intraocular: gentamicin 100 mcg or amikacin 400 mcg and vancomycin 1000 mcg or ceftazidime 2000 mcg
   B. Subconjunctival: gentamicin 40 mg and triamcinolone acetonide (Kenalog) 40 mg*
   C. Topical: gentamicin 9.1 or 13.4 mg/mL and cefazolin 50 mg/mL and prednisolone acetate 1%
   D. Systemic: cefazolin (Ancef or Kefzol) 1000 mg every 6 to 8 hours. (Ceftriaxone has good penetration of the blood ocular barrier and may be used as an alternative.) The use of systemic antibiotics is controversial; many practitioners do not employ them.

3. If cultures are positive for virulent bacteria, consider repeating the above intraocular injections at the bedside on the second and fourth postoperative days. Continue topical treatment every half hour, subconjunctival treatment daily, and systemic therapy. Consider therapeutic vitrectomy with repeat intraocular antibiotics.

4. If cultures are negative after 48 hours, do not repeat intraocular antibiotics. Consider tapering topical, subconjunctival, and systemic antibiotic therapy while continuing topical and subconjunctival corticosteroids.

5. If endophthalmitis presents as a *delayed inflammation* in which a fungal etiology is considered, the vitreous sample should be obtained by a vitreous instrument using membrane filters; intraocular amphotericin B (Fungizone) at a dosage of 5 mcg should be considered.

6. If endophthalmitis presents as a delayed inflammation or chronic indolent infection, a *Propionibacterium acnes* infection should be considered.

Source: Mandelbaum S, Forster RK.
Anonymous. Results of endophthalmitis vitrectomy study. *Arch Ophthalmol*. 1995;113:1479.

*Subconjunctival corticosteroids should be deferred 48 to 72 hours to await culture growth and confirmation if a fungal etiology is suspected or the inflammation is delayed.

TABLE 6
CONCENTRATIONS AND DOSAGE OF PRINCIPAL ANTIBIOTIC AGENTS

DRUG NAME*	TOPICAL	SUBCONJUNCTIVAL	INTRAVITREAL	INTRAVENOUS†
Amikacin sulfate	10 mg/mL	25 mg	400 mcg	15 mg/kg daily in 2–3 doses
Ampicillin sodium	50 mg/mL	50–150 mg	5 mg	4–12 g daily in 4 doses
Bacitracin zinc	10,000 units/mL	5000 units	...	...
Cefazolin sodium	50 mg/mL	100 mg	2250 mcg	2–4 g daily in 3–4 doses
Ceftazidime	50 mg/mL	100 mg	2000 mcg	1 g daily in 2–3 doses
Ceftriaxone	50 mg/mL	...	...	1–4 g daily in 1–2 doses
Clindamycin	50 mg/mL	15–50 mg	1000 mcg	900–1800 mg daily in 2–3 doses
Colistimethate sodium	10 mg/mL	15–25 mg	100 mcg	2.5–5 mg/kg daily in 2–4 doses
Erythromycin	50 mg/mL	100 mg	500 mcg	...
Gentamicin sulfate	8–15 mg/mL	10–20 mg	100–200 mcg	3–5 mg/kg daily in 2–3 doses
Imipenem/Cilastatin sodium	5 mg/mL	...	...	2 g daily in 3–4 doses
Kanamycin sulfate	30–50 mg/mL	30 mg	500 mcg	...
Neomycin sulfate	5–8 mg/mL	125–250 mg	...	...
Penicillin G	100,000 units/mL	0.5–1.0 million units	300 units	12–24 million units daily in 4–6 doses
Piperacillin	12.5 mg/mL	100 mg	...	...
Polymyxin B sulfate	10,000 units/mL	100,000 units	...	...
Ticarcillin disodium	6 mg/mL	100 mg	...	200–300 mg/kg daily 3 x in 4–6 doses
Tobramycin sulfate	8–15 mg/mL	10–20 mg	100–200 mcg	3–5 mg/kg daily in 2–3 doses
Vancomycin hydrochloride‡	20–25 mg/mL	25 mg	1000 mcg	15–30 mg/kg daily in 1–2 doses

*Most penicillins and cephalosporins are physically incompatible when combined in the same bottle with aminoglycosides such as amikacin, gentamicin, or tobramycin. †Adult doses. ‡Usage discouraged by CDC because of increased resistant organisms.

TABLE 7

ANTIFUNGAL AGENTS

GENERIC (TRADE) NAME	ROUTE	DOSAGE	SPECTRUM
Amphotericin B (Fungizone)	Topical	0.1–0.5% solution (most commonly 0.15%); dilute with water for injection or dextrose 5% in water	Blastomyces Candida Coccidioides Histoplasma
	Subconjunctival	0.8–1.0 mg	
	Intravitreal	5 mcg	
	Intravenous	*	
Fluconazole (Diflucan)	Oral	200 mg on day 1, then 100 mg daily in divided doses	Candida
		400 mg on day 1, then 200 mg daily in divided doses	Cryptococcus
Flucytosine (Ancobon)	Oral	50–150 mg/kg daily in 4 divided doses*	Candida Cryptococcus
Itraconazole (Sporanox)	Oral Intravenous	200–400 mg daily* 200 mg IV twice a day for 4 days, then switch to oral daily dosage for 14 days*	Blastomyces Histoplasma Aspergillus Onychomyces
Ketoconazole (Nizoral)	Oral	200–400 mg daily*	Candida Cryptococcus Histoplasma
Natamycin (Natacyn)	Topical	5% suspension	Candida Aspergillus Cephalosporium Fusarium Penicillium

*Because of potential side effects and toxicity, the practitioner should consult the main *PDR* for possible dosage adjustments and warnings.

TABLE 8

ANTIVIRAL AGENTS

GENERIC (TRADE) NAME	TOPICAL CONC.	INTRAVIT. DOSE	SYSTEMIC DOSAGE*
Trifluridine (Viroptic)	1.0% (oph. solution)	...	...
Acyclovir sodium (Zovirax)	...	...	Oral–*Herpes simplex* keratitis: 200 mg 5 times daily for 7–10 days Oral–*Herpes zoster ophthalmicus:* 600–800 mg 5 times daily for 10 days; IV therapy†
Cidofovir (Vistide)	...	...	IV–Induction: 5 mg/kg constant infusion over 1 hour administered once weekly for 2 consecutive weeks Maintenance: 5 mg/kg constant infusion over 1 hour administered once every 2 weeks
Famciclovir (Famvir)	...	...	Oral–*Herpes zoster ophthalmicus:* 500 mg 3 times daily for 7 days
Fomiversen (Vitravene)	...	330 mcg	Every other week for 4 doses, then every 4 weeks. Contains 6.6 mg/mL, in a 0.25-mL vial
Foscarnet sodium (Foscavir)	...	...	IV–by controlled infusion only, either by central vein or by peripheral vein–Induction: 60 mg/kg (adjusted for renal function) given over 1 h every 8 h for 14–21 days Maintenance: 90–120 mg/kg given over 2 hours once daily
Ganciclovir sodium (Cytovene)	...	200 mcg	IV–Induction: 5 mg/kg every 12 h for 14–21 days Maintenance: 5 mg/kg daily for 7 days or 6 mg once daily for 5 days/week Oral–After IV induction: 1000 mg 3 times daily with food or 500 mg 6 times daily every 3 h
Ganciclovir sodium (Vitrasert)	...	4.5 mg	Sterile intravitreal insert designed to release the drug over a 5- to 8-month period
Valacyclovir (Valtrex)	...	...	Oral–*Herpes zoster ophthalmicus:* 1 gram 3 times daily for 7 days

*Because of potential side effects and toxicity, the practitioner should consult the main *PDR* for possible dosage adjustments and warnings.
†IV therapy should be considered if the patient is immunocompromised.

3. OCULAR ANTI-INFLAMMATORY AGENTS

A wide variety of medications are available to treat ocular inflammation. They are listed in **Table 9**. Corticosteroids are the most commonly used. Many are available in combination with antibiotics and/or other medications.

At one time, it was felt that corticosteroids were contraindicated in infectious disease states. However, it is now appreciated that steroids, when used in conjunction with appropriate antimicrobial, antifungal, or antiviral agents, may help prevent more serious ocular damage.

TABLE 9

TOPICAL ANTI-INFLAMMATORY AGENTS

NAME AND DOSAGE FORM	TRADE NAME	CONCENTRATION
Dexamethasone Sodium Phosphate Ophthalmic Solution or Ointment	Decadron Ocu-Dex Available generically	0.1% 0.1% 0.1%
Fluorometholone Ophthalmic Ointment	FML S.O.P.	0.1%
Fluorometholone Ophthalmic Suspension	Fluor-Op FML FML Forte Available generically	0.1% 0.1% 0.25% 0.1%
Fluorometholone Acetate Ophthalmic Suspension	Flarex Eflone	0.1% 0.1%
Loteprednol Etabonate Ophthalmic Suspension	Alrex Lotemax	0.2% 0.5%
Medrysone Ophthalmic Suspension	HMS	1%
Prednisolone Acetate Ophthalmic Suspension	Pred Mild Econopred Econopred Plus Pred Forte Available generically	0.12% 0.125% 1% 1% 1%
Prednisolone Sodium Phosphate Ophthalmic Solution	Inflamase Mild Available generically AK-Pred Inflamase Forte Available generically	0.125% 0.125% 1% 1% 1%
Rimexolone Ophthalmic Suspension	Vexol	1%
NONSTEROIDAL ANTI-INFLAMMATORY DRUGS		
Diclofenac Sodium Ophthalmic Solution	Voltaren	0.1%
Flurbiprofen Sodium Ophthalmic Solution	Ocufen Available generically	0.03% 0.03%
Ketorolac Tromethamine Ophthalmic Solution	Acular LS Acular Acular PF	0.4% 0.5% 0.5%

Steroids may be administered by four different routes in the treatment of ocular inflammation. **Table 10** lists the preferred route in various conditions.

Topical corticosteroids can elevate intraocular pressure and, in susceptible individuals, can induce glaucoma. Some corticosteroids, such as fluorometholone acetate, medrysone, and loteprednol cause less elevation of intraocular pressure than others. Corticosteroids may also cause cataract formation, a complication more likely with high-dose, long-term systemic use.

There are also three nonsteroidal anti-inflammatory drugs (NSAIDs) available. They are: diclofenac (Voltaren); flurbiprofen (Ocufen); and ketorolac (Acular). Flurbiprofen is indicated solely for inhibition of intraoperative miosis. Diclofenac has an official indication for the postoperative prophylaxis and treatment of ocular inflammation. Ketorolac is indicated for the treatment of postoperative inflammation and for relief of ocular itching due to seasonal allergic conjunctivitis. It has also shown some success in alleviating the pain associated with keratotomy, although unapproved for this use. Both diclofenac and ketorolac have also been used successfully to prevent and treat cystoid macular edema. NSAIDs cause little, if any, rise in intraocular pressure. However, in rare instances, topical NSAIDs have been associated with corneal melts and perforations, especially in older patients with ocular surface disease such as dry eyes.

TABLE 10

USUAL ROUTE OF STEROID ADMINISTRATION IN OCULAR INFLAMMATION

CONDITION	ROUTE
Anterior uveitis	Topical and/or periocular
Blepharitis	Topical
Conjunctivitis	Topical
Cranial arteritis	Systemic
Endophthalmitis	Systemic-periocular, and/or intravitreal
Episcleritis	Topical
Keratitis	Topical
Optic neuritis	Systemic or periocular
Posterior uveitis	Systemic and/or periocular
Scleritis	Topical and/or systemic
Sympathetic ophthalmia	Systemic and topical

Other useful agents include mast-cell inhibitors, antihistamines, low-concentration steroids, and decongestants to treat vernal conjunctivitis or allergic keratoconjunctivitis. Tetracycline, taken orally, in doses of 250 mg 4 times daily for 4 weeks, then 250 mg once daily, is useful in treating ocular rosacea. Alternatively, doxycycline or minocycline, taken orally, in doses of 100 mg twice daily for 1 to 2 weeks, then 100 mg once daily, may be used.

Agents useful in treatment of seasonal allergic conjunctivitis are listed in **Table 11**.

TABLE 11

AGENTS FOR RELIEF OF SEASONAL ALLERGIC CONJUNCTIVITIS

GENERIC NAME	TRADE NAME	CLASS	TYPICAL DAILY DOSE
Azelastine	Optivar	H_1-Antagonist/Mast-cell inhibitor	2
Cromolyn	Crolom	Mast-cell inhibitor	4-6
Emedastine	Emadine	H_1-Antagonist	4
Epinastine HCl	Elestat	H_1- and H_2-antagonist/ Mast-cell inhibitor	2
Ketorolac	Acular	NSAID	4
Ketotifen	Zaditor	H_1-Antagonist/Mast-cell inhibitor	2
Levocabastine	Livostin	H_1-Antagonist	4
Lodoxamide	Alomide	Mast-cell inhibitor	4
Loteprednol	Alrex Lotemax	Corticosteroid	4
Naphazoline/antazoline	Vasocon-A	Antihistamine/decongestant	4
Naphazoline/pheniramine	Naphcon-A Opcon-A Visine-A	Antihistamine/decongestant	4
Nedocromil	Alocril	H_1-Antagonist/Mast-cell inhibitor	2
Olopatadine	Patanol	H_1-Antagonist/Mast-cell inhibitor	2
Pemirolast	Alamast	Mast-cell inhibitor	4

4. ANESTHETIC AGENTS

A. Topical anesthetics

The agents listed in **Table 12** permit the clinician to perform ocular procedures such as tonometry, removal of foreign bodies from the surface of the eye, and lacrimal canalicular manipulation and irrigation. Cocaine, the prototype topical anesthetic, is a natural compound; the others are synthetic.

Cocaine is rarely used as an anesthetic agent because it causes damage to the corneal epithelium, produces pupillary dilation, and may affect intraocular pressure. However, it is considered useful when removal of the corneal epithelium is desired, as in epithelial debridement for dendritic keratitis.

The table lists available agents and concentrations. Most begin working within a minute and continue acting for 10 to 20 minutes. A transient, superficial punctate keratitis may develop rapidly after instillation of the agent.

B. Regional anesthetics

The actions, benefits, and drawbacks of the most common regional anesthetic agents used in ophthalmic surgery are summarized in **Table 13**.

TABLE 12

TOPICAL ANESTHETIC AGENTS

USP OR NF NAME	TRADE NAME	CONCENTRATION
Cocaine hydrochloride*	. . .	1%–4%
Proparacaine hydrochloride	Alcaine	0.5%
	Ocu-Caine	0.5%
	Ophthetic	0.5%
	Parcaine	0.5%
Tetracaine hydrochloride	Pontocaine	0.5%
	Available generically	0.5%

*Extemporaneous formulation.

TABLE 13

REGIONAL ANESTHETICS*

USP OR NF NAME	CONCENTRATION/ MAXIMUM DOSE	ONSET OF ACTION	DURATION OF ACTION	MAJOR ADVANTAGES/ DISADVANTAGES
Bupivacaine[†,‡]	0.25%–0.75%	5–11 min	480–720 min (with epinephrine)	
Etidocaine[†]	1%	3 min	300–600 min	
Lidocaine[†]	1%–2%/500 mg	4–6 min	40–60 min 120 min (with epinephrine)	Spreads readily without hyaluronidase
Mepivacaine[†]	1%–2%/500 mg	3–5 min	120 min	Duration of action greater without epinephrine[2]
Prilocaine[†]	1%–2%/600 mg	3–4 min	90–120 min (with epinephrine)	As effective as lidocaine
Procaine[§]	1%–4%/500 mg	7–8 min	30–45 min 60 min (with epinephrine)	Short duration. Poor absorption from mucous membranes
Tetracaine[§]	0.25%	5–9 min	120–140 min (with epinephrine)	

*Retrobulbar injection has been reported to cause apnea.
[†]Amide type compound.
[‡]A mixture of bupivacaine, lidocaine, and epinephrine has been shown to be effective in retinal detachment surgery under local anesthesia.[1]
[§]Ester type compound.

REFERENCES

1. Holekamp TLR, Arribas NP, Boniuk I. Bupivacaine anesthesia in retinal detachment surgery. *Arch Ophthalmol.* 1979;97:109.
2. Everett WG, Vey EK, Finlay JW. Duration of oculomotor akinesia of injectable anesthetics. *Trans Am Acad Ophthalmol.* 1961;65:308.

5. AGENTS FOR TREATMENT OF GLAUCOMA

A. Miotics — see **Table 14**
Parasympathomimetic agents (miotics) are used primarily as topical therapy for glaucoma. A secondary use is the control of accommodative esotropia. This class of agents mimics the effect of acetylcholine on parasympathomimetic postganglionic nerve endings within the eye. The class is subdivided into direct-acting (cholinergic) agents and indirect-acting (anticholinesterase) agents, based on their respective abilities to bind acetylcholine receptors and inhibit the enzymatic hydrolysis of acetylcholine. **Table 14** lists the parasympathomimetics approved for topical use in this country. In addition, two agents are available for intraocular use: Miochol-E, a 1% solution of acetylcholine, and Miostat or Carbastat, a 0.01% solution of carbachol.

B. Sympathomimetics — see **Table 15**
These medications work by improving aqueous outflow and, to a lesser extent, improving uveoscleral output. The prodrug dipivefrin causes fewer systemic side effects than epinephrine and can sometimes be used in patients who have developed a sensitivity to epinephrine.

C. β-Adrenergic blocking agents — see **Table 16**
These medications work by blocking β-adrenergic receptor sites and decreasing aqueous production, thereby reducing intraocular pressure. Because β-adrenergic receptors occur in a number of organ systems, systemic side effects of these drugs may include slowed heart rate, decreased blood pressure, and exacerbation of intrinsic bronchial asthma and emphysema. These agents can also enhance the effects of a number of systemic medications including β-blockers, digitalis alkaloids, and reserpine. Since betaxolol is a cardioselective β-blocker, it has significantly less effect on the respiratory system and can be used in some patients with respiratory illnesses.

D. Hyperosmotic agents — see **Table 17**
These medications decrease intraocular pressure by creating an osmotic gradient between the blood and intraocular fluid, causing fluid to move out of the aqueous and vitreous humors into the bloodstream. Though not usually used in open-angle glaucoma, these medications are employed to decrease pressure in an attack of angle-closure glaucoma, and to give a "soft" eye during surgery.

E. Carbonic anhydrase inhibitors — see **Table 18**
Used both topically and systemically, these drugs decrease the formation and secretion of aqueous humor. The systemic forms are usually used to supplement various topical agents (but not topical CAIs). Use of the systemic agents is limited by their side effects, which include paresthesias, anorexia, gastrointestinal disturbances, headaches, altered taste and smell, sodium and potassium depletion, ureteral colic, a predisposition to form renal calculi, and, rarely, bone marrow suppression. The most commonly reported adverse effects of the topical solution are superficial punctate keratitis and ocular allergic reactions. Less frequently reported are blurred vision, tearing, ocular dryness, and photophobia. Infrequent are headache, nausea, asthenia, and fatigue. Rarely, skin rashes, urolithiasis, and iridocyclitis may occur.

F. α_2 Selective agonists — see **Table 19**
There are two medications in this class: apraclonidine and brimonidine. Apraclonidine is available as a single-dose applicator of a 1% solution for suppression of the acute intraocular pressure spikes that occur after laser treatments. A 0.5% concentration is also available, supplied in a multiple-dose bottle for use with other glaucoma medications to control pressure in patients who are not responding adequately to maximally tolerated glaucoma therapy. The medication is generally useful only for short-term therapy, since it has been associated with tachyphylaxis within 3 months in up to 48% of patients. Brimonidine, the second agent in this class, is 23 to 32 times more selective for alpha$_2$ versus alpha$_1$ adrenoreceptors than is apraclonidine. This allows the medication to be used on a chronic basis with reduced risk of tachyphylaxis. Brimonidine ophthalmic solution is available in concentrations of 0.2% (generic) and 0.15% (Alphagan-P).

G. Prostaglandins — see **Table 20**
The prostaglandin latanoprost was developed specifically for the treatment of glaucoma. A single daily dose has been shown to be more effective in reducing IOP than timolol 0.5% administered twice daily. Ocular side effects—hyperemia, itching, tearing, foreign-body sensation, and stinging appear to be minimal, and systemic side effects have not been observed. An increase in pigmentation in the iris occurs in 7.2% of patients with mixed-color irises, and the change appears to be permanent. Its clinical significance is unknown. Other prostaglandin analogues are also available, such as travoprost, unoprostone, and bimatoprost.

H. Another option for the treatment of glaucoma is the brand Cosopt, which is a combination of the β-adrenergic blocker timolol with the carbonic anhydrase inhibitor dorzolamide (see **Table 21**).

REFERENCE

Fiscella RG, Winarko T. Glaucoma—new therapeutic options. *U.S. Pharmacist*, December 1996.

TABLE 14
MIOTICS

GENERIC NAME	TRADE NAME	STRENGTHS	SIZES
CHOLINERGIC AGENTS			
Carbachol	Isopto Carbachol	0.75%, 1.5%, 3%	15, 30 mL
Pilocarpine hydrochloride	Isopto Carpine	1%, 2%, 4%, 6%, 8%	15 & 30 mL
	Pilocar	0.5%, 1%, 2%, 4%, 6%	15 & 2 x 15 mL
	Pilopine-HS gel	4%	3.5 g
	Piloptic	0.5%, 1%, 2%, 3%, 4%, 6%	15 mL
	Available generically	0.5%, 1%, 2%, 3%, 4%, 6%	15 mL

TABLE 15
SYMPATHOMIMETICS

GENERIC NAME	TRADE NAME	CONCENTRATION	SIZES (mL)
Dipivefrin hydrochloride	Propine	0.1%	5, 10, 15
	Available generically	0.1%	5, 10, 15
Epinephrine hydrochloride	Epifrin	0.5%, 1%, 2%	5, 10, 15

TABLE 16
β-ADRENERGIC BLOCKING AGENTS

GENERIC NAME	TRADE NAME	CONCENTRATION	SIZES (mL)
Betaxolol hydrochloride	Betoptic-S	0.25%	2.5, 5, 15
	Available generically	0.5%	5, 10, 15
Carteolol hydrochloride	Ocupress	1%	5, 10
	Available generically	1%	5, 10, 15
Levobunolol hydrochloride	Betagan	0.25%, 0.5%	2, 5, 10, 15
	Available generically	0.25%, 0.5%	5, 10, 15
Metipranolol	OptiPranolol	0.3%	5, 10
	Available generically	0.3%	5, 10
Timolol	Betimol	0.25%, 0.5%	2.5, 5, 10, 15
Timolol maleate	Timoptic	0.25%, 0.5%	2.5, 5, 10, 15
	Available generically	0.25%, 0.5%	5, 10, 15
Timolol maleate (gel)	Timoptic - XE	0.25%, 0.5%	2.5, 5
	Available generically	0.25%, 0.5%	2.5, 5

TABLE 17
HYPEROSMOTIC AGENTS

USP OR NF NAME	TRADE NAME	PREPARATION	DOSE	ROUTE	ONSET/DURATION OF ACTION
Glycerin	Osmoglyn	50%	1–1.5 g/kg	Oral	. . .
Mannitol*	Osmitrol	5%–20%	0.5–2 g/kg	IV	30–60 min/6 h
Urea	Ureaphil	Powder (4 g) for reconstitution to 30% soln	0.5–2 g/kg	IV	30–45 min/5–6 h

*Do not confuse with mannitol hexanitrate, an antianginal agent.

TABLE 18
CARBONIC ANHYDRASE INHIBITORS

USP OR NF NAME	TRADE NAME	PREPARATION	ONSET/DURATION OF ACTION
Acetazolamide	Diamox	125, 250 mg tablets 500 mg (timed-release) capsules	2 h/4–6 h
	Available generically	125, 250 mg tablets	
Brinzolamide	Azopt	1% ophthalmic suspension	...
Dorzolamide HCl	Trusopt	2% ophthalmic solution	...
Methazolamide	Neptazane Available generically	25, 50 mg tablets 25, 50 mg tablets	2 h/4–6 h

TABLE 19
α_2 SELECTIVE AGONISTS

GENERIC NAME	TRADE NAME	CONCENTRATION	SIZES (mL)
Apraclonidine	Iopidine	0.5% 1.0%	5, 10 single-use container
Brimonidine	Alphagan P Available generically	0.15% 0.2%	5, 10, 15 5, 10, 15

TABLE 20
PROSTAGLANDINS

GENERIC NAME	TRADE NAME	CONCENTRATION	SIZES (mL)
Bimatoprost	Lumigan	0.03%	2.5
Latanoprost	Xalatan	0.005%	2.5
Travoprost	Travatan	0.004%	2.5
Unoprostone	Rescula	0.15%	5

TABLE 21
COMBINATION AGENT

GENERIC NAME	TRADE NAME	CONCENTRATION	SIZES (mL)
Dorzolamide HCl and timolol maleate	Cosopt	2% dorzolamide/0.5% timolol	5, 10

6. MEDICATIONS FOR DRY EYE

Dry eye refers to a deficiency in either the aqueous or mucin components of the precorneal tear film. The most commonly encountered aqueous-deficient dry eye in the United States is keratoconjunctivitis sicca, while mucin-deficient dry eyes may be seen in cases of hypovitaminosis A, Stevens-Johnson syndrome, ocular pemphigoid, extensive trachoma, and chemical burns.

Dry eye is treated with artificial tear preparations (see **Table 22**), prescription medication (see **Table 23**) and ophthalmic lubricants (see **Table 24**). The lubricants form an occlusive film over the ocular surface and protect the eye from drying. Administered as a nighttime medication, they are useful both for dry eye and in cases of recurrent corneal erosion.

TABLE 22

ARTIFICIAL TEAR PREPARATIONS

MAJOR COMPONENT(S)	CONCENTRATION	TRADE NAME	PRESERVATIVE/EDTA*
Carboxymethylcellulose	0.5%	Refresh Plus	None
		Refresh Tears	Purite
	1%	Celluvisc	None
	1%	Refresh Liquigel	Purite
	0.25%	TheraTears	None
Glycerin	0.3%	Moisture Eyes	Benzalkonium chloride
	1.0%	Computer Eye Drops	Benzalkonium chloride, EDTA
Glycerin, polysorbate 80	1% (both)	Refresh Endura	None
Hydroxypropyl cellulose	5 mg/insert	Lacrisert (biodegradable insert)	None
Hydroxypropyl methylcellulose	0.3%	GenTeal	Sodium perborate
		GenTeal Gel	Sodium perborate
		GenTeal PF	None
	0.2%	GenTeal Mild	Sodium perborate
	0.5%	Tearisol	Benzalkonium chloride, EDTA
Hydroxypropyl methylcellulose, dextran 70		Bion Tears	None
		Tears Renewed	Benzalkonium chloride, EDTA
Hydroxypropyl methylcellulose, glycerin		Clear Eyes CLR	Sorbic acid, EDTA
		Visine for Contacts	Potassium sorbate, EDTA
Hydroxypropyl methylcellulose, glycerin, dextran 70		Tears Naturale Forte	Polyquaternium-1
		Tears Naturale Free	None
Hydroxypropyl methylcellulose, glycerin, PEG-400		Visine Tears	Benzalkonium chloride
		Visine Tears PF	None
Hypromellose, dextran 70	0.8%, 0.1%	Moisture Eyes	None
Methylcellulose	1%	Murocel	Methylparabens, propylparabens
Polycarbophil, PEG-400, dextran 70		AquaSite	EDTA
		AquaSite multi-dose	EDTA, sorbic acid
Polyvinyl alcohol	1.4%	AKWA Tears	Benzalkonium chloride, EDTA
Polyvinyl alcohol, PEG-400, dextrose	1%	HypoTears	Benzalkonium chloride, EDTA
		HypoTears PF	EDTA
Polyvinyl alcohol, povidone	1.4%	Murine Tears	Benzalkonium chloride, EDTA
Propylene glycol, PEG-400	0.3%, 0.4%	Systane	Polyquaternium-1

*EDTA = ethylenediaminetetraacetic acid.

TABLE 23

PRESCRIPTION MEDICINE FOR DRY EYE SYNDROME

MAJOR COMPONENT	CONCENTRATION	DOSE	TRADE NAME	PRESERVATIVE
Cyclosporine	0.05%	q12h	Restasis	None

TABLE 24
OPHTHALMIC LUBRICANTS

TRADE NAME	COMPOSITION OF STERILE OINTMENT
AKWA Tears Ointment	White petrolatum, liquid lanolin, and mineral oil
HypoTears Ointment Tears Renewed	White petrolatum and light mineral oil
Lacri-Lube S.O.P.	White petrolatum, mineral oil, chlorobutanol, and lanolin alcohols
Refresh P.M.	42.5% mineral oil, 57.3% white petrolatum, and lanolin alcohols

7. OCULAR DECONGESTANTS

These topically applied adrenergic medications are commonly used to whiten the eye. Those containing naphazoline and tetrahydrozoline are more stable than those with phenylephrine. Usual dosage is 1 or 2 drops no more than 4 times a day (see **Table 25**).

TABLE 25
OCULAR DECONGESTANTS

DRUG	TRADE NAME	ADDITIONAL COMPONENTS
Naphazoline hydrochloride	AK-Con (0.1%)	Benzalkonium chloride, edetate disodium
	Albalon (0.1%)	Benzalkonium chloride, edetate disodium
	All Clear (0.012%)	Benzalkonium chloride, edetate disodium, PEG-300
	All Clear AR (0.03%)	Benzalkonium chloride, edetate disodium, hydroxypropyl methylcellulose 0.5%
	Clear Eyes (0.012%)	Benzalkonium chloride, edetate disodium
	Available generically	Benzalkonium chloride, EDTA[†]
Oxymetazoline hydrochloride	Visine L.R. (0.025%)	Benzalkonium chloride, edetate disodium
Phenylephrine hydrochloride	AK-Nefrin (0.12%)	Benzalkonium chloride, edetate disodium
Tetrahydrozoline hydrochloride	EyeSine (0.05%)	Benzalkonium chloride, edetate disodium
	Murine Tears Plus (0.05%)	Benzalkonium chloride, edetate disodium, polyvinyl alcohol, povidone
	Visine (0.05%)	Benzalkonium chloride, edetate disodium
	Visine Advanced Relief (0.05%)	Benzalkonium chloride, edetate disodium, PEG-400, povidone, dextran 70
	Available generically	Benzalkonium chloride, edetate disodium, PEG-400, povidone, dextran 70
DECONGESTANT/ASTRINGENT COMBINATIONS		
Naphazoline hydrochloride plus antazoline phosphate	Visine-A	Benzalkonium chloride, edetate disodium
	Naphcon-A	Benzalkonium chloride, edetate disodium
Naphazoline hydrochloride plus pheniramine maleate	Vasocon-A	Benzalkonium chloride, edetate disodium
Naphazoline hydrochloride plus zinc sulfate	Clear Eyes ACR (0.125%) (allergy/cold relief)	Benzalkonium chloride, edetate disodium, glycerin
Tetrahydrozoline plus zinc sulfate	Visine A.C.	Benzalkonium chloride, edetate disodium

[†]EDTA = ethylenediaminetetraacetic acid.

8. OPHTHALMIC IRRIGATING SOLUTIONS

Listed in **Table 26** are sterile isotonic solutions for general ophthalmic use. They are all over-the-counter products. There are also intraocular irrigating solutions available for use during surgical procedures. They include prescription medications such as Bausch & Lomb's Balanced Salt Solution, Alcon's BSS and BSS Plus, and Iolab's Iocare Balanced Salt Solution.

TABLE 26

OPHTHALMIC IRRIGATING SOLUTIONS

TRADE NAME	COMPONENTS	ADDITIONAL COMPONENTS
AK-Rinse	Sodium, potassium, calcium, and magnesium chlorides, sodium acetate, and sodium citrate	Benzalkonium chloride
Collyrium Fresh Eyes	Boric acid and sodium borate	Benzalkonium chloride
Dacriose	Sodium and potassium chlorides, and sodium phosphate	Benzalkonium chloride, edetate disodium
Eye Wash Solution	Boric acid and sodium borate	EDTA*, sorbic acid

*EDTA = ethylenediaminetetraacetic acid.

9. HYPEROSMOLAR AGENTS

Hyperosmolar (hypertonic) agents are used to reduce corneal edema. They act through osmotic attraction of water through the semipermeable corneal epithelium.

TABLE 27

HYPEROSMOLAR AGENTS

GENERIC NAME	TRADE NAME	CONCENTRATION
Sodium chloride	Muro-128	2% or 5% (solution), 5% (ointment)
	Available generically	5% (solution and ointment)

10. DIAGNOSTIC AGENTS

Some of the more common diagnostic agents and tests used in ophthalmologic practice are listed below.

A. Examination of the Conjunctiva, Cornea, and Lacrimal Apparatus

Fluorescein, applied primarily as a 2% alkaline solution, and with impregnated paper strips, is used to examine the integrity of the conjunctival and corneal epithelia. Defects in the corneal epithelium will appear bright green in ordinary light and bright yellow when a cobalt blue filter is used in the light path. Similar lesions of the conjunctiva appear bright orange-yellow in ordinary illumination.

Fluorescein has also come into wide use in the fitting of rigid contact lenses, though it cannot be used for soft lenses, which absorb the dye. Proper fit is determined by examining the pattern of fluorescein beneath the contact lens.

In addition, fluorescein is used in performing applanation tonometry. Also, one test of lacrimal apparatus patency (Jones test) uses 1 drop of 1% fluorescein instilled into the conjunctival sac. If the dye appears in the nose, drainage is normal.

Rose bengal, available as 1% solution or in impregnated strips, is particularly useful for demonstrating abnormal conjunctival or corneal epithelium. Devitalized cells stain bright red, while normal cells show no change. *Lissamine green,* available as 1% solution or in impregnated strips, also stains abnormal conjunctival and corneal cells. It is less irritating to the eye than rose bengal. The abnormal epithelial cells that present in dry eye disorders are effectively revealed by these stains.

The *Schirmer* test is a valuable method of assessing tear production. It employs prepared strips of filter paper 5 by 30 mm in size. The strips are inserted into the topically anesthetized conjunctival sac at the junction of the middle and outer third of the lower lid, with approximately 25 mm of paper exposed. After 5 minutes, the strip is removed and the amount of moistening measured. The normal range is 10 to 25 mm. If inadequate production of tears is found on the initial test, a Schirmer II test can be performed by repeating the procedure while stimulating the nasal mucosa. A number of variations of the Schirmer test can be found in textbooks and journals.

B. Examination of Acquired Ptosis or Extraocular Muscle Palsy

To confirm myasthenia gravis as the cause of ptosis or muscle palsy, an intravenous injection of 2 mg of *edrophonium chloride* is administered, followed 45 seconds later by an additional 8 mg if there is no response to the first dose. (In case of a severe reaction to the edrophonium, immediately give atropine sulfate, 0.6 mg intravenously.)

C. Examination of the Retina and Choroid

Sodium fluorescein solution, in concentrations of 5%, 10%, and 25%, is injected intravenously to study the retinal and choroidal circulation. It has been used primarily in examination of lesions at the posterior pole of the eye, but anterior segment fluorescein angiography (wherein the vessels of the iris, sclera, and conjunctiva are studied) is also a useful clinical tool.

Intravascular fluorescein is normally prevented from entering the retina by the intact retinal vascular endothelium (blood-retinal barrier) and the intact retinal pigment epithelium. Defects in either the retinal vessels or the pigment epithelium will allow leakage of fluorescein, which can then be studied by either direct observation or photography. For good results, appropriate filters are needed to excite the fluorescein and exclude unwanted wavelengths. The peak frequencies for excitation lie between 485 and 500 nm and, for emission, between 520 and 530 nm.

Fluorescein has proved to be a safe diagnostic agent, the most common side effects being nausea and vomiting. However, occasional allergic and vagal reactions do occur, so oxygen and emergency equipment should be readily available when angiography is performed. Patients should also be warned that the dye will temporarily stain their skin and urine; in the average patient this lasts no more than a day.

Indocyanine green (IC-Green) has been used in recent years, either alone or with fluorescein, to obtain better frames of choroid neovascularization.

D. Examination of Abnormal Pupillary Responses

Methacholine, as a 2.5% solution instilled into the conjunctival sac, will cause the tonic pupil (Adie's pupil) to contract, but will leave a normal pupil unchanged. A similar pupillary response is seen following instillation of 2.5% methacholine in patients with familial dysautonomia (Riley-Day syndrome).

Table 28 shows the effects of several drugs on miosis due to interruption of the sympathetic nervous system (Horner's syndrome). The effect depends on the location of the lesion in the sympathetic chain.

TABLE 28

HORNER'S SYNDROME

TOPICAL DROP (CENTRAL)	NEURON III (POST-GANGLIONIC)	NEURON II (PRE-GANGLIONIC)	NEURON I
Cocaine 2%–10%	–	–	+/–
Epinephrine (Adrenalin) 1:1000	+++	+	–
Phenylephrine 1%	+++	+	+/–

Pilocarpine may be used to determine whether a fixed dilated pupil is due to an atropine-like drug or interruption of the pupil's parasympathetic innervation.[3] If an atropine-like drug is involved, the pupil will not react to pilocarpine. If dilation is due to interruption of the parasympathetic innervation (compression by aneurysm, Adie's tonic pupil) instillation of pilocarpine will cause the pupil to constrict.

REFERENCES

Hecht SD. Evaluation of the lacrimal drainage system. *Ophthalmology*. 1978;85:1250.

Thompson HS, Mensher JH. Adrenergic mydriasis in Horner's syndrome: hydroxyampheta mine test for diagnosis of post-ganglionic defects. *Am J Ophthalmol*. 1971;72:472.

Thompson HS, Newsome DA, Lowenfeld IE. The fixed dilated pupil. Sudden iridoplegia or mydriatic drops; a simple diagnostic test. *Arch Ophthalmol*. 1971;86:12.

11. VISCOELASTIC MATERIALS USED IN OPHTHALMOLOGY

Viscoelastic substances are used in ophthalmic surgery to maintain the anterior chamber, hydraulically dissect tissues, act as a vitreous substitute/tamponade, and prevent mechanical damage to tissue, especially the corneal endothelium. The individual characteristics of the various viscoelastic materials are the result of the chain length and intra- and interchain molecular interactions of the compounds comprising the viscoelastic substance. All viscoelastic materials have the potential to produce a large postoperative increase in pressure if they are not adequately removed from the anterior chamber following surgery.

AMVISC (Bausch and Lomb) – Composed of sodium hyaluronate 1.2% in physiologic saline. The viscosity is 40,000 cSt (@25°C, 1/sec shear rate), and molecular weight is ≥2,000,000 daltons. Its shelf life is estimated at 2 years.

AMVISC PLUS (Bausch and Lomb) – Composed of sodium hyaluronate 1.6% in physiologic saline. The viscosity is 55,000 cSt (@25°C, 1/sec shear rate), and molecular weight is approximately 1,500,000 daltons. The greater viscosity is obtained by increasing total concentration and using sodium hyaluronate of lower molecular weight. Its shelf life is estimated at 1 year.

BIOLON (Akorn) – Composed of sodium hyaluronate 1%. The viscosity is 215,000 cps, and the molecular weight is approximately 3,000,000 daltons. The product does not require refrigeration and its shelf life is estimated to be approximately 2 years.

DUOVISC (Alcon) – Package contains two separate syringes. One syringe containing Provisc; the other containing Viscoat. Please see individual descriptions below for details of each.

HEALON (Pfizer) – Composed of sodium hyaluronate 1% in physiologic saline. The viscosity is 200,000 (@ 0/sec shear rate), and the molecular weight is approximately 4,000,000 daltons.

HEALON GV (Pfizer) – Composed of sodium hyaluronate 1.4% in physiologic saline. The viscosity is 2,000,000 (@ 0/sec shear rate), and the molecular weight is approximately 5,000,000 daltons. In the presence of high positive vitreous pressure, Healon GV has 3 times more resistance to pressure than does Healon.

HEALON 5 (Pfizer) – Composed of sodium hyaluronate 2.3%. The viscosity is 7,000,000 cP (@ 25°C, 1/sec shear rate), and the molecular weight is 4,000,000 daltons.

OCUCOAT (Storz – Bausch and Lomb) – Composed of hydroxypropylmethylcellulose 2% in balance salt solution (BSS). The viscosity is 4,000 cSt (@ 37°C measured on Cannon-Fenske Viscometer), and the molecular weight is approximately 80,000 daltons. Occucoat is termed a viscoadherent rather than a viscoelastic because of its coating ability, which is related to its contact angle and low surface tension.

PROVISC (Alcon) – Composed of sodium hyaluronate 1% in physiologic saline. The viscosity is 39,000 cps (@ 25°C, 2/sec shear rate) and the molecular weight is approximately 1,900,000 daltons. Clinical studies demonstrate that ProVisc functions in a similar fashion to Healon.

VISCOAT (Alcon) – Composed of a 1:3 mixture of chondroitin sulfate 4% (CS) and sodium hyaluronate 3% (SH) in physiologic saline. The viscosity is 40,000 cps (@ 25°C, 2/sec shear rate), and the molecular weight is 22,500 daltons for CS and 500,000 daltons for SH.

VITRAX (Allergan) – Composed of sodium hyaluronate 3% in balanced salt solution (BSS). The viscosity is 30,000 cps (@ 2/sec shear rate) and the molecular weight is 500,000 daltons. It is highly concentrated to produce a significantly viscous material. It does not require refrigeration and has a shelf life of 18 months.

12. OFF-LABEL DRUG APPLICATIONS IN OPHTHALMOLOGY

A. Acetylcysteine
This agent is used to treat corneal conditions such as alkali burns, corneal melts, and keratoconjunctivitis sicca. It is thought to improve healing by inhibiting the action of collagenase, which may contribute to delay in healing. The drug is available generically or under the trade name Mucomyst in 10% and 20% solutions. Though none of the commercially available solutions are approved for use in ophthalmology, they have been administered as frequently as hourly in acute cases, and up to 4 times a day in maintenance therapy.

B. Alteplase (tissue plasminogen activator)
This thrombolytic agent, available under the trade name Activase, is used to treat fibrin formation in postvitrectomy patients. Though initial studies were based on intraocular injections of 25 mcg, more recent work has shown the drug to be effective in doses of as little as 3 to 6 mcg. Because by-products of alteplase activity may mediate endothelial cell toxicity, the lower doses are preferred. This agent has also been used for submacular hemorrage, but this use is controversial.

C. Antimetabolites
5-Fluorouracil (5-FU). This drug inhibits fibroblast proliferation and diminishes scarring after glaucoma filtering surgery. Initial recommendations of the 5-FU study group called for subconjunctival injections of 5 mg twice daily for 7 days postoperatively and once daily for the next 7 days (total 21 injections). Other physicians achieve success with five injections over 15 days. Many physicians are using an intraoperative application of 50 mg/mL solution soaked into a murocell sponge lasting for 3 to 5 minutes, with a body of literature supporting its effectiveness (see references listed at the end of this section). Use of this drug is associated with a number of complications, including conjunctival wound leak, corneal epithelial defects, hypotony associated with permanently reduced vision acuity, serious corneal infections in eyes with preexistent corneal epithelial edema, and increased susceptibility to late-onset bleb infections. The drug should be considered only when there is a high risk of surgical failure.

Mitomycin. This potent chemotherapeutic agent, available under the trade name Mutamycin, is being used in filtering surgery for the same purpose and on the same type of patients as 5-FU. It is applied once during surgery on a small piece of Gelfilm or Weck Cell in a concentration of 0.2 to 0.4 mg/mL. Reported side effects are similar to those of 5-FU. However, some serious side effects may go unreported, since there is a possibility of delayed reactions 6 to 24 months after surgery. Mitomycin has also been administered in a 0.02% to 0.04% solution 2 to 4 times a day — and more recently as a one-time application in the operating room — to prevent recurrence after pterygium surgery and reduce scarring after corneal surgery, especially excimer laser surgery. Serious side effects associated with this therapy include corneal melts and scleral ulceration and calcification.

Physicians should bear in mind the possibility of major side effects from all antineoplastic agents and carefully weigh the risks and benefits of their use. Remember, too, that these agents should always be handled and discarded in accordance with OSHA, AMA, ASHP, and/or hospital policies regarding the safe use of antineoplastics.

D. Cyclosporine
This potent immunosuppressant has a high degree of selectivity for T lymphocytes. Available under the trade name Sandimmune, it's been used in a 0.5–2% topical solution as prophylaxis against rejection in high-risk, penetrating keratoplasty and for treating severe vernal conjunctivitis resistant to conventional therapy, ligneous conjunctivitis unresponsive to other topical therapy, and noninfectious peripheral ulcerative keratitis associated with systemic autoimmune disorders.

E. Doxycycline
This derivative of tetracycline is used for the treatment of ocular rosacea and meibomianitis. The usual dose is 100 mg PO daily for 6 to 12 weeks. It has the same side effects, contraindications, and interactions as tetracycline.

F. Edetate disodium
This chelating agent plays a role in treating band keratopathy. After removal of the corneal epithelium, it's used to remove calcium from Bowman's membrane.

REFERENCES
Dietze PJ, Feldman RM, Gross RL. Intraoperative application of 5-fluorouracil during trabeculectomy. *Ophthalmic Surg Lasers*. 1992;23(10):662.
Dunn J, Seamone S, Ostler H. Development of scleral ulceration and calcification after pterygium excision and mitomycin therapy. *Am J Ophthalmol*. 1991;112:343.
Feldman RM, Dietze PJ, Gross RL, et al. Intraoperative 5 fluorouracil administration in trabeculectomy. *J Glaucoma*. 1994;3:302.
Frucht-Perry J, et al. The effect of doxycycline on ocular rosacea. *Am J Ophthalmol*. 1989;170(4):434.
Jaffe G, Abrams G, et al. Tissue plasminogen activator for post vitrectomy fibrin formation. *Ophthalmology*. 1990;97:189.
Goldenfeld M, Krupin T, Ruderman JM, et al. 5-Fluorouracil in initial trabeculectomy. A prospective, randomized, multicenter study. *Ophthalmology*. 1994;101(6):1024.
Lanigan L, Sturmer J, Baez KA, Hitchings RA, Khaw PT. Single intraoperative applications of 5-fluorouracil during filtration surgery: early results. *Br J Ophthalmol*. 1994;78(1):33.
Lish A, Camras C, Podos S. Effect of apraclonidine on intraocular pressure in glaucoma patients receiving maximally tolerated medications. *Glaucoma*. 1992;1:19.
McDermott M, Edelhauser H, et al. Tissue plasminogen activator and corneal endothelium. *Am J Ophthalmol*. 1989;108:91-92.
Mora JS, Nguyen N, Iwach AG, et al. Trabeculectomy with intraoperative sponge 5-fluorouracil. *Ophthalmology*. 1996;103(6):963. Review.
Perry HD, Donnenfeld ED. Medications for dry eye syndrome: a drug-therapy review. *Manag Care*. 2003;12(suppl 12):26.
Pflugfelder SC. Antiinflammatory therapy for dry eye. *Am J Ophthalmol*. 2004;137:337.
Quarterman MJ, et al. Signs, symptoms, and tear studies before and after treatment with doxycycline. *Arch Dermatol*. 1997;133:89.
Rothman RF, Liebmann JM, Ritch R. Low-dose 5-fluorouracil trabeculectomy as initial surgery in uncomplicated glaucoma: long-term followup. *Ophthalmology*. 2000;107(6):1184.
Rubinfeld R, Pfister R, et al. Serious complications of topical mitomycin-C after pterygium surgery. *Ophthalmology*. 1992;99:1647.
Sall K, Stevenson OD, Nundorf TK, Reis BL. Two multicenter, randomized studies of the efficacy and safety of cyclosporine ophthalmic emulsion in moderate to severe dry eye disease. CsA Phase 3 Study Group. *Ophthalmology*. 2000;107:631. Erratum in: *Ophthalmology*. 2000;107:1220.
Smith MF, Sherwood MB, Doyle JW, Khaw PT. Results of intraoperative 5-fluorouracil supplementation on trabeculectomy for open-angle glaucoma. *Am J Ophthalmol*. 1992;114(6):737.
Stevenson D, Tauber J, Reis BL. Efficacy and safety of cyclosporine A ophthalmic emulsion in the treatment of moderate-to-severe dry eye disease: a dose-ranging, randomized trial. The Cyclosporin A Phase 2 Study Group. *Ophthalmology*. 2000;107:967.
Three-year follow-up of the Fluorouracil Filtering Surgery Study. *Am J Ophthalmol*. 1993;115(1):82.
Williams D, Benett S, et al. Low-dose intraocular tissue plasminogen activator for treatment of postvitrectomy fibrin formations. *Am J Opthalmol*. 1990;109:606.

---

13. OCULAR TOXICOLOGY — F. W. Fraunfelder, MD

The table on the following pages lists recently reported ocular side effects of systemic drugs in general, as well as systemic and ocular side effects of ophthalmic medications. The list is not intended to be comprehensive but should provide clinicians with an overview of some of the more clinically relevant side effects that have been reported. For more extensive information, please consult the reference list.

Toxicology data are cataloged by the National Registry of Drug-Induced Ocular Side Effects. To report a suspected adverse drug response, or to obtain references for the information listed in the table, please contact:

F.W. Fraunfelder, MD, Director, National Registry of Drug-Induced Ocular Side Effects
Casey Eye Institute
Oregon Health & Science University
3375 SW Terwilliger Blvd.
Portland, OR 97201-4197
Phone: (503) 494-4318
Fax: (503) 494-4286
E-mail: eyedrug@ohsu.edu
Website: www.eyedrugregistry.com

REFERENCES
Fraunfelder FT, Fraunfelder FW. *Drug-Induced Ocular Side Effects*, ed 5. Woburn, Mass: Butterworth-Heinemann; 2001.
Fraunfelder FT, Fraunfelder FW, Edwards R: Ocular side effects possibly associated with isotretinoin usage. *Am J Ophthalmol*. 2001;132(3):299-305.
Fraunfelder FW: Ocular side effects associated with bisphosphonates. *Drugs of Today*. 2003;39(11):829-835.
Fraunfelder FW: Twice-yearly exams not necessary for patients taking Seroquel. *Am J Ophthalmol*. June 2004 (in press).
Fraunfelder FW, Fraunfelder FT: Topiramate associated acute, bilateral, secondary angle-closure glaucoma. *Ophthalmol*. 2004;111(1):109-111.
Fraunfelder FW, Fraunfelder FT: Oculogyric crisis in patients taking cetirizine. *Am J Ophthalmol*. 2004;137(2):355-57.
Fraunfelder FW, Fraunfelder FT: Bisphosphonates and ocular inflammation. *N Engl J Med*. 2003;348(12):1187-1188.
Fraunfelder FW, Fraunfelder FT: Scleritis associated with pamidronate disodium use. *Am J Ophthalmol*. 2003;135(2):219-222.
Fraunfelder FW, Fraunfelder FT, Corbett JJ: Isotretinoin-associated intracranial hypertension. *Ophthalmology*. 2004;111(6):1248-1250.
Fraunfelder FW, Rich LF: Possible adverse effects of drugs used in refractive surgery. *J Cataract Refractive Surg*. 2003;29(1):170-175.
Fraunfelder FW, Solomon J, Druker BJ, et al: Ocular side effects associated with imatinib mesylate (Gleevec®). *J Ocular Pharmacol Therapeutics*. 2003;19(4):371-375.
Wheeler D, Fraunfelder FW: Ocular motility dysfunction associated with chemotherapeutic agents. *J Am Assoc Pediatr Ophthalmol Strabismus*. 2004;8(1):15-17.

TABLE 29

ADVERSE DRUG EFFECTS

GENERIC NAME	PRINCIPAL GENERAL USE	POSSIBLE ADVERSE EFFECTS
I. MEDICATION BY INJECTION		
Adrenal Corticosteroids		
Depo-steroids	Allergic disorders Anti-inflammatory disorders	If injected into a blood vessel, eg, the tonsillar fossa, may cause unilateral or bilateral retinal arterial occlusions due to emboli of depo-steroid. Permanent bilateral blindness may ensue.
Triamcinolone	Allergic disorders Anti-inflammatory disorders	Fatty atrophy in area of injection, ie, enophthalmus if given retrobulbar or, if given in periocular skin, some deformity can occur in area due to loss of fat.
Antifungals		
Amphotericin B	Aspergillosis, blastomycosis, candidiasis, coccidioidomycosis, histoplasmosis	Ischemic necrosis after subconjunctival injection Subconjunctival nodule, yellow discoloration
Antineoplastics		
Carmustine	Brain tumors Multiple myeloma	Optic neuritis Retinal vascular disorders
Cisplatin	Metastatic testicular or ovarian tumors. Advanced bladder carcinoma	Cortical blindness Papilledema, retrobulbar or optic neuritis
Fluorouracil	Carcinoma of the colon, rectum, breast, stomach, and pancreas	Ocular irritation with tearing, conjunctival hyperemia, canalicular fibrosis, ocular motility dysfunction
Ophthalmic Dyes		
Fluorescein	Ocular diagnostic tests	Nausea, vomiting, urticaria, rhinorrhea, dizziness, hypotension, pharyngoedema, anaphylactic reaction
Parasympathomimetics		
Acetylcholine	Produces prompt, short-term miosis	Hypotension and bradycardia with intraocular injection
II. ORAL		
Anthelmintics		
Levamisol hydrochloride	Connective tissue disorders Ascaris infestation	Patients with Sjögren's syndrome and possibly keratitis sicca have marked increase in systemic side effects, including pruritus and muscle weakness
Antiarrhythmics		
Amiodarone hydrochloride	Cardiac abnormalities Ventricular arrhythmias	Keratopathy Lens opacities, optic neuropathy, color vision defects Discoloration of conjunctiva and eyelids
Propranolol	Cardiovascular abnormalities Certain hypertensive states	May precipitate latent myotonia May mask hyperthyroidism; when taken off drug, thyroid stare and exophthalmos may occur
Antibiotics and Antituberculars		
Chloramphenicol	Typhoid fever	Aplastic anemia
Ethambutol hydrochloride	Pulmonary tuberculosis	Optic neuropathy
Rifampin	Asymptomatic carriers of meningococcus Many gram-negative and gram-positive cocci, including *Neisseria* and *Haemophilus influenzae* Pulmonary tuberculosis	Conjunctival hyperemia Exudative conjunctivitis Increased lacrimation
Minocycline	Useful against gram-negative and gram-positive bacteria Members of lymphogranuloma-psittacosis group *Mycoplasma* Acne rosacea	Pseudotumor cerebri and papilledema as early as 3 days after onset of medication in infants and in young adults Transient myopia Permanent pigmentation of sclera
Antihistamines		
Cetirizine	Treatment of perennial allergic rhinitis, chronic urticaria, and allergic rhinitis	Oculogyric crisis (primarily in children)

GENERIC NAME	PRINCIPAL GENERAL USE	POSSIBLE ADVERSE EFFECTS
Antihypertensives		
Sodium nitroprusside	Provides controlled hypertension during anesthesia Management of severe hypertension	Contraindicated in Leber's hereditary optic atrophy and tobacco amblyopia
Antileprotics		
Clofazimine	Dermatologic diseases—psoriasis, pyoderma gangrenosum Leprosy	Conjunctival, corneal, and macular pigmentation
Antimalarials and Anti-inflammatories		
Hydroxychloroquine	Malaria Lupus erythematosus Rheumatoid arthritis	Disturbance of accommodation Corneal changes Bull's-eye maculopathy—central, pericentral, or paracentral scotomas
Antineoplastics		
Busulfan	Chronic myelogenous leukemia	Cataracts Decreased lacrimation
Tamoxifen	Metastatic breast carcinoma	Corneal opacities Refractile retinal deposits Posterior subcapsular cataracts Decreased color perception
Bisphosphonates	Osteoporosis Hypercalcemia of malignancy	Scleritis, uveitis, conjunctivitis, episcleritis (reversible)
Imatinib mesylate	Treatment of chronic myelogenous leukemia and gastrointestinal stromal tumors	Periorbital edema, epiphora, conjunctivitis
Antipsychotics		
Lithium carbonate	Manic phase of manic/depressive exophthalmos psychosis	Oculogyric crisis Myoclonus
Antiseizure		
Topiramate	Refractory epilepsy	Acute angle-closure glaucoma, myopia, uveal effusion
Antispasmodics		
Baclofen	Muscle spasms in multiple sclerosis and disorders associated with increased muscular tone	Blurred vision Hallucinations
Carbonic Anhydrase Inhibitors		
Acetazolamide Methazolamide	Glaucoma	Aggravation of metabolic acidosis, primarily in known CO_2-retaining diseases such as emphysema and bronchiectasis, and in patients with poor vital capacity Aplastic anemia, various blood disorders Decreased libido Impotency
Chelating Agents		
Penicillamine	Cystinuria Heavy metal antagonist—iron, lead, copper, mercury poisoning Wilson's disease	Facial or ocular myasthenia, including extraocular muscle paralysis, ptosis, and diplopia Ocular pemphigoid Optic neuritis and color-vision problems
Erectile Dysfunction Agents		
Sildenafil	Erectile dysfunction	Transitory changes in color perception, blurred vision, changes in light perception, electroretinography (ERG) changes, conjunctival hyperemia, ocular pain, photophobia, subconjunctival hemorrhages
Hormonal Agents		
Oral contraceptives	Amenorrhea Dysfunctional uterine bleeding Dysmenorrhea Hypogonadism Oral contraception Premenstrual tension	Contraindicated in patients with preexisting retinal vascular diseases Decrease in color vision with chronic use Macular edema

GENERIC NAME	PRINCIPAL GENERAL USE	POSSIBLE ADVERSE EFFECTS
Hydantoins		
Phenytoin	Chronic epilepsy	Optic nerve hypoplasia in infants with epileptic mothers on the drug; ocular teratogenic effects, including strabismus, ptosis, hypertelorism, epicanthus
Nonsteroidal Anti-inflammatory Drugs		
Ibuprofen	Rheumatoid arthritis Osteoarthritis	Decreased color vision Optic neuritis Visual field defects
Naproxen	Rheumatoid arthritis Osteoarthritis Ankylosing spondylitis	Corneal opacity Periorbital edema
Sulindac	Rheumatoid arthritis Osteoarthritis Ankylosing spondylitis	Keratitis Stevens-Johnson syndrome
Psychedelics		
Marijuana	Cerebral sedative or narcotic	Conjunctival hyperemia; decreased lacrimation; decreased intraocular pressure; dyschromatopsia with chronic long-term use
Sedatives and Hypnotics		
Ethanol	Antiseptic Used as a beverage	Fetal alcohol syndrome: offspring of alcoholic mothers may have epicanthus, small palpebral fissures, and microphthalmia
Synthetic Retinoids		
Isotretinoin	Severe recalcitrant nodular acne	Permanent night blindness, color vision defects, keratitis sicca. **Note:** All retinoids, in rare instances, can cause intracranial hypertension.
III. TOPICAL		
Anticholinergics		
Cyclopentolate hydrochloride	Used as a cycloplegic and mydriatic	Central nervous system toxicity, including slurred speech, ataxia, hallucinations, hyperactivity, seizures, syncope, and paralytic ileus
Tropicamide	Used as a cycloplegic and mydriatic	Cyanosis, muscle rigidity, nausea, pallor, vomiting, vasomotor collapse
Parasympathomimetics or Anticholinesterases		
Echothiophate iodide Pilocarpine	Glaucoma	Retinal detachments primarily in eyes with peripheral retinal or retinal-vitreal disease. (Patients need to be warned of this possible effect when first placed on this medication.) Miotic upper respiratory infection—rhinorrhea, sensation of chest constriction, cough, conjunctival hyperemia; seen primarily in young children on anticholinesterase agents
Prostaglandins		
Latanoprost	Open-angle glaucoma	Flu-like syndrome; increased pigmentation of iris, eyelid skin, eyelid and eyelash; eyelashes—increased number, growth, and curling; iritis
Sympathomimetics		
Dipivefrin Epinephrine	Open-angle glaucoma Used as a bronchodilator Open-angle glaucoma Used as a vasoconstrictor to prolong anesthetic action	Follicular blepharoconjunctivitis, keratitis Cicatricial pemphigoid Stains soft contact lenses black Hypertension, headache
10% Phenylephrine	Used as a mydriatic and vasoconstrictor	Cardiac arrhythmias and cardiac arrests with pledget form or subconjunctival injection, possible myocardial infarcts, systemic hypertension
Betaxolol Levobunolol hydrochloride Timolol	Open-angle glaucoma	Cardiac syncope, bradycardia, light-headedness, fatigue, congestive heart failure; In diabetics—hyperglycemia; in myasthenia gravis—severe dysarthria

SECTION 3
SUTURE MATERIALS

Although sutureless cataract surgery is diminishing the need for certain sutures, there is still no other discipline that requires as many specialized needles and suture materials as ophthalmic surgery. To meet this need, manufacturers offer the ophthalmologist a comprehensive array of precisely manufactured reverse-cutting and spatula needles swaged to suture materials of collagen (plain and chromic), silk (black and white braided), virgin silk (black and white twisted), Nylon, Dacron, and synthetics.

Suture material intended for use in ophthalmic surgery can be either absorbable or nonabsorbable. Following is a list of various suture materials available with a brief description of each.

Absorbable
The absorption of sutures occurs in two distinct phases. After implantation, the suture's tensile strength diminishes during the early postoperative period. When most of the strength is lost, the remaining suture mass begins to decrease in what may be termed the second phase of absorption. The mass-loss phase then proceeds until the entire suture has been absorbed.

Plain Catgut—Prepared from the submucosal or mucosal layers of sheep or beef intestine, respectively, this material consists primarily of collagen—a fibrous protein—which is absorbed by the body. The material is chemically purified to minimize tissue reaction. Available in sizes 4–0 through 6–0.

Chromic Catgut—same as plain catgut except that it is treated with chromium salts to delay the absorption time. Available in sizes 4–0 through 7–0.

Plain Collagen—prepared from bovine deep flexor tendon. The tendon is purified and converted to a uniform suspension of collagen fibril. This fibrillar suspension is then extruded into suture strands and chemically treated to accurately control absorption rate. Available in sizes 4–0 through 7–0.

TABLE 1

COMPARISON OF OPHTHALMIC SUTURE MATERIALS

SUTURE MATERIAL	RELATIVE TENSILE STRENGTH*	RELATIVE HOLDING DURATION†	RELATIVE TISSUE REACTION‡	EASE OF HANDLING	SPECIAL KNOT REQUIRED	BEHAVIOR OF EXPOSED ENDS	AVAILABLE SIZES§
ABSORBABLE							
Surgical gut or collagen							
Plain	6	1 week	4+	Fair	No	Stiff	4–0 to 7–0
Chromic	6	<2 weeks	3+	Fair	No	Stiff	4–0 to 8–0
SYNTHETIC ABSORBABLE							
Polyglactin 910							
Braided	9	2 weeks	2+	Good	Yes	Stiff	4–0 to 9–0
Monofilament	9	2 weeks	2+	Good	Yes	Stiff	9–0 to 10–0
Polyglycolic acid	9	2 weeks	2+	Good	Yes	Stiff	4–0 to 10–0
NONABSORBABLE							
Silk							
Virgin	7	2 months	3+	Excellent	No	Softest	8–0 to 9–0
Braided	8	2 months	3+	Good	No	Soft	4–0 to 9–0
Polyamide (Nylon)	9	6 months	1+	Fair	Yes	Stiff, sharp	8–0 to 11–0
Polypropylene	10	>12 months	1+	Fair	Yes	Stiff, sharp	4–0 to 6–0 / 9–0 to 10–0

*The higher the number, the greater the relative tensile strength. Strength varies with size of material; estimates apply mainly to size 8–0 sutures.
† Holding duration will vary with location and size of suture, health of patient, medications employed, etc. The time given in this table is an average of the time at which about 30% of tensile strength is lost.
‡ 1+ indicates least inflammatory response, 4+ greatest.
§ With needles appropriate for ophthalmic use. Sizes available will vary from time to time.
Adapted from Spaeth GL. *Ophthalmic Surgery, Principles and Practice*. Philadelphia, Pa: WB Saunders; 1982:64.

Chromic Collagen—prepared in the same way as plain collagen except that chromium salts are added during the chemical treatment to further delay absorption. Available in sizes 4–0 through 8–0.

Synthetic Absorbable Sutures—Products include Vicryl (Polyglactin 910, a copolymer of lactide and glycolide) and Dexon (polyglycolic acid). These materials offer high tensile strength and minimal tissue reaction during the critical postoperative healing period, followed by predictable absorption. Coated Vicryl sutures are also available. Manufactured in size 4–0 through 10–0 (coated 4–0 through 8–0).

Nonabsorbable
Virgin Silk—twisted with the individual silk filaments still embedded in their natural sericin coating, providing a smooth, uniform suture in very fine sizes. The suture is offered in black or white, permitting optimum contrast with tissues. Available in sizes 8–0 and 9–0.

Black Braided Silk Suture—braided under controlled conditions to maximize strength and assure resistance to breaking while knots are tied. Gums and other impurities are removed, resulting in a suture that remains tightly braided, with virtually no loose filaments and minimal tendency to broom. Available in sizes 4–0 through 9–0.

Monofilament Nylon Sutures (Ethilon, Dermalon, and Supramid)—These sutures offer high tensile strength and minimal tissue reaction. Nylon has been reported to lose tensile strength postoperatively at a rate of approximately 15% per year. Available in sizes 8–0 through 11–0.

Polypropylene Suture (Prolene)—a monofilament suture with high tensile strength and minimal tissue reaction. The material is not degraded or weakened by tissue enzymes. Available in sizes 4-0 to 6-0 and 9-0 to 10-0.

Polyester Fiber Sutures—Products include Mersilene and Ti Cron. They exhibit minimal tissue reaction and are braided by a special method for tightness, uniformity, and a smooth surface that minimizes trauma. Available in sizes 4–0 through 6–0.

A variety of physical characteristics of different sutures have been published. In addition, the United States Pharmacopeia has established specifications for various suture materials. Some of the useful parameters measured have been: (1) tensile strength, (2) elasticity, (3) suture diameters, and (4) weight per unit length. Data are summarized in **Tables 1** through **3**.

TABLE 2

ELASTICITY OF SELECTED SUTURES

SUTURE MATERIAL	ELONGATION OF STANDARD 30.5-cm SEGMENT	INCREASE IN LENGTH	WEIGHT AT BREAKING POINT
6–0 plain gut	4.7 cm	15.4%	264 g
6–0 chromic gut	4.3 cm	14.1%	257 g
6–0 Mersilene	1.9 cm	6.3%	254 g
6–0 braided silk	1.2 cm	3.9%	237 g
7–0 chromic gut	3.6 cm	1.8%	118 g
7–0 braided silk	0.9 cm	3.0%	126 g
8–0 virgin silk	0.8 cm	2.6%	53 g
10–0 Nylon	8.7 cm	28.5%	23 g

From Middleton DG, McCulloch C. *Adv Ophthalmol.* 1970;22:35.

TABLE 3

WEIGHT OF SELECTED SUTURE MATERIAL

SUTURE MATERIAL	WEIGHT/LENGTH (mg/cm)
6–0 plain gut (wet)	0.170
6–0 chromic gut (wet)	0.176
6–0 Mersilene	0.116
6–0 braided silk	0.165
7–0 chromic gut (wet)	0.062
7–0 braided silk	0.065
8–0 virgin silk	0.025
10–0 Nylon	0.007

SECTION 4
OPHTHALMIC LENSES

1. COMPARISON AND CONVERSION TABLES

TABLE 1

RELATIVE MAGNIFICATION PRODUCED BY CONTACT AND SPECTACLE LENSES

The percentage increase (or decrease) in the size of the retinal image afforded by contact lenses in comparison with orthodox spectacles fitted at 12 mm from the cornea.

SPECTACLE REFRACTION	EQUIVALENT POWER OF CONTACT LENS SYSTEM	PERCENTAGE INCREASE AFFORDED BY CONTACT LENS	SPECTACLE REFRACTION	EQUIVALENT POWER OF CONTACT LENS SYSTEM	PERCENTAGE INCREASE AFFORDED BY CONTACT LENS	SPECTACLE REFRACTION	EQUIVALENT POWER OF CONTACT LENS SYSTEM	PERCENTAGE INCREASE AFFORDED BY CONTACT LENS
−20	−15.73	27.2	−8	−7.07	12.9	+6	+6.10	−4.7
−18	−14.41	24.8	−6	−5.42	10.5	+8	+8.29	−7.4
−16	−13.06	22.5	−4	−3.69	7.8	+10	+10.62	−10.3
−14	−11.65	20.1	−2	−1.88	5.4	+12	+13.07	−13.8
−12	−10.19	17.8	+2	+1.96	1.2	+14	+15.64	−17.3
−10	−8.66	15.3	+4	+3.99	−1.7			

Bennet AG. *Optics of Contact Lenses,* ed 4. London: Hatton Press; 1966.

TABLE 2

INDEX OF REFRACTION OF LENS MATERIAL

	CROWN GLASS	1.6-INDEX CROWNLITE GLASS	HILITE GLASS	8-INDEX GLASS	CR–39 PLASTIC	HIRI PLASTIC	1.6-INDEX PLASTIC	POLY-CARBONATE THIN–LITE PLASTIC
INDEX OF REFRACTION The higher the number, the thinner the material	1.523	1.601	1.701	1.805	1.498	1.56	1.6	1.586
SPECIFIC GRAVITY The higher the number, the heavier the material	2.5	2.67	2.99	3.37	1.32	1.216	1.34	1.20
DISPERSION The higher the number, the less chromatic aberration (Abbe value)	59	42.24	31	25	58	38	37	31
PERSONALITY	Temperable, coatable, ease in handling, vast availability	Chemically temperable, ease in handling, limited availability	Chemically temperable, fairly easy to handle, SV and multifocals; vacuum coatings cause lens to become highly sensitive to scratching	SV, difficult to temper, highly reflective so A/R coatings recommended, but have same problems as hilite; mfrs suggest having patient sign liability waiver when ground thin. Multifocal available in laminate.	Strong, tintable, coatable, ease in handling, vast availability	SV and bifocal, tints well before SRC, edges well, must be SRC, extremely brittle	SV only, tints well before SRC, edges well, must be SRC	SV and multifocal, strongest lens material available, limited tintability, must be SPC, no fast fabrication, special edging equipment needed, a must for children and athletes

SV = single-vision lenses. A/R = antireflective. SRC = scratch-resistant coating. SPC = scratch-proof coating.

TABLE 3

CORNEAL RADIUS EQUIVALENCE DIOPTERS/MILLIMETERS

DIOPTERS	mm	DIOPTERS	mm	DIOPTERS	mm	DIOPTERS	mm	DIOPTERS	mm	DIOPTERS	mm	DIOPTERS	mm	DIOPTERS	mm
20.00	16.875	36.00	9.375	39.00	8.653	42.00	8.035	45.00	7.500	48.00	7.031	51.00	6.617	54.00	6.250
22.00	15.340	36.12	9.343	39.12	8.627	42.12	8.012	45.12	7.480	48.12	7.013	51.12	6.602	54.12	6.236
24.00	14.062	36.25	9.310	39.25	8.598	42.25	7.988	45.25	7.458	48.25	6.994	51.25	6.585	54.25	6.221
26.00	12.980	36.37	9.279	39.37	8.572	42.37	7.965	45.37	7.438	48.37	6.977	51.37	6.569	54.37	6.207
27.00	12.500	36.50	9.246	39.50	8.544	42.50	7.941	45.50	7.417	48.50	6.958	51.50	6.553	54.50	6.192
28.00	12.053	36.62	9.216	39.62	8.518	42.62	7.918	45.62	7.398	48.62	6.941	51.62	6.538	54.62	6.179
29.00	11.638	36.75	9.183	39.75	8.490	42.75	7.894	45.75	7.377	48.75	6.923	51.75	6.521	54.75	6.164
29.50	11.441	36.87	9.153	39.87	8.465	42.87	7.872	45.87	7.357	48.87	6.906	51.87	6.506	54.87	6.150
30.00	11.250	37.00	9.121	40.00	8.437	43.00	7.848	46.00	7.336	49.00	6.887	52.00	6.490	55.00	6.136
30.50	11.065	37.12	9.092	40.12	8.412	43.12	7.826	46.12	7.317	49.12	6.870	52.12	6.475	55.12	6.123
31.00	10.887	37.25	9.060	40.25	8.385	43.25	7.803	46.25	7.297	49.25	6.852	52.25	6.459	55.25	6.108
31.50	10.714	37.37	9.031	40.37	8.360	43.37	7.781	46.37	7.278	49.37	6.836	52.37	6.444	55.37	6.095
32.00	10.547	37.50	9.000	40.50	8.333	43.50	7.758	46.50	7.258	49.50	6.818	52.50	6.428	55.50	6.081
32.50	10.385	37.62	8.971	40.62	8.308	43.62	7.737	46.62	7.239	49.62	6.801	52.62	6.413	55.62	6.068
33.00	10.227	37.75	8.940	40.75	8.282	43.75	7.714	46.75	7.219	49.75	6.783	52.75	6.398	55.75	6.054
33.50	10.075	37.87	8.912	40.87	8.257	43.87	7.693	46.87	7.200	49.87	6.767	52.87	6.383	55.87	6.041
34.00	9.926	38.00	8.881	41.00	8.231	44.00	7.670	47.00	7.180	50.00	6.750	53.00	6.367	56.00	6.027
34.25	9.854	38.12	8.853	41.12	8.207	44.12	7.649	47.12	7.162	50.12	6.733	53.12	6.353	56.50	5.973
34.50	9.783	38.25	8.823	41.25	8.181	44.25	7.627	47.25	7.142	50.25	6.716	53.25	6.338	57.00	5.921
34.75	9.712	38.37	8.795	41.37	8.158	44.37	7.606	47.37	7.124	50.37	6.700	53.37	6.323	57.50	5.869
35.00	9.643	38.50	8.766	41.50	8.132	44.50	7.584	47.50	7.105	50.50	6.683	53.50	6.308	58.00	5.819
35.25	9.574	38.62	8.738	41.62	8.109	44.62	7.563	47.62	7.087	50.62	6.667	53.62	6.294	58.50	5.769
35.50	9.507	38.75	8.708	41.75	8.083	44.75	7.541	47.75	7.068	50.75	6.650	53.75	6.279	59.00	5.720
35.75	9.440	38.87	8.682	41.87	8.060	44.87	7.521	47.87	7.050	50.87	6.634	53.87	6.265	60.00	5.625

TABLE 4

VERTEX DISTANCE CONVERSION SCALE (mm)

SPECTACLE LENS POWER	PLUS LENSES								MINUS LENSES							
	8	9	10	11	12	13	14	15	8	9	10	11	12	13	14	15
4.00	4.12	4.12	4.12	4.12	4.25	4.25	4.25	4.25	3.87	3.87	3.87	3.87	3.87	3.75	3.75	3.75
4.50	4.62	4.75	4.75	4.75	4.75	4.75	4.75	4.87	4.37	4.37	4.25	4.25	4.25	4.25	4.25	4.25
5.00	5.25	5.25	5.25	5.25	5.25	5.37	5.37	5.37	4.75	4.75	4.75	4.75	4.75	4.75	4.62	4.62
5.50	5.75	5.75	5.75	5.87	5.87	5.87	6.00	6.00	5.25	5.25	5.25	5.12	5.12	5.12	5.12	5.12
6.00	6.25	6.37	6.37	6.37	6.50	6.50	6.50	6.62	5.75	5.62	5.62	5.62	5.62	5.50	5.50	5.50
6.50	6.87	6.87	7.00	7.00	7.00	7.12	7.12	7.25	6.12	6.12	6.12	6.00	6.00	6.00	6.00	5.87
7.00	7.37	7.50	7.50	7.62	7.62	7.75	7.75	7.75	6.62	6.62	6.50	6.50	6.50	6.37	6.37	6.37
7.50	8.00	8.00	8.12	8.12	8.25	8.25	8.37	8.50	7.12	7.00	7.00	6.87	6.87	6.87	6.75	6.75
8.00	8.50	8.62	8.75	8.75	8.87	8.87	9.00	9.12	7.50	7.50	7.37	7.37	7.25	7.25	7.25	7.25
8.50	9.12	9.25	9.25	9.37	9.50	9.50	9.62	9.75	8.00	7.87	7.87	7.75	7.75	7.62	7.62	7.50
9.00	9.75	9.75	9.87	10.00	10.12	10.25	10.37	10.37	8.37	8.37	8.25	8.25	8.12	8.00	8.00	8.00
9.50	10.25	10.37	10.50	10.62	10.75	10.87	11.00	11.12	8.87	8.75	8.62	8.62	8.50	8.50	8.37	8.37
10.00	10.87	11.00	11.12	11.25	11.37	11.50	11.62	11.75	9.25	9.12	9.12	9.00	8.87	8.87	8.75	8.75
10.50	11.50	11.62	11.75	11.87	12.00	12.12	12.25	12.50	9.62	9.62	9.50	9.37	9.37	9.25	9.12	9.12
11.00	12.00	12.25	12.37	12.50	12.75	12.87	13.00	13.12	10.12	10.00	9.87	9.75	9.75	9.62	9.50	9.50
11.50	12.62	12.87	13.00	13.12	13.37	13.50	13.75	13.87	10.50	10.37	10.37	10.25	10.12	10.00	9.87	9.87
12.00	13.25	13.50	13.62	13.87	14.00	14.25	14.50	14.62	11.00	10.87	10.75	10.62	10.50	10.37	10.25	10.12
12.50	13.87	14.12	14.25	14.50	14.75	15.00	15.25	15.37	11.37	11.25	11.12	11.00	10.87	10.75	10.62	10.50
13.00	14.50	14.75	15.00	15.25	15.50	15.62	16.00	16.12	11.75	11.62	11.50	11.37	11.25	11.12	11.00	10.87
13.50	15.12	15.37	15.62	15.87	16.12	16.37	16.62	16.87	12.25	12.00	11.87	11.75	11.62	11.50	11.37	11.25
14.00	15.75	16.00	16.25	16.50	16.75	17.12	17.50	17.75	12.62	12.50	12.25	12.12	12.00	11.87	11.75	11.50
14.50	16.50	16.75	17.00	17.25	17.50	17.87	18.25	18.50	13.00	12.75	12.62	12.50	12.37	12.25	12.00	11.87
15.00	17.00	17.37	17.75	18.00	18.25	18.62	19.00	19.37	13.37	13.25	13.00	12.87	12.75	12.50	12.37	12.25
15.50	17.75	18.00	18.25	18.75	19.00	19.37	19.75	20.25	13.75	13.62	13.50	13.25	13.00	12.87	12.75	12.62
16.00	18.25	18.75	19.00	19.37	19.75	20.25	20.50	21.00	14.25	14.00	13.75	13.62	13.50	13.25	13.00	12.87
16.50	19.00	19.37	19.75	20.25	20.50	21.00	21.50	21.87	14.50	14.37	14.12	14.00	13.75	13.62	13.50	13.25
17.00	19.75	20.25	20.50	21.00	21.50	22.00	22.25	22.87	15.00	14.75	14.50	14.25	14.12	14.00	13.75	13.50
17.50	20.50	20.75	21.25	21.75	22.25	22.75	23.25	23.75	15.37	15.12	14.87	14.75	14.50	14.25	14.00	13.87
18.00	21.00	21.50	22.00	22.50	23.00	23.50	24.00	24.62	15.75	15.50	15.25	15.00	14.75	14.62	14.37	14.12
18.50	21.75	22.25	22.75	23.25	23.75	24.50	25.00	25.62	16.12	15.87	15.62	15.37	15.12	14.87	14.75	14.50
19.00	22.50	23.00	23.50	24.00	24.75	25.25	26.00	26.50	16.50	16.25	16.00	15.75	15.50	15.25	15.00	14.75

OPHTHALMIC LENSES / **27**

TABLE 5

MJK SPHEROCYLINDRICAL VERTEX CHART

VERTEX DISTANCE = 13.00 mm		SPHERE INCREMENT = 0.125 DIOPTER								CYLINDER INCREMENT = 0.25 DIOPTER		
SR	SRV	−0.25	−0.50	−0.75	−1.00	−1.25	−1.50	−1.75	−2.00	−2.25	−2.50	−2.75	−3.00
−3.00	−2.87	−0.25	−0.50	−0.75	−1.00	−1.25	−1.25	−1.50	−1.75	−2.00	−2.25	−2.50	−2.75
−3.25	−3.12	−0.25	−0.50	−0.75	−1.00	−1.25	−1.25	−1.50	−1.75	−2.00	−2.25	−2.50	−2.75
−3.50	−3.37	−0.25	−0.50	−0.75	−1.00	−1.25	−1.25	−1.50	−1.75	−2.00	−2.25	−2.50	−2.75
−3.75	−3.62	−0.25	−0.50	−0.75	−1.00	−1.00	−1.25	−1.50	−1.75	−2.00	−2.25	−2.50	−2.75
−4.00	−3.75	−0.25	−0.50	−0.75	−1.00	−1.00	−1.25	−1.50	−1.75	−2.00	−2.25	−2.50	−2.50
−4.25	−4.00	−0.25	−0.50	−0.75	−1.00	−1.00	−1.25	−1.50	−1.75	−2.00	−2.25	−2.50	−2.50
−4.50	−4.25	−0.25	−0.50	−0.75	−1.00	−1.00	−1.25	−1.50	−1.75	−2.00	−2.25	−2.25	−2.50
−4.75	−4.50	−0.25	−0.50	−0.75	−1.00	−1.00	−1.25	−1.50	−1.75	−2.00	−2.25	−2.25	−2.50
−5.00	−4.75	−0.25	−0.50	−0.75	−0.75	−1.00	−1.25	−1.50	−1.75	−2.00	−2.25	−2.25	−2.50
−5.25	−4.87	−0.25	−0.50	−0.75	−0.75	−1.00	−1.25	−1.50	−1.75	−2.00	−2.25	−2.25	−2.50
−5.50	−5.12	−0.25	−0.50	−0.75	−0.75	−1.00	−1.25	−1.50	−1.75	−2.00	−2.00	−2.25	−2.50
−5.75	−5.37	−0.25	−0.50	−0.75	−0.75	−1.00	−1.25	−1.50	−1.75	−2.00	−2.00	−2.25	−2.50
−6.00	−5.62	−0.25	−0.50	−0.75	−0.75	−1.00	−1.25	−1.50	−1.75	−2.00	−2.00	−2.25	−2.50
−6.25	−5.75	−0.25	−0.50	−0.75	−0.75	−1.00	−1.25	−1.50	−1.75	−1.75	−2.00	−2.25	−2.50
−6.50	−6.00	−0.25	−0.50	−0.75	−0.75	−1.00	−1.25	−1.50	−1.75	−1.75	−2.00	−2.25	−2.50
−6.75	−6.25	−0.25	−0.50	−0.75	−0.75	−1.00	−1.25	−1.50	−1.75	−1.75	−2.00	−2.25	−2.50
−7.00	−6.37	−0.25	−0.50	−0.50	−0.75	−1.00	−1.25	−1.50	−1.75	−1.75	−2.00	−2.25	−2.50
−7.25	−6.62	−0.25	−0.50	−0.50	−0.75	−1.00	−1.25	−1.50	−1.75	−1.75	−2.00	−2.25	−2.50
−7.50	−6.87	−0.25	−0.50	−0.50	−0.75	−1.00	−1.25	−1.50	−1.50	−1.75	−2.00	−2.25	−2.50
−7.75	−7.00	−0.25	−0.50	−0.50	−0.75	−1.00	−1.25	−1.50	−1.50	−1.75	−2.00	−2.25	−2.50
−8.00	−7.25	−0.25	−0.50	−0.50	−0.75	−1.00	−1.25	−1.50	−1.50	−1.75	−2.00	−2.25	−2.50
−8.25	−7.50	−0.25	−0.50	−0.50	−0.75	−1.00	−1.25	−1.50	−1.50	−1.75	−2.00	−2.25	−2.25
−8.50	−7.62	−0.25	−0.50	−0.50	−0.75	−1.00	−1.25	−1.50	−1.50	−1.75	−2.00	−2.25	−2.25
−8.75	−7.87	−0.25	−0.50	−0.50	−0.75	−1.00	−1.25	−1.50	−1.50	−1.75	−2.00	−2.25	−2.25
−9.00	−8.00	−0.25	−0.50	−0.50	−0.75	−1.00	−1.25	−1.25	−1.50	−1.75	−2.00	−2.25	−2.25
−9.25	−8.25	−0.25	−0.50	−0.50	−0.75	−1.00	−1.25	−1.25	−1.50	−1.75	−2.00	−2.00	−2.25
−9.50	−8.50	−0.25	−0.50	−0.50	−0.75	−1.00	−1.25	−1.25	−1.50	−1.75	−2.00	−2.00	−2.25
−9.75	−8.62	−0.25	−0.50	−0.50	−0.75	−1.00	−1.25	−1.25	−1.50	−1.75	−2.00	−2.00	−2.25
−10.00	−8.87	−0.25	−0.50	−0.50	−0.75	−1.00	−1.25	−1.25	−1.50	−1.75	−2.00	−2.00	−2.25
−10.25	−9.00	−0.25	−0.50	−0.50	−0.75	−1.00	−1.25	−1.25	−1.50	−1.75	−2.00	−2.00	−2.25
−10.50	−9.25	−0.25	−0.50	−0.50	−0.75	−1.00	−1.25	−1.25	−1.50	−1.75	−2.00	−2.00	−2.25
−10.75	−9.37	−0.25	−0.50	−0.50	−0.75	−1.00	−1.25	−1.25	−1.50	−1.75	−2.25	−2.00	−2.25
+4.00	+4.25	−0.25	−0.50	−0.75	−1.00	−1.25	−1.75	−2.00	−2.25	−2.50	−2.75	−3.00	−3.25
+4.25	+4.50	−0.25	−0.50	−0.75	−1.00	−1.50	−1.75	−2.00	−2.25	−2.50	−2.75	−3.00	−3.25
+4.50	+4.75	−0.25	−0.50	−0.75	−1.00	−1.50	−1.75	−2.00	−2.25	−2.50	−2.75	−3.00	−3.25
+4.75	+5.12	−0.25	−0.50	−0.75	−1.00	−1.50	−1.75	−2.00	−2.25	−2.50	−2.75	−3.00	−3.25
+5.00	+5.37	−0.25	−0.50	−0.75	−1.00	−1.50	−1.75	−2.00	−2.25	−2.50	−2.75	−3.00	−3.25
+5.25	+5.62	−0.25	−0.50	−0.75	−1.00	−1.50	−1.75	−2.00	−2.25	−2.50	−2.75	−3.00	−3.25
+5.50	+5.87	−0.25	−0.50	−0.75	−1.00	−1.50	−1.75	−2.00	−2.25	−2.50	−2.75	−3.00	−3.25
+5.75	+6.25	−0.25	−0.50	−0.75	−1.00	−1.50	−1.75	−2.00	−2.25	−2.50	−2.75	−3.00	−3.25
+6.00	+6.50	−0.25	−0.50	−0.75	−1.00	−1.50	−1.75	−2.00	−2.25	−2.50	−2.75	−3.00	−3.50
+6.25	+6.75	−0.25	−0.50	−1.00	−1.00	−1.50	−1.75	−2.00	−2.25	−2.50	−2.75	−3.25	−3.50
+6.50	+7.12	−0.25	−0.50	−1.00	−1.00	−1.50	−1.75	−2.00	−2.25	−2.50	−3.00	−3.25	−3.50
+6.75	+7.37	−0.25	−0.50	−1.00	−1.00	−1.50	−1.75	−2.00	−2.25	−2.50	−3.00	−3.25	−3.50
+7.00	+7.75	−0.25	−0.50	−1.00	−1.00	−1.50	−1.75	−2.00	−2.25	−2.75	−3.00	−3.25	−3.50
+7.25	+8.00	−0.25	−0.50	−1.00	−1.00	−1.50	−1.75	−2.00	−2.25	−2.75	−3.00	−3.25	−3.50
+7.50	+8.25	−0.25	−0.50	−1.00	−1.00	−1.50	−1.75	−2.00	−2.25	−2.50	−2.75	−3.00	−3.25	−3.50
+7.75	+8.62	−0.25	−0.50	−1.00	−1.00	−1.50	−1.75	−2.00	−2.50	−2.75	−3.00	−3.25	−3.50
+8.00	+8.87	−0.25	−0.50	−1.00	−1.00	−1.50	−1.75	−2.25	−2.50	−2.75	−3.00	−3.25	−3.50
+8.25	+9.25	−0.25	−0.50	−1.00	−1.00	−1.50	−1.75	−2.25	−2.50	−2.75	−3.00	−3.25	−3.50
+8.50	+9.25	−0.25	−0.75	−1.00	−1.25	−1.50	−1.75	−2.25	−2.50	−2.75	−3.00	−3.25	−3.75
+8.75	+9.87	−0.25	−0.75	−1.00	−1.25	−1.50	−1.75	−2.25	−2.50	−2.75	−3.00	−3.25	−3.75
+9.00	+10.25	−0.25	−0.75	−1.00	−1.25	−1.50	−2.00	−2.25	−2.50	−2.75	−3.00	−3.50	−3.75
+9.25	+10.50	−0.25	−0.75	−1.00	−1.25	−1.50	−2.00	−2.25	−2.50	−2.75	−3.00	−3.50	−3.75
+9.50	+10.87	−0.25	−0.75	−1.00	−1.25	−1.50	−2.00	−2.25	−2.50	−2.75	−3.25	−3.50	−3.75
+9.75	+11.12	−0.25	−0.75	−1.00	−1.25	−1.50	−2.00	−2.25	−2.50	−2.75	−3.25	−3.50	−3.75
+10.00	+11.50	−0.25	−0.75	−1.00	−1.25	−1.50	−2.00	−2.25	−2.50	−3.00	−3.25	−3.50	−3.75
+10.25	+11.87	−0.25	−0.75	−1.00	−1.25	−1.75	−2.00	−2.25	−2.50	−3.00	−3.25	−3.50	−3.75
+10.50	+12.12	−0.25	−0.75	−1.00	−1.25	−1.75	−2.00	−2.25	−2.50	−3.00	−3.25	−3.50	−3.75
+10.75	+12.50	−0.25	−0.75	−1.00	−1.25	−1.75	−2.00	−2.25	−2.50	−3.00	−3.25	−3.50	−4.00
+11.00	+12.87	−0.25	−0.75	−1.00	−1.25	−1.75	−2.00	−2.25	−2.75	−3.00	−3.25	−3.50	−4.00
+11.25	+13.12	−0.25	−0.75	−1.00	−1.25	−1.75	−2.00	−2.25	−2.75	−3.00	−3.25	−3.50	−4.00
+11.50	+13.50	−0.25	−0.75	−1.00	−1.25	−1.75	−2.00	−2.25	−2.75	−3.00	−3.25	−3.75	−4.00
+11.75	+13.87	−0.25	−0.75	−1.00	−1.25	−1.75	−2.00	−2.25	−2.75	−3.00	−3.25	−3.75	−4.00

Example: Spectacle refraction (SR) at 13 mm = −5.75 − 2.50 × 180.
  Matching up −5.75 (see highlighted boxes) on the left, gives effective spherical power (SRV) of −5.37.
  Following values to the right and reading in the −2.50 cylinder column gives a cylinder value of −2.00.

  Corneal plane refraction − −5.37 − 2.00 × 180.

Legend: In this chart of spherocylindrical corneal plane refractions, the spherical value is calculated and rounded off to the nearest 0.125 diopter, while the cylinder value is rounded off to the nearest 0.25 diopter.

2. SOFT CONTACT LENSES MANUFACTURER DIRECTORY

This section provides a convenient list of the companies that manufacture soft contact lenses, together with the types they provide and the information needed if you have further inquiries.

ACCU-LENS, INC.
- Toric

5353 West Colfax Avenue
Denver, CO 80214
Phone: (303) 232-6244
Toll-free: (800) 525-2470
Fax: 303-235-0472
Website: www.accu-lens.com

ACUITY ONE, LLC.
- Spherical Daily Wear
- Bifocal/Multifocal
- Bifocal/Multifocal Disposable/Planned Replacement
- Toric

7642 East Gray Road, Suite 103
Scottsdale, AZ 85260
Phone: (480) 607-2998
Toll-free: (877) 228-4891
Fax: (877) 607-2871
E-mail: visions@acuityone.com
Website: acuityone.com

AERO CONTACT LENS, INC.
- Bifocal/Multifocal
- Bifocal/Multifocal Disposable/Planned Replacement

2958 Business One Drive
Kalamazoo, MI 49048
Phone: (269) 345-3202
Toll-free: (800) 237-2376
Fax: (269) 345-3806
Website: a-contactlens.com

ALDEN OPTICAL LABORATORIES, INC.
- Bifocal/Multifocal
- Enhancer Tints
- Planned Replacement
- Prosthetic/Therapeutic
- Toric

13295 Broadway
Alden, NY 14004
Phone: (716) 937-9181
Toll-free: (800) 253-3669
Fax: (800) 899-5612
E-mail: ccreighton@aol.com
Website: www.aldenoptical.com

BAUSCH & LOMB
- Spherical Daily Wear
- Extended/Flexible Wear
- Aphakic
- Bifocal/Multifocal
- Disposable
- Enhancer Tints
- Planned Replacement
- Toric

1400 North Goodman Street
Rochester, NY 14603
Phone: (585) 338-6000
Toll-free: (800) 553-5340
Fax: (585) 338-6007
Website: www.bausch.com

BLANCHARD CONTACT LENS
- Spherical Daily Wear
- Bifocal/Multifocal
- Bifocal/Multifocal Disposable/Planned Replacement
- Toric Bifocal/Multifocal

8025 S. Willow St.
Manchester, NH 03103
Toll-free: (800) 367-4009
Fax: (603) 627-3280

E-mail: blanchardlabs@prodigy.net
Website: www.blanchardlab.com

CIBA VISION CORPORATION
- Spherical Daily Wear
- Extended/Flexible Wear
- Aphakic
- Bifocal/Multifocal
- Disposable
- Enhancer Tints
- Opaque Tints
- Planned Replacement
- Prosthetic/Therapeutic
- Toric

11460 Johns Creek Parkway
Duluth, GA 30097
Phone: (678) 415-3937
Toll-free: (800) 241-5999
Fax: (800) 845-8842
Website: www.cibavision.com

CONTACT LENS LABORATORIES, INC.
- Spherical Daily Wear

2465 Dixie Highway
Fort Mitchell, KY 41017
Phone: (859) 331-3980
Toll-free: (800) 354-9853
Fax: (859) 344-3163
E-mail: colinc@fuse.net

CONTINENTAL SOFT LENS, INC.
- Spherical Daily Wear
- Prosthetic/Therapeutic
- Toric

P.O. Box 621029
Littleton, CO 80162
Phone: (303) 795-2130
Toll-free: (800) 637-3845
Fax: (303) 795-6984

COOPERVISION, INC.
- Spherical Daily Wear
- Extended/Flexible Wear
- Aphakic
- Enhancer Tints
- Opaque Tints
- Planned Replacement
- Prosthetic/Therapeutic
- Toric

200 WillowBrook Office Park
Fairport, NY 14450
Phone: (585) 385-6810
Toll-free: (800) 341-2020
Fax: (888) 385-3217
E-mail: info@coopervision.com
Website: www.coopervision.com

CUSTOM COLOR CONTACTS
- Prosthetic/Therapeutic

55 West 49th Street
New York, NY 10020
Phone: (212) 765-4444
Toll-free: (800) 598-2020
Fax: (212) 765-4459
E-mail: dr.cassel@verizon.net
Website: www.customcontacts.com

EXTREME H2O
- Spherical Daily Wear
- Disposable

6447 Parkland Drive
Sarasota, FL 34243
Phone: (941) 758-8256
Fax: (941) 758-1191
Website: www.extreme-h2o.com

IDEAL OPTICS, INC.
- Spherical Daily Wear
- Bifocal/Multifocal

2255 Cumberland Parkway
Building 500
Atlanta, GA 30339
Phone: (770) 432-0048
Toll-free: (800) 554-7353
Fax: (770) 434-8291

KONTUR KONTACT LENS CO.
- Spherical Daily Wear
- Aphakic
- Toric

3033 Richmond Parkway
Richmond, CA 94806
Phone: (510) 758-7180
Toll-free: (800) 227-1320
Fax: (800) 650-6525
E-mail: kontur55@aol.com

LENS DYNAMICS, INC.
- Bifocal/Multifocal

14998 West 6th Avenue, Suite 830
Golden, CO 80401
Phone: (303) 237-6927
Toll-free: (800) 228-2691
Fax: (800) 661-6707
   (303) 274-6707
E-mail: al.vaske@lensdynamics.com
Website: www.lensdynamics.com

THE LIFESTYLE COMPANY, INC.
- Bifocal/Multifocal
- Toric Bifocal/Multifocal

712 Ginesi Drive
Morganville, NJ 07751
Phone: (732) 972-8585
Toll-free: (800) 622-0777
Fax: (732) 972-9205
Website: www.lifestylecompany.com

METRO OPTICS, INC.
- Spherical Daily Wear
- Bifocal/Multifocal
- Enhancer Tints
- Planned Replacement
- Toric
- Toric Bifocal/Multifocal

P.O. Box 14847
Austin, TX 78761
Phone: (512) 251-2382
Toll-free: (800) 223-1858
Fax: (512) 251-6554
E-mail: sjwebb@metro-optics.com
Website: www.metro-optics.com

OCU-EASE OPTICAL PRODUCTS, INC.
- Spherical Daily Wear
- Bifocal/Multifocal
- Prosthetic
- Toric
- Toric Bifocal/Multifocal

629 Tennent Avenue
Pinole, CA 94564
Phone: (510) 724-0384
Toll-free: (800) 521-8984
Fax: (800) 628-3273
E-mail: custom@ocuease.com
Website: www.ocuease.com

OCULAR SCIENCES, INC.
- Spherical Daily Wear
- Extended/Flexible Wear
- Bifocal/Multifocal
- Disposable
- Enhancer Tints

OPHTHALMIC LENSES / 29

- Planned Replacement
- Toric

1855 Gateway Boulevard, Suite 700
Concord, CA 94520-3200
Phone: (925) 969-7000
Toll-free: (800) 628-5367
Fax: (925) 969-7123
Website: www.ocularsciences.com

OPTECH, INC.
- Spherical Daily Wear
- Aphakic
- Bifocal/Multifocal
- Enhancer Tints
- Toric
- Toric Bifocal/Multifocal

6341 South Troy Circle, Unit-E
Englewood, CO 80111-6415
Phone: (303) 708-1390
Toll-free: (800) 525-7465
Fax: (303) 708-1392
E-mail: optechpolyvue@email.MSN.com

PC OPTICAL PRODUCTS, INC.
- Bifocal/Multifocal
- Keratoconus
- Postsurgical
- Spherical Daily Wear
- Toric

7338 Ohms Lane
Edina, MN 55439
Phone: (612) 835-7373
Toll-free: (800) 433-4885
Fax: (800) 895-8235 or (612) 835-2524
Website: www.pcoptical.com

PRECISION VISION, LTD.
- Bifocal/Multifocal
- Keratoconus
- Planned Replacement
- Spherical Daily Wear
- Toric

535-A Nucla Way
Aurora, CO 80011
Phone: (303) 343-0494
Toll-free: (800) 843-5367
Fax: (303) 343-0971
E-mail: frank@precisionvision.com
Website: www.precisionvision.com

PREFERRED OPTICS, INC.
- Bifocal/Multifocal

127 Margaret Avenue
Marietta, GA 30060
Phone: (770) 426-4015
Toll-free: (800) 253-0351
Fax: (770) 424-4341

SODERBERG CONTACT LENS
- Spherical Daily Wear
- Aphakic
- Bifocal/Multifocal
- Bifocal/Multifocal Disposable/Planned Replacement
- Prosthetic/Therapeutic
- Toric
- Toric Bifocal/Multifocal

230 Eva Street
Saint Paul, MN 55107
Phone: (651) 291-1200
Toll-free: (800) 755-5655
Fax: (651) 291-7764
E-mail: info@soderberginc.com
Website: www.soseyes.com

SUNSOFT/BRANCH OF OCULAR SCIENCES
- Spherical Daily Wear
- Extended/Flexible Wear
- Aphakic
- Bifocal/Multifocal Disposable/Planned Replacement
- Toric

6805 Academy Parkway West, Northeast
Albuquerque, NM 87109
Phone: (505) 345-7967
Toll-free: (800) 526-2020
Fax: (888) 301-0264
Website: www.ocularsciences.com

TRU-FORM OPTICS
- Bifocal/Multifocal
- Keratoconus
- Spherical Daily Wear
- Toric

400 South Euless Boulevard, Suite 100
Euless, TX 76040
Phone: (817) 267-9261
Toll-free: (800) 792-1095
Fax: (817) 354-8319
Website: www.tfoptics.com

UNILENS CORPORATION, USA
- Spherical Daily Wear
- Extended/Flexible Wear
- Aphakic
- Bifocal/Multifocal
- Toric

10431 72nd Street North
Largo, FL 33777
Phone: (727) 544-2531
Toll-free: (800) 446-2020
Fax: (727) 545-1883
   (800) 808-8264
E-mail: unilens@aol.com or information@unilens.com
Website: www.unilens.com

UNITED CONTACT LENS, INC.
- Spherical Daily Wear
- Bifocal/Multifocal
- Enhancer Tints
- Planned Replacement
- Toric
- Toric Bifocal/Multifocal

917 134th Street Southwest, Suite A-4
Everett, WA 98204
Phone: (425) 743-7343
Toll-free: (800) 446-1666
Fax: (425) 743-8795
Website: www.unitedcontactlens.com

VALLEY CONTAX
- Spherical Daily Wear
- Bifocal/Multifocal
- Planned Replacement
- Prosthetic/Therapeutic
- Toric
- Toric Bifocal/Multifocal

1110 North 18th Street, Suite 1
Springfield, OR 97477
Phone: (541) 744-9393
Toll-free: (800) 547-8815
Fax: (541) 744-9399
E-mail: contax@valleycontax.com
Website: www.valleycontax.com

VISTAKON
- Bifocal/Multifocal Disposable/Planned Replacement
- Disposable
- Planned Replacement

7500 Centurion Parkway, Suite 100
Mail Stop D-CREL
Jacksonville, FL 32256
Phone: (904) 443-1000
Toll-free: (800) 874-5278
Fax: (800) 456-2733
Website: www.acuvue.com

WESTCON CONTACT LENS COMPANY, INC.
- Spherical Daily Wear
- Bifocal/Multifocal
- Toric
- Toric Bifocal/Multifocal

611 Eisenhauer Street
Grand Junction, CO 81505
Phone: (970) 245-3845
Toll-free: (800) 346-4303
Fax: (970) 245-4516
   (800) 715-3388
E-mail: westcon@westconlens.com
Website: www.westconlens.com

WORLD OPTICS, INC.
- Spherical Daily Wear
- Bifocal/Multifocal
- Disposable

2445 Kanan Road
Agoura, CA 91301
Phone: (818) 707-9061
Toll-free: (800) 421-4657
Fax: (818) 707-9179
E-mail: woptics@aol.com

X-CEL CONTACTS/A WALMAR COMPANY
- Spherical Daily Wear
- Aphakic
- Planned Replacement
- Toric

2775 Premiere Parkway, Suite 600
Duluth, GA 30097
(See website for more office locations.)
Phone: (770) 622-9235
Toll-free: (800) 241-9312
Fax: (800) 622-8989
Website: www.walman.com

SECTION 5
VISION STANDARDS AND LOW-VISION AIDS

1. VISION STANDARDS

TABLE 1

VISION STANDARDS FOR PILOTS

	WITHOUT RX[1]	REQUIRING RX[1] CORRECTED TO	NEAR VISION WITH/ WITHOUT RX	PHORIAS[2]	FIELDS	COLOR	PATHOLOGY
1st class	20/20	20/100 to 20/20	20/40 (J_3)	6 D eso/exo 1 Δ hyper	Normal	Normal	4
2nd class	20/20	20/100 to 20/20	20/40 (J_3)	6 D eso/exo 1 Δ hyper	Normal	3	5
3rd class	20/50	To 20/30	20/60 (J_6)	...	...	3	5

1. Each eye.
2. If exceeded, further evaluation required to determine bifoveal fixation and adequate vergence phoria relationship.
3. Able to distinguish aviation signal red, aviation signal green, and white.
4. No acute or chronic pathologic condition of either eye of adnexa that might interfere with its proper function, might progress to that degree, or be aggravated by flying.
5. No serious pathology.

Note: By amendment regulations (12/21/76) correction may be by spectacles or contact lenses.

TABLE 2

VISION STANDARDS FOR ADMISSION TO SERVICE ACADEMIES

US Coast Guard Academy	Minimum uncorrected 20/200 each eye; correctable to 20/20 each eye; refractive error not more than ±5.50 D any meridian; astigmatism not over 3.00 D; anisometropia not exceeding 3.50 D; full visual fields; normal color vision; no chronic, disfiguring, disabling, ocular pathology.
US Merchant Marine Academy	Minimum uncorrected 20/100 each eye; correctable to 20/20 each eye; refractive error as for Coast Guard Academy; color vision normal by Farnsworth lantern test or pseudoisochromatic plates; certain pathologies may disqualify.
US Naval Academy	Uncorrected vision 20/20 each eye; limited waivers if correctable to 20/20 each eye and to refraction standards, Coast Guard Academy; color vision normal–no waivers; no chronic, disfiguring, disabling ocular pathology.
US Military Academy	Distance vision correctable to 20/20 each eye; refractive error as for Coast Guard Academy; able to distinguish vivid red and green; ET less than 15 prism diopters; XT less than 10 prism diopters; hypertropia less than 2 prism diopters; certain pathologies may disqualify.
US Air Force Academy	*Pilot:* Uncorrected vision 20/20 or better each eye, far and near; refractive error hyperopia no greater than +1.75 D and nearsightedness less than plano in any one meridian; the astigmatic error must not exceed 0.75 D. *Navigator:* Uncorrected vision 20/70 or better correctable with ordinary glasses to 20/20 each eye; near acuity 20/20 or better each eye, uncorrected; hyperopia not greater than +3.00 D and myopia not greater than –1.50 D any meridian; astigmatism not to exceed 2.00 D. *Commission:* Distance acuity correctable 20/40 one eye and 20/70 other, or 20/30 one eye and 20/100 other; near acuity correctable to 20/20 (J_1) one eye and 20/30 (J_2) in other; refractive error of equivalent sphere not more than ±8.00 D; no chronic, disfiguring, disabling ocular pathology.

Based on information as of May 17, 1983, Medical Examination Review Board, Department of Defense.

TABLE 3

VISION STANDARDS FOR COMMERCIAL DRIVERS

	VISUAL ACUITY BINOC	VISUAL FIELD MONOC	VISUAL FIELD BINOC	COLOR	OTHER	RETEST
Alabama	20/70	No	No	No	No	No
Alaska	20/40	No	No	No	No	Periodic
Arizona	20/40	No	No	No	No	Periodic
Arkansas	20/50	NS	NS	NS	NS	NS
California	20/40	70, 70	NS	R,G,A	NS	Periodic
Colorado	20/40	Yes	Yes	Yes	ST	Periodic
Connecticut	20/40	Yes	Yes	Yes	ST	No
Delaware	20/40	No	No	No	No	Periodic
Florida	20/70	No	No	No	No	Periodic
Georgia	20/60	140, 140	140	No	No	Periodic
Hawaii	20/40	70, 70	140	R,G,A	ST, EC	Periodic
Idaho	20/40	NS	NS	NS	NS	Periodic
Illinois	20/40	70, 70	140	NS	NS	Periodic
Indiana	20/50	No	No	No	NS	Periodic
Iowa	20/70	No	No	No	NS	Periodic
Kansas	20/40	NS	NS	NS	NS	Periodic
Kentucky	20/45, PV	No	No	No	No	No
Louisiana	20/40	No	No	No	No	Periodic
Maine	20/40	NS	NS	NS	NS	No
Maryland	20/40	140, 140	140	No	No	Periodic
Massachusetts	20/40	90, 90	120	Yes	No	Periodic
Michigan	20/40	70, 70	140	NS	NS	Periodic
Minnesota	20/40	NS	NS	NS	NS	Periodic
Mississippi	20/40	90, 90	180	No	ST	No
Missouri	20/40	55, 55	No	No	No	Periodic
Montana	20/40	75, 75	No	Yes	ST	Periodic
Nebraska	20/40	70, 70	140	Yes	No	Periodic
Nevada	20/40	No	No	No	No	Periodic
New Hampshire	20/40	NS	NS	NS	NS	Periodic
New Jersey	20/40	70, 70	No	R,G,A	No	NS
New Mexico	20/40	NS	NS	NS	NS	Periodic
New York	20/40	NS	NS	NS	NS	Periodic
North Carolina	20/50	No	70	Yes	No	Periodic
North Dakota	20/40	70, 70	140	No	No	Periodic
Ohio	20/40	70, 70	No	No	No	Periodic
Oklahoma	20/40	No	No	No	No	No
Oregon	20/40	No	110	No	No	No
Pennsylvania	20/40	No	140	No	No	No
Rhode Island	20/40	60, 60	120	Yes	No	Periodic
South Carolina	PV	NS	NS	NS	NS	Periodic
South Dakota	20/40	No	No	No	No	Periodic
Tennessee	20/40	No	No	No	No	No
Texas	20/50	No	No	No	No	Periodic
Utah	20/40	NS	NS	Yes	ST	Periodic
Vermont	20/40	NS	NS	NS	NS	No
Virginia	20/40	100, 100	100	No	NS	Periodic
Washington	20/40	No	140	R,G,A	No	Periodic
West Virginia	20/40	No	No	No	No	No
Wisconsin	20/40	70, 70	140	No	No	Periodic
Wyoming	20/40	No	No	No	No	Periodic

Key: Visual acuity is expressed in Snellen notation; visual field is given in degrees along the horizontal meridian; color abbreviations: R = red, G = green, A = amber; abbreviations for other conditions: EC = eye coordination; ST = stereopsis (absence of); NS = standard not specified; No = no standard; PV = default to private vehicle standard.

Source: US Dept of Transportation. *Visual Disorders and Commercial Drivers*. Washington, DC: Federal Highway Administration, Office of Motor Carriers; Nov 1991. US Dept of Transportation publication FHWA-MC-92-003, HCS-10/1-92(200)E.

2. LOW-VISION AIDS

Under federal regulation, a patient is considered legally blind when the best vision attained in the better eye is 20/200 or less, or when, whatever the acuity achieved, the field of vision of the better eye is 20° or less. While most states have adopted these standards, individual variations may exist at the local level.

Patients whose vision is reduced or inadequate for their visual tasks — those whose best corrected vision ranges from 20/50 downward toward the 20/200 level — can frequently be aided by the same techniques and devices used for the legally blind and visually rehabilitated. These modalities include rehabilitation training programs and optical and nonoptical aids. They often can help restore independence and mobility, allowing the patient to remain productive.

For those patients considered partially sighted rather than partially blind, increased vision is obtained by magnification or approximation. For distance, this may be accomplished by telescopic devices. Although difficult to use while moving about, these instruments may be quite effective for distinguishing a street sign or the number of a house or bus. They are also useful aids in the theater or classroom and at sporting events.

Telescopic devices can be obtained in magnifications of 2.2, 2.5, 3.0, 3.5, 4.0, 6.0, 8.0, and 10× from suppliers such as Designs for Vision, Keeler, Nikon, Selsi, Walters, and Zeiss. Some are fixed focus; others may be refocused for viewing closer material. Telescopes fitted with reading cap lenses permit reading at greater distances than high-plus aids. A familiar example of this system is the surgical loupe.

Because the field diminishes as the power increases, the magnification of telescopic devices should be kept to the minimum needed to secure desired acuity. Differences in design and construction of these devices may cause slight variations in the fields produced at a given magnification. A representative sample may be drawn from the devices produced by Designs for Vision:

MAGNIFICATION	FIELD AT 20 FEET
2.2 standard	12°
2.2 wide angle	17°
3.0 standard	8°
3.0 wide angle	12°
4.0 standard	6°

Near vision can be augmented by higher adds, high-plus "Micro" lenses (American Optical, Lucerne Optical), binocular loupes, and handheld or stand magnifiers. The higher plus values permit approximation to increase the angle subtended with little or no demand on accommodation. The add to obtain J_5 can be estimated by the inverse of the best distance vision obtained. For example, if best distance vision is 20/200, the add is 200/20, or 10 D.

Greater detail can be obtained through increased add power or supplementary magnifiers. If the patient will not read at extremely close range, lower adds may be used in combination with magnifiers. Required magnification at desired working distance can also be provided by a telemicroscope system modified with a reading cap or objective lens, as in a surgical loupe.

When binocular function is present, prism base-in may be required in the near prescription (about 1 prism diopter per diopter of add). Plastic-lens, half-eye spectacles of 6, 8, or 10 D with incorporated prism are available from American Optical and Lucerne Optical. Handheld magnifiers ranging from 23 to 83 are available from Bausch & Lomb, Coburn, Coil, Eschenbach, McLeod, and Selsi. Once again, the higher powers have reduced fields of view. Patients with physical infirmities can use stand magnifiers that rest on the material and remain in focus as they are moved across the page.

Nonoptical aids include reading masks, large-print publications, heavily ruled stationery, check-writing guides, large playing cards, and easy-to-thread needles. Also available are fixed-power opaque projection magnifiers (Nesbit Co) and closed-circuit television devices with variable magnification.

Television permits a greater range of magnification and can, when polarity is reversed, provide a white-on-black image instead of the usual black-on-white. This effect, for many, is an additional aid. Products are available from Telesensory Systems and Visualtek. Advances in electronics have also made possible talking clocks, calculators, computers, and word processors whose "voices" open the way to gainful employment for the visually impaired.

For those with clouded vision, absorptive lenses provide glare protection and can help improve acuity. Neutral gray lenses with 5–15% transmission are specifically recommended for achromatopes, who may also require the protection of wide side-shield frames. Albinotic patients are aided by brown tints with 75% transmission indoors and 25% outdoors. Retinitis pigmentosa patients generally require daytime outdoor protection with the darker sunglass tints. Many are aided in night vision by the Kalichrome lenses (Bausch & Lomb) and the Hazemaster line (American Optical).

For more information on optical aids and other resources for the visually impaired, contact:

American Council of the Blind
Phone: 800-424-8666, 202-467-5081
Website: www.acb.org

American Foundation for the Blind
Phone: 800-232-5463, 212-502-7600
Website: www.afb.org

Library of Congress, National Library Service for the Blind and Physically Handicapped
Phone: 800-424-8567, 202-707-5100
Website: www.loc.gov/nls

SECTION 6
PRODUCT IDENTIFICATION GUIDE

To aid in quick identification, manufacturers participating in this section have furnished full-color photographs of selected ophthalmic products. Capsules and tablets are shown in actual size. Tubes, bottles, boxes, and other types of packaging appear in reduced size to fit available space.

For more information on any of the products in this section, please turn to the Pharmaceutical and Equipment Product Information Section, or check directly with the manufacturer. The page number of each product's text entry appears above its photograph.

While every effort has been made to guarantee faithful reproduction of the products in this section, changes in size, color, and design are always a possibility. Be sure to confirm a product's identity with the manufacturer or your pharmacist.

102/PDR FOR OPHTHALMIC MEDICINES™

MANUFACTURERS INDEX

Allergan, Inc. 103	Novartis Ophthalmics 105
Bausch & Lomb Pharmaceuticals, Inc. 104	Pfizer Consumer Health Care 106
King Pharamceuticals. 104	Pharmacia & Upjohn 106
Merck & Co., Inc. 104	Vistakon Pharmaceuticals LLC 106

PRODUCT INDEX

Acular (Allergan, Inc.) 103
Acular LS (Allergan, Inc.) 103
Acular PF (Allergan, Inc.) 103
Alamast (Vistakon Pharmaceuticals LLC) . . .106
Alphagan P (Allergan, Inc.) 103
Alrex (Bausch & Lomb, Inc.) 104
Betimol (Vistakon Pharmaceuticals LLC) . . .106
Blephamide (Allergan, Inc.) 103
Brimonidine Tartrate Ophthalmic Solution 0.2%
    (Bausch & Lomb, Inc.) 104
Cortisporin Ophthalmic Suspension
    (King Pharmaceuticals) 104
Cosopt (Merck & Co., Inc.) 104
Crolom
    (Bausch & Lomb, Inc.) 104
Daranide (Merck & Co., Inc.) 104
Fluor-I-Strip
    (Bausch & Lomb, Inc.) 104
Fluor-I-Strip-A.T.
    (Bausch & Lomb, Inc.) 104
FML Ointment (Allergan, Inc.) 103
GenTeal Lubricant Eye Drops
    (Novartis Ophthalmics) 105
GenTeal PF Lubricant Eye Drops with Natural
    Tear Ions (Novartis Ophthalmics) 105
GenTeal Lubricant Eye Gel
    (Novartis Ophthalmics) 105
Lacrisert (Merck & Co., Inc.) 105
Lotemax
    (Bausch & Lomb, Inc.) 104
Lumigan (Allergan, Inc.) 103
Muro 128
    (Bausch & Lomb, Inc.) 104

Ocuvite
    (Bausch & Lomb, Inc.) 104
Ocuvite extra
    (Bausch & Lomb, Inc.) 104
Ocuvite Lutein
    (Bausch & Lomb, Inc.) 104
Ocuvite PreserVision
    (Bausch & Lomb, Inc.) 104
OptiPranolol
    (Bausch & Lomb, Inc.) 104
Pred Forte (Allergan, Inc.) 103
Quixin (Vistakon Pharmaceuticals LLC) 106
Refresh Celluvisc (Allergan, Inc.) 103
Refresh Endura (Allergan, Inc.) 103
Refresh Liquigel (Allergan, Inc.) 103
Refresh Plus (Allergan, Inc.) 103
Refresh P.M. (Allergan, Inc.) 103
Refresh Tears (Allergan, Inc.) 103
Restasis (Allergan, Inc.) 103
Rev-Eyes
    (Bausch & Lomb, Inc.) 104
Timoptic (Merck & Co., Inc.) 105
Timoptic-XE (Merck & Co., Inc.) 105
Trusopt (Merck & Co., Inc.) 105
Visine (Pfizer Consumer Health Care) 105
Visine-A (Pfizer Consumer Health Care) 106
Visine For Contacts
    (Pfizer Consumer Health Care) 106
Visine Tears (Pfizer Consumer Health Care) . .106
Visudyne (Novartis Ophthalmics) 105
Xalatan (Pharmacia & Upjohn) 106
Zaditor (Novartis Ophthalmics) 105
Zymar (Allergan, Inc.) 103

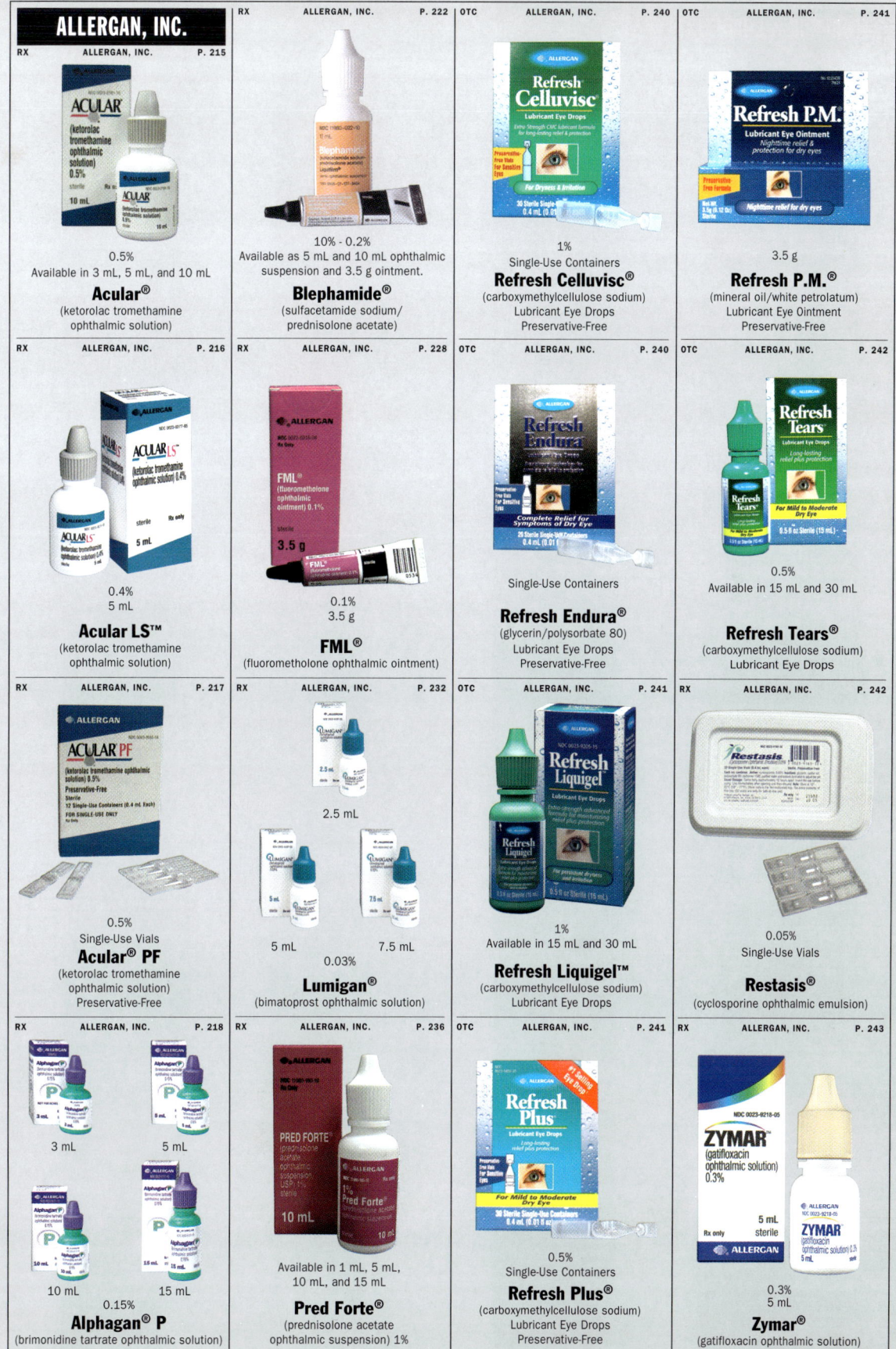

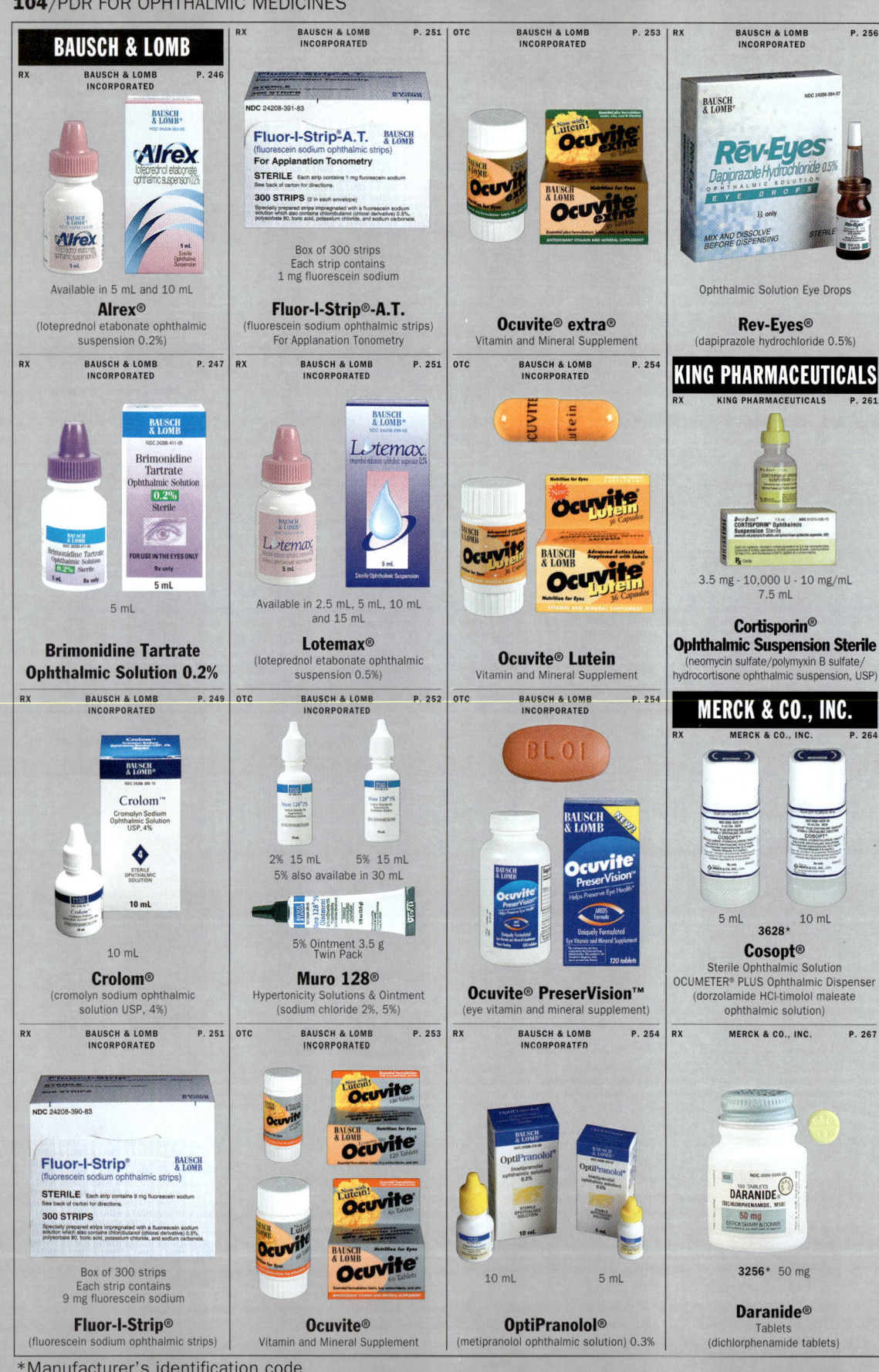

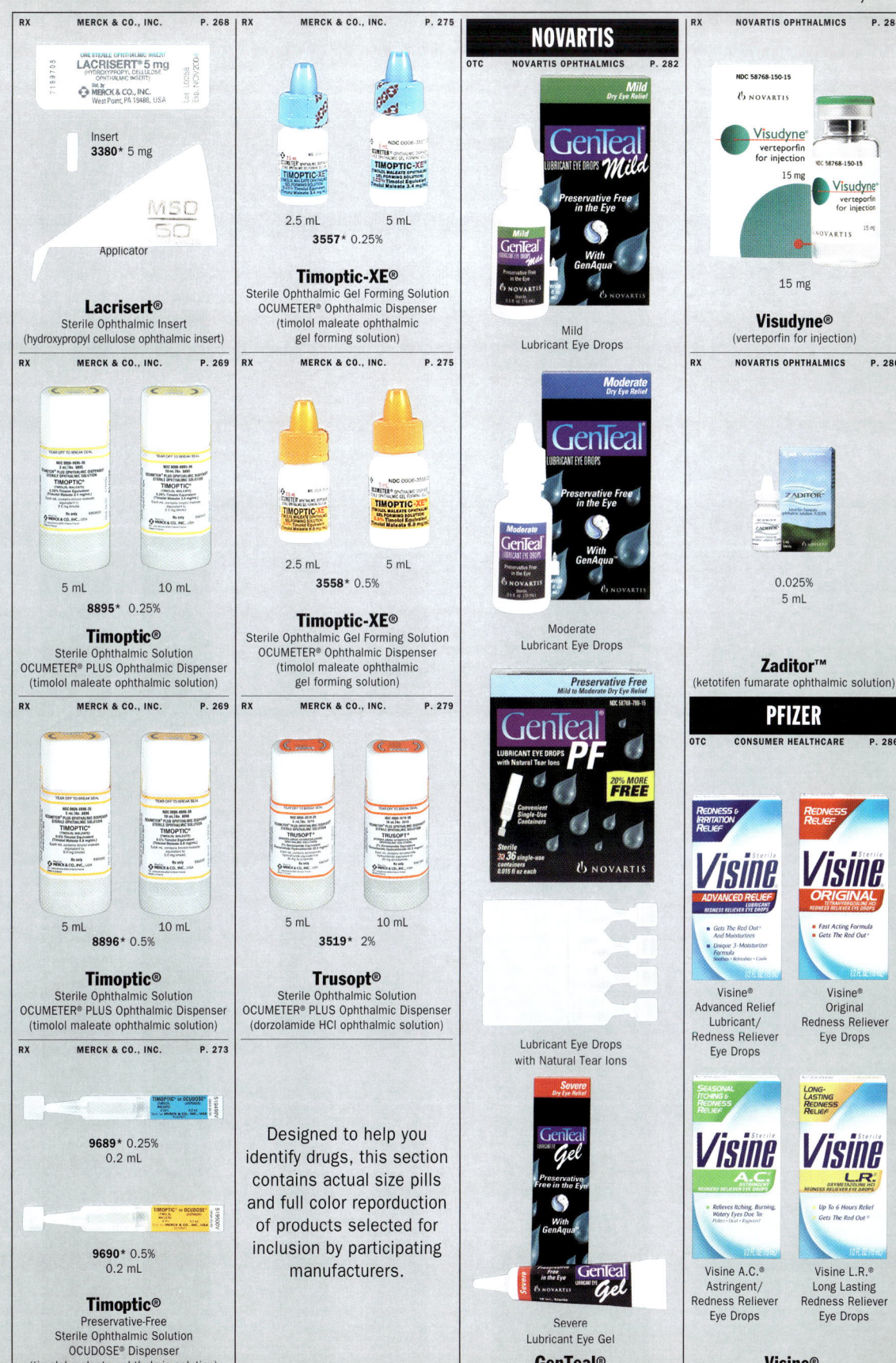

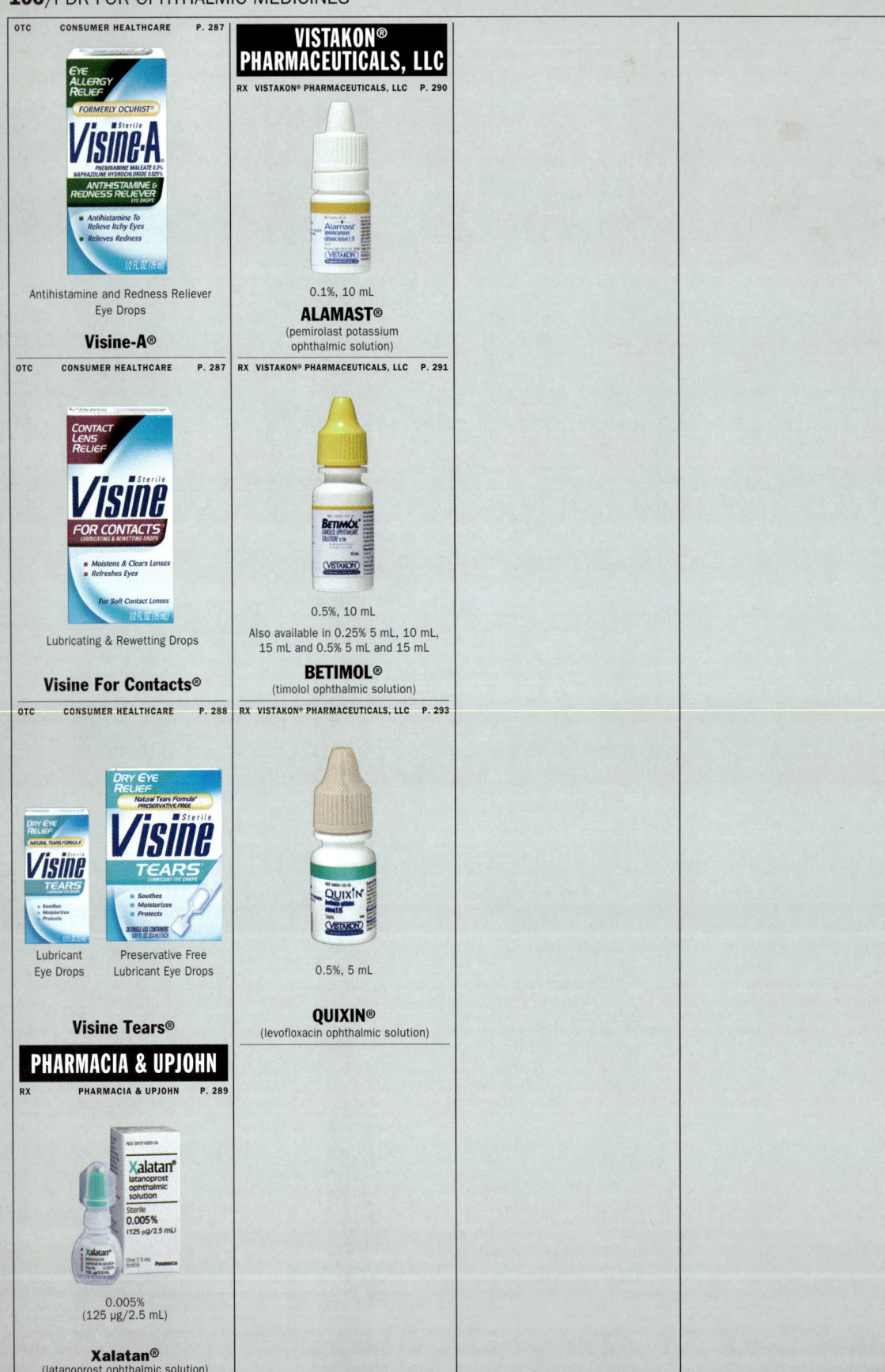

SECTION 7

PRODUCT INFORMATION ON PHARMACEUTICALS AND EQUIPMENT

This book is made possible through the courtesy of the manufacturers whose products appear in this and the following section. The information concerning each pharmaceutical product has been prepared by the manufacturer, and edited and approved by the manufacturer's medical department, medical director, or medical counsel.

For those products that have official package circulars, the descriptions in *Physicians' Desk Reference For Ophthalmic Medicines* must be in full compliance with Food and Drug Administration regulations pertaining to the labeling of prescription drugs. For more information, please turn to the Foreword. In presenting the following material, the publisher is not necessarily advocating the use of any product listed.

Alcon Laboratories, Inc.
and its affiliates
CORPORATE HEADQUARTERS:
6201 SOUTH FREEWAY
FORT WORTH, TX 76134

Address Inquiries to:
Pharmaceuticals/Consumer
Products   800-451-3937
(Therapeutic Drugs/Lens Care)
Surgical   800-862-5266
(Instrumentation/Surgical Meds)

AZOPT® ℞
(brinzolamide ophthalmic suspension) 1%

Description: AZOPT® (brinzolamide ophthalmic suspension) 1% contains a carbonic anhydrase inhibitor formulated for multidose topical ophthalmic use. Brinzolamide is described chemically as: (R)-(+)-4-Ethylamino-2-(3-methoxypropyl)-3,4-dihydro-2H-thieno[3,2-e]-1,2-thiazine-6-sulfonamide-1,1-dioxide. Its empirical formula is $C_{12}H_{21}N_3O_5S_3$. Brinzolamide has a molecular weight of 383.5 and a melting point of about 131°C. It is a white powder, which is insoluble in water, very soluble in methanol and soluble in ethanol.
AZOPT® (brinzolamide ophthalmic suspension) 1% is supplied as a sterile, aqueous suspension of brinzolamide which has been formulated to be readily suspended and slow settling, following shaking. It has a pH of approximately 7.5 and an osmolality of 300 mOsm/kg. Each mL of AZOPT® (brinzolamide ophthalmic suspension) 1% contains 10 mg brinzolamide. Inactive ingredients are mannitol, carbomer 974P, tyloxapol, edetate disodium, sodium chloride, hydrochloric acid and/or sodium hydroxide (to adjust pH), and purified water. Benzalkonium chloride 0.01% is added as a preservative.

Clinical Pharmacology: Carbonic anhydrase (CA) is an enzyme found in many tissues of the body including the eye. It catalyzes the reversible reaction involving the hydration of carbon dioxide and the dehydration of carbonic acid. In humans, carbonic anhydrase exists as a number of isoenzymes, the most active being carbonic anhydrase II (CA-II), found primarily in red blood cells (RBCs), but also in other tissues. Inhibition of carbonic anhydrase in the ciliary processes of the eye decreases aqueous humor secretion, presumably by slowing the formation of bicarbonate ions with subsequent reduction in sodium and fluid transport.
The result is a reduction in intraocular pressure (IOP).
AZOPT® (brinzolamide ophthalmic suspension) 1% contains brinzolamide, an inhibitor of carbonic anhydrase II (CA-II). Following topical ocular administration, brinzolamide inhibits aqueous humor formation and reduces elevated intraocular pressure. Elevated intraocular pressure is a major risk factor in the pathogenesis of optic nerve damage and glaucomatous visual field loss.
Following topical ocular administration, brinzolamide is absorbed into the systemic circulation. Due to its affinity for CA-II, brinzolamide distributes extensively into the RBCs and exhibits a long half-life in whole blood (approximately 111 days). In humans, the metabolite N-desethyl brinzolamide is formed, which also binds to CA and accumulates in RBCs. This metabolite binds mainly to CA-I in the presence of brinzolamide. In plasma, both parent brinzolamide and N-desethyl brinzolamide concentrations are low and generally below assay quantitation limits (<10 ng/mL). Binding to plasma proteins is approximately 60%. Brinzolamide is eliminated predominantly in the urine as unchanged drug. N-Desethyl brinzolamide is also found in the urine along with lower concentrations of the N-desmethoxypropyl and O-desmethyl metabolites.
An oral pharmacokinetic study was conducted in which healthy volunteers received 1 mg capsules of brinzolamide twice per day for up to 32 weeks. This regimen approximates the amount of drug delivered by topical ocular administration of AZOPT® (brinzolamide ophthalmic suspension) 1% dosed to both eyes three times per day and simulates systemic drug and metabolite concentrations similar to those achieved with long-term topical dosing. RBC CA activity was measured to assess the degree of systemic CA inhibition. Brinzolamide saturation of RBC CA-II was achieved within 4 weeks (RBC concentrations of approximately 20 µM). N-Desethyl brinzolamide accumulated in RBCs to steady-state within 20–28 weeks reaching concentrations ranging from 6–30 µM. The inhibition of CA-II activity at steady-state was approximately 70–75%, which is below the degree of inhibition expected to have a pharmacological effect on renal function or respiration in healthy subjects.
In two, three-month clinical studies, AZOPT® (brinzolamide ophthalmic suspension) 1% dosed three times per day (TID) in patients with elevated intraocular pressure (IOP), produced significant reductions in IOPs (4–5 mmHg). These IOP reductions are equivalent to the reductions observed with TRUSOPT* (dorzolamide hydrochloride ophthalmic solution) 2% dosed TID in the same studies.
In two clinical studies in patients with elevated intraocular pressure, AZOPT® (brinzolamide ophthalmic suspension) 1% was associated with less stinging and burning upon instillation than TRUSOPT* 2%.

Indications and Usage: AZOPT® (brinzolamide ophthalmic suspension) 1% is indicated in the treatment of elevated intraocular pressure in patients with ocular hypertension or open-angle glaucoma.
Contraindications: AZOPT® (brinzolamide ophthalmic suspension) 1% is contraindicated in patients who are hypersensitive to any component of this product.
Warnings: AZOPT® (brinzolamide ophthalmic suspension) 1% is a sulfonamide and although administered topically it is absorbed systemically. Therefore, the same types of adverse reactions that are attributable to sulfonamides may occur with topical administration of AZOPT® (brinzolamide ophthalmic suspension) 1%. Fatalities have occurred, although rarely, due to severe reactions to sulfonamides including Stevens-Johnson syndrome, toxic epidermal necrolysis, fulminant hepatic necrosis, agranulocytosis, aplastic anemia, and other blood dyscrasias. Sensitization may recur when a sulfonamide is re-administered irrespective of the route of administration. If signs of serious reactions or hypersensitivity occur, discontinue the use of this preparation.
Precautions
General:
Carbonic anhydrase activity has been observed in both the cytoplasm and around the plasma membranes of the corneal endothelium. The effect of continued administration of AZOPT® (brinzolamide ophthalmic suspension) 1% on the corneal endothelium has not been fully evaluated. The management of patients with acute angle-closure glaucoma requires therapeutic interventions in addition to ocular hypotensive agents. AZOPT® (brinzolamide ophthalmic suspension) 1% has not been studied in patients with acute angle-closure glaucoma.
AZOPT® (brinzolamide ophthalmic suspension) 1% has not been studied in patients with severe renal impairment (CrCl <30 mL/min). Because AZOPT® (brinzolamide ophthalmic suspension) 1% and its metabolite are excreted predominantly by the kidney, AZOPT® (brinzolamide ophthalmic suspension) 1% is not recommended in such patients.
AZOPT® (brinzolamide ophthalmic suspension) 1% has not been studied in patients with hepatic impairment and should be used with caution in such patients.
There is a potential for an additive effect on the known systemic effects of carbonic anhydrase inhibition in patients receiving an oral carbonic anhydrase inhibitor and AZOPT® (brinzolamide ophthalmic suspension) 1%. The concomitant administration of AZOPT®

Continued on next page

Azopt—Cont.

(brinzolamide ophthalmic suspension) 1% and oral carbonic anhydrase inhibitors is not recommended.

Information For Patients:
AZOPT® (brinzolamide ophthalmic suspension) 1% is a sulfonamide and although administered topically, it is absorbed systemically; therefore, the same types of adverse reactions attributable to sulfonamides may occur with topical administration. Patients should be advised that if serious or unusual ocular or systemic reactions or signs of hypersensitivity occur, they should discontinue the use of the product and consult their physician (see **Warnings**).

Vision may be temporarily blurred following dosing with AZOPT® (brinzolamide ophthalmic suspension) 1%. Care should be exercised in operating machinery or driving a motor vehicle.

Patients should be instructed to avoid allowing the tip of the dispensing container to contact the eye or surrounding structures or other surfaces, since the product can become contaminated by common bacteria known to cause ocular infections. Serious damage to the eye and subsequent loss of vision may result from using contaminated solutions.

Patients should also be advised that if they have ocular surgery or develop an intercurrent ocular condition (e.g., trauma or infection), they should immediately seek their physician's advice concerning the continued use of the present multidose container.

If more than one topical ophthalmic drug is being used, the drugs should be administered at least ten minutes apart. The preservative in AZOPT® (brinzolamide ophthalmic suspension) 1% Ophthalmic Suspension, benzalkonium chloride, may be absorbed by soft contact lenses. Contact lenses should be removed during instillation of AZOPT® (brinzolamide ophthalmic suspension) 1%, but may be reinserted 15 minutes after instillation.

Drug Interactions:
AZOPT® (brinzolamide ophthalmic suspension) 1% contains a carbonic anhydrase inhibitor. Acid-base and electrolyte alterations were not reported in the clinical trials with brinzolamide. However, in patients treated with oral carbonic anhydrase inhibitors, rare instances of drug interactions have occurred with high-dose salicylate therapy. Therefore, the potential for such drug interactions should be considered in patients receiving AZOPT® (brinzolamide ophthalmic suspension) 1%.

Carcinogenesis, Mutagenesis, Impairment of Fertility:
Carcinogenicity data on brinzolamide are not available. The following tests for mutagenic potential were negative: (1) *in vivo* mouse micronucleus assay; (2) *in vivo* sister chromatid exchange assay; and (3) Ames *E. coli* test. The *in vitro* mouse lymphoma forward mutation assay was negative in the absence of activation, but positive in the presence of microsomal activation.

In reproduction studies of brinzolamide in rats, there were no adverse effects on the fertility or reproductive capacity of males or females at doses up to 18 mg/kg/day (375 times the recommended human ophthalmic dose).

Pregnancy:
Teratogenic Effects: Pregnancy Category C. Developmental toxicity studies with brinzolamide in rabbits at oral doses of 1, 3, and 6 mg/kg/day (20, 62, and 125 times the recommended human ophthalmic dose) produced maternal toxicity at 6 mg/kg/day and a significant increase in the number of fetal variations, such as accessory skull bones, which was only slightly higher than the historic value at 1 and 6 mg/kg. In rats, statistically decreased body weights of fetuses from dams receiving oral doses of 18 mg/kg/day (375 times the recommended human ophthalmic dose) during gestation were proportional to the reduced maternal weight gain, with no statistically significant effects on organ or tissue development. Increases in unossified sternebrae, reduced ossification of the skull, and unossified hyoid that occurred at 6 and 18 mg/kg were not statistically significant. No treatment-related malformations were seen. Following oral administration of ^{14}C-brinzolamide to pregnant rats, radioactivity was found to cross the placenta and was present in the fetal tissues and blood.

There are no adequate and well-controlled studies in pregnant women. AZOPT® (brinzolamide ophthalmic suspension) 1% should be used during pregnancy only if the potential benefit justifies the potential risk to the fetus.

Nursing Mothers:
In a study of brinzolamide in lactating rats, decreases in body weight gain in offspring at an oral dose of 15 mg/kg/day (312 times the recommended human ophthalmic dose) were seen during lactation. No other effects were observed. However, following oral administration of ^{14}C-brinzolamide to lactating rats, radioactivity was found in milk at concentrations below those in the blood and plasma.

It is not known whether this drug is excreted in human milk. Because many drugs are excreted in human milk and because of the potential for serious adverse reactions in nursing infants from AZOPT® (brinzolamide ophthalmic suspension) 1%, a decision should be made whether to discontinue nursing or to discontinue the drug, taking into account the importance of the drug to the mother.

Pediatric Use:
Safety and effectiveness in pediatric patients have not been established.

Geriatric Use: No overall differences in safety or effectiveness have been observed between elderly and younger patients.

Adverse Reactions:
In clinical studies of AZOPT® (brinzolamide ophthalmic suspension) 1%, the most frequently reported adverse events associated with AZOPT® (brinzolamide ophthalmic suspension) 1% were blurred vision and bitter, sour or unusual taste. These events occurred in approximately 5–10% of patients. Blepharitis, dermatitis, dry eye, foreign body sensation, headache, hyperemia, ocular discharge, ocular discomfort, ocular keratitis, ocular pain, ocular pruritus and rhinitis were reported at an incidence of 1–5%.

The following adverse reactions were reported at an incidence below 1%: allergic reactions, alopecia, chest pain, conjunctivitis, diarrhea, diplopia, dizziness, dry mouth, dyspnea, dyspepsia, eye fatigue, hypertonia, keratoconjunctivitis, keratopathy, kidney pain, lid margin crusting or sticky sensation, nausea, pharyngitis, tearing and urticaria.

Overdosage: Although no human data are available, electrolyte imbalance, development of an acidotic state, and possible nervous system effects may occur following oral administration of an overdose. Serum electrolyte levels (particularly potassium) and blood pH levels should be monitored.

Dosage and Administration: Shake well before use. The recommended dose is 1 drop of AZOPT® (brinzolamide ophthalmic suspension) 1% in the affected eye(s) three times daily.

AZOPT® (brinzolamide ophthalmic suspension) 1% may be used concomitantly with other topical ophthalmic drug products to lower intraocular pressure.

If more than one topical ophthalmic drug is being used, the drugs should be administered at least ten minutes apart.

How Supplied: AZOPT® (brinzolamide ophthalmic suspension) 1% is supplied in plastic DROP-TAINER® dispensers with a controlled dispensing-tip as follows:

NDC 0065-0275-24	2.5 mL
NDC 0065-0275-05	5 mL
NDC 0065-0275-10	10 mL
NDC 0065-0275-15	15 mL

Storage: Store AZOPT® (brinzolamide ophthalmic suspension) 1% at 4–30°C (39–86°F).
℞ Only
U.S. Patent Numbers: 5,240,923; 5,378,703; 5,461,081; 6,071,904.
*TRUSOPT is a registered trademark of Merck & Co., Inc.

BETADINE® 5%
Sterile Ophthalmic Prep Solution ℞
[bē'tă-dīne]
(povidone-iodine ophthalmic solution)
(0.5% available iodine)

Description: Povidone-Iodine is a broad-spectrum microbicide with the chemical formulas: 2-pyrrolidinone, 1- ethenyl-, homopolymer, compound with iodine; 1-vinyl-2-pyrrolidinone polymer, compound with iodine. The structural formula is as follows:

$$\left[\begin{array}{c} CHCH_2 \\ | \\ N \\ \diagdown \diagup \\ O \end{array} \right]_n \cdot xI$$

BETADINE® 5% Sterile Ophthalmic Prep Solution contains 5% povidone-iodine (0.5% available iodine) as a sterile dark brown solution stabilized by glycerin. Inactive Ingredients: citric acid, glycerin, nonoxynol-9, sodium chloride, sodium hydroxide, and dibasic sodium phosphate.

Clinical Pharmacology: A placebo-controlled study in 38 normal volunteers yielded data for 36 subjects who showed a mean $\log_{10}$ reduction of 3.05 $\log_{10}$ units in total aerobes at 10 minutes following prepping the skin with BETADINE 5% Sterile Ophthalmic Prep Solution compared with reduction of 1.58 $\log_{10}$ units after prepping with vehicle free of the iodine complex. This placebo-controlled study indicates a mean $\log_{10}$ reduction by the iodine complex compared with the control solution of 1.47 $\log_{10}$ units at 10 minutes and 1.79 $\log_{10}$ units at 45 minutes. The base-line mean aerobic bacterial count was 7,586 organisms per square cm.

Indications and Usage: BETADINE 5% Sterile Ophthalmic Prep Solution for the eye is indicated for prepping of the periocular region (lids, brow, and cheek) and irrigation of the ocular surface (cornea, conjunctiva, and palpebral fornices).

Contraindications: Do not use on individuals known to be sensitive to iodine, or other components of this product.

Warnings: FOR EXTERNAL USE ONLY. NOT FOR INTRAOCULAR INJECTION OR IRRIGATION.

Precautions:
General: No studies are available in patients with thyroid disorders; therefore, caution is advised in using BETADINE 5% Sterile Ophthalmic Prep Solution in these patients due to the possibility of iodine absorption.

Carcinogenesis, Mutagenesis, Impairment of Fertility: No long term studies in animals have been performed to evaluate the carcinogenic or mutagenic potential of povidone-iodine. One report of the mutagenic potential of povidone-iodine indicated that it was positive in a modification of the Ames S. **typhimurium** model, but these results could not be reproduced by another researcher. Another test using mouse lymphoma and Balb/3T3 cells showed that povidone-iodine has no significant mutagenic or transformation capabilities. Other data indicated that it does not produce mutagenic effects in mice or hamsters according to the dominant lethal test, micronucleus test, and chromosome analysis.

Pregnancy Category C: Animal reproduction studies have not been conducted with BETADINE® 5% Sterile Ophthalmic Prep Solution. It is also not known whether BETADINE 5% Sterile Ophthalmic Prep Solution can cause fetal harm when administered to a pregnant woman or can affect reproductive capacity. BETADINE 5% Sterile Ophthalmic Prep Solution should only be used on a pregnant woman if clearly needed.

Nursing Mothers: Because of the potential for serious adverse reactions in nursing infants from BETADINE 5% Sterile Ophthalmic Prep Solution, a decision should be made to discontinue nursing or discontinue the drug, taking into account the importance of the drug to the mother.

Pediatric Use: Safety and effectiveness in pediatric patients have not been established.

Geriatric Use:

Adverse Reactions: Local sensitivity has been exhibited by some individuals to povidone-iodine ophthalmic solution.

Dosage and Administration: While the inner surface and contents of the immediate container (i.e. bottle) are sterile, the outer surface of the bottle is not sterile. The use of the bottle in a sterile field should be avoided.

BETADINE 5% Sterile Ophthalmic Prep Solution is used as follows:

1. Make sure container is intact before use. To open, COMPLETELY TWIST OFF TAB, do not pull off. Gently squeeze entire contents of bottle into a sterile prep cup.
2. Saturate sterile cotton-tipped applicator to prep lashes and lid margins using one or more applicators per lid; repeat once.
3. Saturate sterile prep sponge or other suitable material to prep lids, brow and cheek in a circular ever-expanding fashion until the entire field is covered; repeat prep three (3) times.
4. While separating the lids, irrigate the cornea, conjunctiva and palpebral fornices with BETADINE 5% Sterile Ophthalmic Prep Solution using a sterile bulb syringe.
5. After the BETADINE 5% Sterile Ophthalmic Prep Solution has been left in contact for two minutes, sterile saline solution in a bulb syringe should be used to flush the residual prep solution from the cornea, conjunctiva, and the palpebral fornices.

How Supplied: BETADINE 5% Sterile Ophthalmic Prep Solution is packaged under sterile conditions and supplied in 1 fl.oz. (30 mL) form sealed blue HDPE bottles (NDC #0065 0411 30). Twenty-four (24) bottles are packed in each shipper.

Store at 15-25°C (59-77°F).

℞ Only

Single use only

BETADINE® is a registered trademark of The Purdue Frederick Company.

BETOPTIC S®
(betaxolol HCl)
0.25% as base
Sterile Ophthalmic Suspension   ℞

Description: BETOPTIC S® Ophthalmic Suspension 0.25% contains betaxolol hydrochloride, a cardioselective beta-adrenergic receptor blocking agent, in a sterile resin suspension formulation. Betaxolol hydrochloride is a white, crystalline powder, with a molecular weight of 343.89.

Empirical Formula: $C_{18}H_{29}NO_3 \cdot HCl$

Chemical Name:
(±)-1-[p-[2-(cyclopropylmethoxy)ethyl]phenoxy]-3-(isopropylamino)-2-propanol hydrochloride.

Each mL of BETOPTIC S Ophthalmic Suspension contains: **Active:** betaxolol HCl 2.8 mg equivalent to 2.5 mg of betaxolol base. **Preservative:** benzalkonium chloride 0.01%. **Inactive:** Mannitol, Poly(Styrene-Divinyl Benzene) sulfonic acid, Carbomer 934P, edetate disodium, hydrochloric acid or sodium hydroxide (to adjust pH) and purified water.

Clinical Pharmacology: Betaxolol HCl, a cardioselective (beta-1-adrenergic) receptor blocking agent, does not have significant membrane-stabilizing (local anesthetic) activity and is devoid of intrinsic sympathomimetic action. Orally administered beta-adrenergic blocking agents reduce cardiac output in healthy subjects and patients with heart disease. In patients with severe impairment of myocardial function, beta-adrenergic receptor antagonists may inhibit the sympathetic stimulatory effect necessary to maintain adequate cardiac function.

When instilled in the eye, BETOPTIC S Ophthalmic Suspension 0.25% has the action of reducing elevated intraocular pressure, whether or not accompanied by glaucoma. Ophthalmic betaxolol has minimal effect on pulmonary and cardiovascular parameters.

Elevated IOP presents a major risk factor in glaucomatous field loss. The higher the level of IOP, the greater the likelihood of optic nerve damage and visual field loss. Betaxolol has the action of reducing elevated as well as normal intraocular pressure and the mechanism of ocular hypotensive action appears to be a reduction of aqueous production as demonstrated by tonography and aqueous fluorophotometry. The onset of action with betaxolol can generally be noted within 30 minutes and the maximal effect can usually be detected 2 hours after topical administration. A single dose provides a 12-hour reduction in intraocular pressure.

In controlled, double-masked studies, the magnitude and duration of the ocular hypotensive effect of BETOPTIC S® Ophthalmic Suspension 0.25% and BETOPTIC® Ophthalmic Solution 0.5% were clinically equivalent. BETOPTIC S Suspension was significantly more comfortable than BETOPTIC Solution.

Ophthalmic betaxolol solution at 1% (one drop in each eye) was compared to placebo in a crossover study challenging nine patients with reactive airway disease. Betaxolol HCl had no significant effect on pulmonary function as measured by FEV_1, Forced Vital Capacity (FVC), FEV_1/FVC and was not significantly different from placebo. The action of isoproterenol, a beta stimulant, administered at the end of the study was not inhibited by ophthalmic betaxolol.

No evidence of cardiovascular beta adrenergic-blockade during exercise was observed with betaxolol in a double-masked, crossover study in 24 normal subjects comparing ophthalmic betaxolol and placebo for effects on blood pressure and heart rate.

Indications and Usage: BETOPTIC S Ophthalmic Suspension 0.25% has been shown to be effective in lowering intraocular pressure and may be used in patients with chronic open-angle glaucoma and ocular hypertension. It may be used alone or in combination with other intraocular pressure lowering medications.

Contraindications: Hypersensitivity to any component of this product. BETOPTIC S Ophthalmic Suspension 0.25% is contraindicated in patients with sinus bradycardia, greater than a first degree atrioventricular block, cardiogenic shock, or patients with overt cardiac failure.

Warning: FOR TOPICAL OPHTHALMIC USE ONLY. Topically applied beta adrenergic blocking agents may be absorbed systemically. The same adverse reactions found with systemic administration of beta-adrenergic blocking agents may occur with topical administration. For example, severe respiratory reactions and cardiac reactions, including death due to bronchospasm in patients with asthma, and rarely death in association with cardiac failure, have been reported with topical application of beta-adrenergic blocking agents. BETOPTIC S® Ophthalmic Suspension 0.25% has been shown to have a minor effect on heart rate and blood pressure in clinical studies. Caution should be used in treating patients with a history of cardiac failure or heart block. Treatment with BETOPTIC S® Ophthalmic Suspension 0.25% should be discontinued at the first signs of cardiac failure.

Precautions:

General: Diabetes Mellitus. Beta-adrenergic blocking agents should be administered with caution in patients subject to spontaneous hypoglycemia or to diabetic patients (especially those with labile diabetes) who are receiving insulin or oral hypoglycemic agents. Beta-adrenergic receptor blocking agents may mask the signs and symptoms of acute hypoglycemia.

Thyrotoxicosis. Beta-adrenergic blocking agents may mask certain clinical signs (e.g., tachycardia) of hyperthyroidism. Patients suspected of developing thyrotoxicosis should be managed carefully to avoid abrupt withdrawal of beta-adrenergic blocking agents, which might precipitate a thyroid storm.

Muscle Weakness. Beta-adrenergic blockade has been reported to potentiate muscle weakness consistent with certain myasthenic symptoms (e.g., diplopia, ptosis and generalized weakness).

Major Surgery. Consideration should be given to the gradual withdrawal of beta-adrenergic blocking agents prior to general anesthesia because of the reduced ability of the heart to respond to beta-adrenergically mediated sympathetic reflex stimuli.

Pulmonary. Caution should be exercised in the treatment of glaucoma patients with excessive restriction of pulmonary function. There have been reports of asthmatic attacks and pulmonary distress during betaxolol treatment. Although rechallenges of some such patients with ophthalmic betaxolol has not adversely affected pulmonary function test results, the possibility of adverse pulmonary effects in patients sensitive to beta blockers cannot be ruled out.

Information for Patients: Do not touch dropper tip to any surface, as this may contaminate the contents. Do not use with contact lenses in eyes.

Drug Interactions: Patients who are receiving a beta-adrenergic blocking agent orally and BETOPTIC S® Ophthalmic Suspension 0.25% should be observed for a potential additive effect either on the intraocular pressure or on the known systemic effects of beta blockade. Close observation of the patient is recommended when a beta blocker is administered to patients receiving catecholamine-depleting drugs such as reserpine, because of possible additive effects and the production of hypotension and/or bradycardia.

Betaxolol is an adrenergic blocking agent; therefore, caution should be exercised in patients using concomitant adrenergic psychotropic drugs.

Risk from anaphylactic reaction: While taking beta-blockers, patients with a history of atopy or a history of severe anaphylactic reaction to a variety of allergens may be more reactive to repeated accidental, diagnostic, or therapeutic

Continued on next page

Betoptic S—Cont.

challenge with such allergens. Such patients may be unresponsive to the usual doses of epinephrine used to treat anaphylactic reactions.

Ocular: In patients with angle-closure glaucoma, the immediate treatment objective is to reopen the angle by constriction of the pupil with a miotic agent. Betaxolol has little or no effect on the pupil. When BETOPTIC S® Ophthalmic Suspension 0.25% is used to reduce elevated intraocular pressure in angle-closure glaucoma, it should be used with a miotic and not alone.

Carcinogenesis, Mutagenesis, Impairment of Fertility: Lifetime studies with betaxolol HCl have been completed in mice at oral doses of 6, 20 or 60 mg/kg/day and in rats at 3, 12 or 48 mg/kg/day; betaxolol HCl demonstrated no carcinogenic effect. Higher dose levels were not tested.

In a variety of *in vitro* and *in vivo* bacterial and mammalian cell assays, betaxolol HCl was nonmutagenic.

Pregnancy: Pregnancy Category C. Reproduction, teratology, and peri- and postnatal studies have been conducted with orally administered betaxolol HCl in rats and rabbits. There was evidence of drug related postimplantation loss in rabbits and rats at dose levels above 12 mg/kg and 128 mg/kg, respectively. Betaxolol HCl was not shown to be teratogenic, however, and there were no other adverse effects on reproduction at subtoxic dose levels. There are no adequate and well-controlled studies in pregnant women. BETOPTIC S should be used during pregnancy only if the potential benefit justifies the potential risk to the fetus.

Nursing Mothers: It is not known whether betaxolol HCl is excreted in human milk. Because many drugs are excreted in human milk, caution should be exercised when BETOPTIC S® Ophthalmic Suspension 0.25% is administered to nursing women.

Pediatric Use: Safety and effectiveness in pediatric patients have not been established.

Geriatric Use: No overall differences in safety or effectiveness have been observed between elderly and younger patients.

Adverse Reactions:

Ocular: In clinical trials, the most frequent event associated with the use of BETOPTIC S® Ophthalmic Suspension 0.25% has been transient ocular discomfort. The following other conditions have been reported in small numbers of patients: blurred vision, corneal punctate keratitis, foreign body sensation, photophobia, tearing, itching, dryness of eyes, erythema, inflammation, discharge, ocular pain, decreased visual acuity and crusty lashes.

Additional medical events reported with other formulations of betaxolol include allergic reactions, decreased corneal sensitivity, corneal punctate staining which may appear in dendritic formations, edema and anisocoria.

Systemic: Systemic reactions following administration of BETOPTIC S® Ophthalmic Suspension 0.25% or BETOPTIC® Ophthalmic Solution 0.5% have been rarely reported. These include:

Cardiovascular: Bradycardia, heart block and congestive failure.

Pulmonary: Pulmonary distress characterized by dyspnea, bronchospasm, thickened bronchial secretions, asthma and respiratory failure.

Central Nervous System: Insomnia, dizziness, vertigo, headaches, depression, lethargy, and increase in signs and symptoms of myasthenia gravis.

Other: Hives, toxic epidermal necrolysis, hair loss, and glossitis. Perversions of taste and smell have been reported.

Overdosage: No information is available on overdosage of humans. The oral LD50 of the drug ranged from 350–920 mg/kg in mice and 860–1050 mg/kg in rats. The symptoms which might be expected with an overdose of a systemically administered beta-1-adrenergic receptor blocking agent are bradycardia, hypotension and acute cardiac failure.

A topical overdose of BETOPTIC S® Ophthalmic Suspension 0.25% may be flushed from the eye(s) with warm tap water.

Dosage and Administration: The recommended dose is one to two drops of BETOPTIC S® Ophthalmic Suspension 0.25% in the affected eye(s) twice daily. In some patients, the intraocular pressure lowering responses to BETOPTIC S® may require a few weeks to stabilize. As with any new medication, careful monitoring of patients is advised. If the intraocular pressure of the patient is not adequately controlled on this regimen, concomitant therapy with pilocarpine and other miotics, and/or epinephrine and/or carbonic anhydrase inhibitors can be instituted.

How Supplied: BETOPTIC S® Ophthalmic Suspension 0.25% is supplied as follows: 2.5, 5, 10 and 15 mL in plastic ophthalmic DROP-TAINER® dispensers.

2.5 mL: **NDC** 0065-0246-20
5 mL: **NDC** 0065-0246-05
10 mL: **NDC** 0065-0246-10
15 mL: **NDC** 0065-0246-15

Storage: Store upright at room temperature. Shake well before using.
℞ Only
U.S. Patents No. 4,911,920
©2003 Alcon Laboratories, Inc.

BION® TEARS OTC
Lubricant Eye Drops

Description: BION® TEARS are specially designed to be physiologically compatible with the surface of the eye and to treat dry eye symptoms by replacing needed tear components. BION® TEARS advanced formula contains:

The unique DUASORB® polymeric system which combines with natural tears to soothe and lubricate sensitive dry spots.

A special lubricating vehicle designed to match the electrolyte balance of sodium, potassium, calcium, magnesium, zinc and bicarbonate found in natural tears.

No preservatives or decongestants that may cause irritation or limit use. BION® TEARS may be used as often as necessary to provide relief.

BION® TEARS special formula requires special packaging. Airtight foil pouches are used to maintain the delicate balance of ingredients until the product is ready for use in the eye. **To ensure optimal effectiveness once the pouch is opened, the containers inside the pouch must be used within four days (96 hours).**

Active Ingredients: DUASORB® water soluble polymeric system containing:
Dextran 70 0.1% and
Hypromellose 2910 0.3%.

Inactive Ingredients: calcium chloride, magnesium chloride, potassium chloride, purified water, sodium bicarbonate, sodium chloride, zinc chloride, hydrochloric acid and/or sodium hydroxide and/or carbon dioxide to adjust pH.

Warnings: If you experience eye pain, changes in vision, continued redness or irritation of the eye, or if the condition worsens or persists for more than 72 hours, discontinue use and consult a doctor.

If solution changes color or becomes cloudy, do not use. To avoid contamination, do not touch tip of container to any surface. Do not reuse. Once opened, discard. Keep this and all drugs out of the reach of children. In case of accidental ingestion, seek professional assistance or contact a Poison Control Center immediately.

How Supplied: BION® TEARS Lubricant Eye Drops are supplied in boxes of 28 0.015 fl. oz. single-use containers.
Product Code 0065-0419-18

BSS® ℞
Sterile Irrigating Solution
(balanced salt solution)

Description: BSS® Sterile Irrigating Solution is a sterile physiological balanced salt solution.

How Supplied:
15 mL Sterile DROP-TAINER® Bottle—**NDC** 0065-0795-15
30 mL Sterile DROP-TAINER® Bottle—**NDC** 0065-0795-30
250 mL Bottle—**NDC** 0065-0795-25
500 mL Bottle—**NDC** 0065-0795-50

Storage: Store at 46° to 80°F (8° to 27°C).

BSS PLUS® ℞
(balanced salt intraocular irrigating solution enriched with bicarbonate, dextrose, and glutathione)
STERILE
U.S. Patent No. 4,550,022

Description: BSS PLUS® is a sterile intraocular irrigating solution for use during all intraocular surgical procedures, even those requiring a relatively long intraocular perfusion time (e.g., pars plana vitrectomy, phacoemulsification, extracapsular cataract extraction/lens aspiration, anterior segment reconstruction, etc.). The solution does not contain a preservative and should be prepared just prior to use in surgery.

How Supplied: BSS PLUS is supplied in two packages for reconstitution prior to use: a 250 mL bottle containing 240 mL (Part I) and a 10 mL vial (Part II)—NDC 0065-0800-25; a 500 mL bottle containing 480 mL (Part I) and a 20 mL vial (Part II)—NDC 0065-0800-50. See the **Precautions** and **Preparation** sections of the package insert for information concerning reconstitution of the solution.

Storage: Store Part I and Part II at 46°–80°F (8°–27°C). Discard prepared solution after six hours.

CILOXAN® ℞
(ciprofloxacin hydrochloride ophthalmic ointment) 0.3% as Base
Sterile Ophthalmic Ointment

Description: CILOXAN® (ciprofloxacin hydrochloride ophthalmic ointment) Ophthalmic Ointment is a synthetic, sterile, multiple dose, antimicrobial for topical use. Ciprofloxacin is a fluoroquinolone antibacterial. It is available as the monohydrochloride monohydrate salt of 1-cyclopropyl-6-fluoro-1,4-dihydro-4-oxo-7-(1-piperazinyl)-3-quinolinecarboxylic acid. Ciprofloxacin is a faint to light yellow crystalline powder with a molecular weight of 385.82. Its empirical formula is $C_{17}H_{18}FN_3O_3 \cdot HCl \cdot H_2O$ and its chemical structure is as follows:

Ciprofloxacin differs from other quinolones in that it has a fluorine atom at the 6-position, a piperazine moiety at the 7-position, and a cyclopropyl ring at the 1-position.

Each gram of CILOXAN (ciprofloxacin hydrochloride ophthalmic ointment) contains:
Active: Ciprofloxacin HCl 3.33 mg equivalent to 3 mg base. **Inactives:** Mineral Oil, White Petrolatum.

Clinical Pharmacology:
Systemic Absorption: Absorption studies in humans with the ciprofloxacin ointment have not been conducted, however, based on studies with ciprofloxacin solution, 0.3%, mean maximal concentrations are expected to be less than 2.5 ng/mL.
Microbiology: Ciprofloxacin has *in vitro* activity against a wide range of gram-negative and gram-positive organisms. The bactericidal action of ciprofloxacin results from interference with the enzyme DNA gyrase which is needed for the synthesis of bacterial DNA.
Ciprofloxacin has been shown to be active against most strains of the following microorganisms both *in vitro* and in clinical infections **(See Indications and Usage** section).
Aerobic gram-positive microorganisms:
Staphylococcus aureus (methicillin-susceptible strains)
Staphylococcus epidermidis (methicillin-susceptible strains)
Streptococcus pneumoniae
Streptococcus Viridans Group
Aerobic gram-negative microorganisms:
Haemophilus influenzae
The following *in vitro* data are available; **but their clinical significance in ophthalmologic infections is unknown**. The safety and effectiveness of ciprofloxacin in treating conjunctivitis due to these microorganisms have not been established in adequate and well controlled trials.
The following organisms are considered susceptible when evaluated using systemic breakpoints. However, a correlation between the *in vitro* systemic breakpoint and ophthalmological efficacy has not been established.
Ciprofloxacin exhibits *in vitro* minimal inhibitory concentrations (MIC's) of 1μg/mL or less (systemic susceptible breakpoint) against most (≥90%) strains of the following ocular pathogens.
Aerobic gram-positive microorganisms:
Bacillus species
Corynebacterium species
Staphylococcus haemolyticus
Staphylococcus hominis
Aerobic gram-negative microorganisms:
Acinetobacter calcoaceticus
Enterobacter aerogenes
Escherichia coli
Haemophilus parainfluenzae
Klebsielle pneumoniae
Moraxella catarrhalis
Neisseria gonorrhoeae
Proteus mirabilis
Pseudomonas aeruginosa
Serratia marcesens
Most strains of *Burkholderia cepacia* and some strains of *Stenotrophomonas maltophilia* are resistant to ciprofloxacin as are most anaerobic bacteria, including *Bacteroides fragilis* and *Clostridium difficile*.
The minimal bactericidal concentration (MBC) generally does not exceed the minimal inhibitory concentration (MIC) by more than a factor of 2. Resistance to ciprofloxacin *in vitro* usually develops slowly (multiple-step mutation).
Ciprofloxacin does not cross-react with other antimicrobial agents such as beta-lactams or aminoglycosides; therefore, organisms resistant to these drugs may be susceptible to ciprofloxacin. Organisms resistant to ciprofloxacin may be susceptible to beta-lactams or aminoglycosides.

Clinical Studies: In multicenter clinical trials, approximately 75% of the patients with signs and symptoms of bacterial conjunctivitis and positive conjunctival cultures were clinically cured and approximately 80% had presumed pathogens eradicated by the end of treatment (day 7).
Indications and Usage: CILOXAN® (ciprofloxacin hydrochloride ophthalmic ointment) is indicated for the treatment of bacterial conjunctivitis caused by susceptible strains of the microorganisms listed below:
Gram-Positive:
Staphylococcus aureus
Staphylococcus epidermidis
Streptococcus pneumoniae
Streptococcus Viridans Group
Gram-Negative:
Haemophilus influenzae
Contraindications: A history of hypersensitivity to ciprofloxacin or any other component of the medication is a contraindication to its use. A history of hypersensitivity to other quinolones may also contraindicate the use of ciprofloxacin.
Warnings:
FOR TOPICAL OPHTHALMIC USE ONLY. NOT FOR INJECTION INTO THE EYE.
Serious and occasionally fatal hypersensitivity (anaphylactic) reactions, some following the first dose, have been reported in patients receiving systemic quinolone therapy. Some reactions were accompanied by cardiovascular collapse, loss of consciousness, tingling, pharyngeal or facial edema, dyspnea, urticaria, and itching. Only a few patients had a history of hypersensitivity reactions. Serious anaphylactic reactions require immediate emergency treatment with epinephrine and other resuscitation measures, including oxygen, intravenous fluids, intravenous antihistamines, corticosteroids, pressor amines and airway management, as clinically indicated.
Precautions:
General: As with other antibacterial preparations, prolonged use of ciprofloxacin may result in overgrowth of nonsusceptible organisms, including fungi. If superinfection occurs, appropriate therapy should be initiated. Whenever clinical judgment dictates, the patient should be examined with the aid of magnification, such as slit lamp biomicroscopy and, where appropriate, fluorescein staining.
Ciprofloxacin should be discontinued at the first appearance of a skin rash or any other sign of hypersensitivity reaction.
Ophthalmic ointments may retard corneal healing and cause visual blurring.
Patients should be advised not to wear contact lenses if they have signs and symptoms of bacterial conjunctivitis.
Information For Patients: Do not touch tip to any surface as this may contaminate the ointment.
Do not use the product if the imprinted carton seals have been damaged, or removed.
Drug Interactions: Specific drug interaction studies have not been conducted with ophthalmic ciprofloxacin. However, the systemic administration of some quinolones has been shown to elevate plasma concentrations of theophylline, interfere with the metabolism of caffeine, enhance the effects of the oral anticoagulant, warfarin, and its derivatives, and has been associated with transient elevations in serum creatinine in patients receiving cyclosporine concomitantly.
Carcinogenesis, Mutagenesis, Impairment of Fertility: Eight *in vitro* mutagenicity tests have been conducted with ciprofloxacin and the test results are listed below:
Salmonella/Microsome Test (Negative)
E. coli DNA Repair Assay (Negative)
Mouse Lymphoma Cell Forward Mutation Assay (Positive)

Chinese Hamster V79 Cell HGPRT Test (Negative)
Syrian Hamster Embryo Cell Transformation Assay (Negative)
Saccharomyces cerevisiae Point Mutation Assay (Negative)
Saccharomyces cerevisiae Mitotic Crossover and Gene Conversion Assay (Negative)
Rat Hepatocyte DNA Repair Assay (Positive)
Thus, two of the eight tests were positive, but the results of the following three *in vivo* test systems gave negative results:
Rat Hepatocyte DNA Repair Assay
Micronucleus Test (Mice)
Dominant Lethal Test (Mice)
Long-term carcinogenicity studies in mice and rats have been completed. After daily oral dosing for up to two years, there is no evidence that ciprofloxacin had any carcinogenic or tumorigenic effects in these species.
Pregnancy: Pregnancy Category C. Reproduction studies have been performed in rats and mice at doses up to six times the usual daily human oral dose and have revealed no evidence of impaired fertility or harm to the fetus due to ciprofloxacin. In rabbits, as with most antimicrobial agents, ciprofloxacin (30 and 100 mg/kg orally) produced gastrointestinal disturbances resulting in maternal weight loss and an increased incidence of abortion. No teratogenicity was observed at either dose. After intravenous administration, at doses up to 20 mg/kg, no maternal toxicity was produced and no embryotoxicity or teratogenicity was observed. There are no adequate and well controlled studies in pregnant women. CILOXAN® (ciprofloxacin hydrochloride ophthalmic ointment) should be used during pregnancy only if the potential benefit justifies the potential risk to the fetus.
Nursing Mothers: It is not known whether topically applied ciprofloxacin is excreted in human milk. However, it is known that orally administered ciprofloxacin is excreted in the milk of lactating rats and oral ciprofloxacin has been reported in human breast milk after a single 500 mg dose. Caution should be exercised when CILOXAN® (ciprofloxacin hydrochloride ophthalmic ointment) is administered to a nursing mother.
Pediatric Use: Safety and effectiveness of CILOXAN (ciprofloxacin hydrochloride ophthalmic ointment) 0.3% in pediatric patients below the age of two years have not been established. Although ciprofloxacin and other quinolones may cause arthropathy in immature Beagle dogs after oral administration, topical ocular administration of ciprofloxacin to immature animals did not cause any arthropathy and there is no evidence that the ophthalmic dosage form has any effect on the weight bearing joints.
Geriatric Use: No overall clinical differences in safety or effectiveness have been observed between the elderly and other adult patients.
Adverse Reactions: The following adverse reactions (incidences) were reported in 2% of the patients in clinical studies for CILOXAN (ciprofloxacin hydrochloride ophthalmic ointment): discomfort, keratopathy. Other reactions associated with ciprofloxacin therapy occurring in less than 1% of patients included allergic reactions, blurred vision, corneal staining, decreased visual acuity, dry eye, edema, epitheliopathy, eye pain, foreign body sensation, hyperemia, irritation, keratoconjunctivitis, lid erythema, lid margin hyperemia, photophobia, pruritus, and tearing.
Systemic adverse reactions related to ciprofloxacin therapy occurred at an incidence below 1% and included dermatitis, nausea and taste perversion.

Continued on next page

Ciloxan Ointment—Cont.

Dosage and Administration: Apply a 1/2" ribbon into the conjunctival sac three times a day on the first two days, then apply a 1/2" ribbon two times a day for the next five days.
How Supplied: 3.5 g sterile ointment supplied in an aluminum tube with a white polyethylene tip and white polyethylene cap. 3.5 g - NDC 0065-0654-35
Storage: Store at 36°F to 77°F (2°C to 25°C).
Animal Pharmacology: Ciprofloxacin and related drugs have been shown to cause arthropathy in immature animals of most species tested following oral administration. However, a one month topical ocular study using immature Beagle dogs did not demonstrate any articular lesions.
℞ Only
©2002, 2003 Alcon, Inc.

CILOXAN® ℞
(ciprofloxacin HCl ophthalmic solution)
0.3% as base
Sterile

Description: CILOXAN® (ciprofloxacin HCl ophthalmic solution) is a synthetic, sterile, multiple dose, antimicrobial for topical ophthalmic use. Ciprofloxacin is a fluoroquinolone antibacterial active against a broad spectrum of gram-positive and gram-negative ocular pathogens. It is available as the monohydrochloride monohydrate salt of 1-cyclopropyl-6-fluoro-1,4-dihydro-4-oxo-7-(1-piperazinyl)-3-quinoline-carboxylic acid. It is a faint to light yellow crystalline powder with a molecular weight of 385.8. Its empirical formula is $C_{17}H_{18}FN_3O_3 \cdot HCl \cdot H_2O$ and its chemical structure is as follows:

Ciprofloxacin differs from other quinolones in that it has a fluorine atom at the 6-position, a piperazine moiety at the 7-position, and a cyclopropyl ring at the 1-position.
Each mL of CILOXAN Ophthalmic Solution contains: **Active:** Ciprofloxacin HCl 3.5 mg equivalent to 3 mg base. **Preservative:** Benzalkonium Chloride 0.006%. **Inactive:** Sodium Acetate, Acetic Acid, Mannitol 4.6%, Edetate Disodium 0.05%, Hydrochloric Acid and/or Sodium Hydroxide (to adjust pH) and Purified Water. The pH is approximately 4.5 and the osmolality is approximately 300 mOsm. DM-00
Clinical Pharmacology:
Systemic Absorption: A systemic absorption study was performed in which CILOXAN Ophthalmic Solution was administered in each eye every two hours while awake for two days followed by every four hours while awake for an additional 5 days. The maximum reported plasma concentration of ciprofloxacin was less than 5 ng/mL. The mean concentration was usually less than 2.5 ng/mL.
Microbiology: Ciprofloxacin has *in vitro* activity against a wide range of gram-negative and gram-positive organisms. The bactericidal action of ciprofloxacin results from interference with the enzyme DNA gyrase which is needed for the synthesis of bacterial DNA.
Ciprofloxacin has been shown to be active against most strains of the following organisms both *in vitro* and in clinical infections. (See Indications and Usage section).
Gram-Positive:
Staphylococcus aureus (including methicillin-susceptible and methicillin-resistant strains)
Staphylococcus epidermidis
Streptococcus pneumoniae
Streptococcus (Viridans Group)
Gram-Negative:
Haemophilus influenzae
Pseudomonas aeruginosa
Serratia marcescens
Ciprofloxacin has been shown to be active *in vitro* against most strains of the following organisms, however, *the clinical significance of these data is unknown:*
Gram-Positive:
Enterococcus faecalis (Many strains are only moderately susceptible)
Staphylococcus haemolyticus
Staphylococcus hominis
Staphylococcus saprophyticus
Streptococcus pyogenes
Gram-Negative:
Acinetobacter calcoaceticus subsp. anitratus
Aeromonas caviae
Aeromonas hydrophila
Brucella melitensis
Campylobacter coli
Campylobacter jejuni
Citrobacter diversus
Citrobacter freundii
Edwardsiella tarda
Enterobacter aerogenes
Enterobacter cloacae
Escherichia coli
Haemophilus ducreyi
Haemophilus parainfluenzae
Klebsiella pneumoniae
Klebsiella oxytoca
Legionella pneumophila
Moraxella (Branhamella) catarrhalis
Morganella morganii
Neisseria gonorrhoeae
Neisseria meningitidis
Pasteurella multocida
Proteus mirabilis
Proteus vulgaris
Providencia rettgeri
Providencia stuartii
Salmonella enteritidis
Salmonella typhi
Shigella sonnei
Shigella flexneri
Vibrio cholerae
Vibrio parahaemolyticus
Vibrio vulnificus
Yersinia enterocolitica
Other Organisms: *Chlamydia trachomatis* (only moderately susceptible) and *Mycobacterium tuberculosis* (only moderately susceptible).
Most strains of *Pseudomonas cepacia* and some strains of *Pseudomonas maltophilia* are resistant to ciprofloxacin as are most anaerobic bacteria, including *Bacteroides fragilis* and *Clostridium difficile*.
The minimal bactericidal concentration (MBC) generally does not exceed the minimal inhibitory concentration (MIC) by more than a factor of 2. Resistance to ciprofloxacin *in vitro* usually develops slowly (multiple-step mutation).
Ciprofloxacin does not cross-react with other antimicrobial agents such as beta-lactams or aminoglycosides; therefore, organisms resistant to these drugs may be susceptible to ciprofloxacin.
Clinical Studies: Following therapy with CILOXAN® Ophthalmic Solution, 76% of the patients with corneal ulcers and positive bacterial cultures were clinically cured and complete re-epithelialization occurred in about 92% of the ulcers.
In 3 and 7 day multicenter clinical trials, 52% of the patients with conjunctivitis and positive conjunctival cultures were clinically cured and 70–80% had all causative pathogens eradicated by the end of treatment.
Indications and Usage: CILOXAN Ophthalmic Solution is indicated for the treatment of infections caused by susceptible strains of the designated microorganisms in the conditions listed below:
Corneal Ulcers: *Pseudomonas aeruginosa*
  *Serratia marcescens**
  Staphylococcus aureus
  Staphylococcus epidermidis
  Streptococcus pneumoniae
  Streptococcus (Viridans Group)*
Conjunctivitis: *Haemophilus influenzae*
  Staphylococcus aureus
  Staphylococcus epidermidis
  Streptococcus pneumoniae

---

*Efficacy for this organism was studied in fewer than 10 infections.
Contraindications: A history of hypersensitivity to ciprofloxacin or any other component of the medication is a contraindication to its use. A history of hypersensitivity to other quinolones may also contraindicate the use of ciprofloxacin.
Warnings: NOT FOR INJECTION INTO THE EYE.
Serious and occasionally fatal hypersensitivity (anaphylactic) reactions, some following the first dose, have been reported in patients receiving systemic quinolone therapy. Some reactions were accompanied by cardiovascular collapse, loss of consciousness, tingling, pharyngeal or facial edema, dyspnea, urticaria, and itching. Only a few patients had a history of hypersensitivity reactions. Serious anaphylactic reactions require immediate emergency treatment with epinephrine and other resuscitation measures, including oxygen, intravenous fluids, intravenous antihistamines, corticosteroids, pressor amines and airway management, as clinically indicated.
Remove contact lenses before using.
Precautions: General: As with other antibacterial preparations, prolonged use of ciprofloxacin may result in overgrowth of nonsusceptible organisms, including fungi. If superinfection occurs, appropriate therapy should be initiated. Whenever clinical judgment dictates, the patient should be examined with the aid of magnification, such as slit lamp biomicroscopy and, where appropriate, fluorescein staining.
Ciprofloxacin should be discontinued at the first appearance of a skin rash or any other sign of hypersensitivity reaction.
In clinical studies of patients with bacterial corneal ulcer, a white crystalline precipitate located in the superficial portion of the corneal defect was observed in 35 (16.6%) of 210 patients. The onset of the precipitate was within 24 hours to 7 days after starting therapy. In one patient, the precipitate was immediately irrigated out upon its appearance. In 17 patients, resolution of the precipitate was seen in 1 to 8 days (seven within the first 24–72 hours), in five patients, resolution was noted in 10–13 days. In nine patients, exact resolution days were unavailable; however, at follow-up examinations, 18–44 days after onset of the event, complete resolution of the precipitate was noted. In three patients, outcome information was unavailable. The precipitate did not preclude continued use of ciprofloxacin, nor did it adversely affect the clinical course of the ulcer or visual outcome. (See Adverse Reactions).
Information for patients: Do not touch dropper tip to any surface, as this may contaminate the solution.
Drug Interactions: Specific drug interaction studies have not been conducted with ophthalmic ciprofloxacin. However, the systemic administration of some quinolones has been shown to elevate plasma concentrations of theophylline, interfere with the metabolism of caffeine, enhance the effects of the oral anticoagulant, warfarin, and its derivatives and has been associated with transient elevations in

serum creatinine in patients receiving cyclosporine concomitantly.
Carcinogenesis, Mutagenesis, Impairment of Fertility: Eight *in vitro* mutagenicity tests have been conducted with ciprofloxacin and the test results are listed below:
  Salmonella/Microsome Test (Negative)
  E. coli DNA Repair Assay (Negative)
  Mouse Lymphoma Cell Forward Mutation Assay (Positive)
  Chinese Hamster V_{79} Cell HGPRT Test (Negative)
  Syrian Hamster Embryo Cell Transformation Assay (Negative)
  Saccharomyces cerevisiae Point Mutation Assay (Negative)
  Saccharomyces cerevisiae Mitotic Crossover and Gene Conversion Assay (Negative)
  Rat Hepatocyte DNA Repair Assay (Positive)
Thus, two of the eight tests were positive, but the results of the following three *in vivo* test systems gave negative results:
  Rat Hepatocyte DNA Repair Assay
  Micronucleus Test (Mice)
  Dominant Lethal Test (Mice)
Long term carcinogenicity studies in mice and rats have been completed. After daily oral dosing for up to two years, there is no evidence that ciprofloxacin had any carcinogenic or tumorigenic effects in these species.
Pregnancy—Pregnancy Category C: Reproduction studies have been performed in rats and mice at doses up to six times the usual daily human oral dose and have revealed no evidence of impaired fertility or harm to the fetus due to ciprofloxacin. In rabbits, as with most antimicrobial agents, ciprofloxacin (30 and 100 mg/kg orally) produced gastrointestinal disturbances resulting in maternal weight loss and an increased incidence of abortion. No teratogenicity was observed at either dose. After intravenous administration, at doses up to 20 mg/kg, no maternal toxicity was produced and no embryotoxicity or teratogenicity was observed. There are no adequate and well controlled studies in pregnant women. CILOXAN® Ophthalmic Solution should be used during pregnancy only if the potential benefit justifies the potential risk to the fetus.
Nursing Mothers: It is not known whether topically applied ciprofloxacin is excreted in human milk; however, it is known that orally administered ciprofloxacin is excreted in the milk of lactating rats and oral ciprofloxacin has been reported in human breast milk after a single 500 mg dose. Caution should be exercised when CILOXAN Ophthalmic Solution is administered to a nursing mother.
Pediatric Use: Safety and effectiveness in pediatric patients below the age of 1 year have not been established. Although ciprofloxacin and other quinolones cause arthropathy in immature animals after oral administration, topical ocular administration of ciprofloxacin to immature animals did not cause any arthropathy and there is no evidence that the ophthalmic dosage form has any effect on the weight bearing joints.
Adverse Reactions: The most frequently reported drug related adverse reaction was local burning or discomfort. In corneal ulcer studies with frequent administration of the drug, white crystalline precipitates were seen in approximately 17% of patients (See Precautions). Other reactions occurring in less than 10% of patients included lid margin crusting, crystals/scales, foreign body sensation, itching, conjunctival hyperemia and a bad taste following instillation. Additional events occurring in less than 1% of patients included corneal staining, keratopathy/keratitis, allergic reactions, lid edema, tearing, photophobia, corneal infiltrates, nausea and decreased vision.
Overdosage: A topical overdose of CILOXAN® Ophthalmic Solution may be flushed from the eye(s) with warm tap water.

Dosage and Administration:
Corneal Ulcers: The recommended dosage regimen for the treatment of **corneal ulcers** is two drops into the affected eye every 15 minutes for the first six hours and then two drops into the affected eye every 30 minutes for the remainder of the first day. On the second day, instill two drops in the affected eye hourly. On the third through the fourteenth day, place two drops in the affected eye every four hours. Treatment may be continued after 14 days if corneal re-epithelialization has not occurred.
Bacterial Conjunctivitis: The recommended dosage regimen for the treatment of **bacterial conjunctivitis** is one or two drops instilled into the conjunctival sac(s) every two hours while awake for two days and one or two drops every four hours while awake for the next five days.
How Supplied: As a sterile ophthalmic solution: 2.5 mL, 5 mL and 10 mL in plastic DROP-TAINER® dispensers.
  2.5 mL – **NDC** 0065-0656-25
  5 mL – **NDC** 0065-0656-05
  10 mL – **NDC** 0065-0656-10
Storage: Store at 2° to 25°C (36° to 77°F). Protect from light.
Animal Pharmacology: Ciprofloxacin and related drugs have been shown to cause arthropathy in immature animals of most species tested following oral administration. However, a one-month topical ocular study using immature Beagle dogs did not demonstrate any articular lesions.
Rx Only
U.S. Patent No. 4,670,444

FLUORESCITE® INJECTION ℞
(fluorescein injection)

Description: FLUORESCITE® Injection is a sterile aqueous solution in two strengths for use intravenously as a diagnostic aid.
  Established name:
    Fluorescein Sodium
  Chemical name:
    Spiro[isobenzofuran-1(3*H*),9′-[9*H*] xanthene]-3-one, 3′6′ dihydroxy, disodium salt.

The solution contains Fluorescein Sodium (equivalent to Fluorescein 10% or 25%), Sodium Hydroxide and/or Hydrochloric Acid (to adjust pH), and Water for Injection.
Clinical Pharmacology: The yellowish-green fluorescence of the drug demarcates the vascular area under observation, distinguishing it from adjacent areas.
Indications and Usage: Indicated in diagnostic fluorescein angiography or angioscopy of the fundus and of the iris vasculature.
Contraindications: Contraindicated in those persons who have shown hypersensitivity to any component of this preparation.
Warning:

> **NOT FOR INTRATHECAL USE**

FOR OPHTHALMIC USE ONLY. Care must be taken to avoid extravasation during injection as the high pH of fluorescein solution can result in severe local tissue damage. The following complications resulting from extravasation of fluorescein have been noted to occur: sloughing of the skin, superficial phlebitis, subcutaneous granuloma, and toxic neuritis along the median curve in the antecubital area. Complications resulting from extravasation can cause severe pain in the arm for up to several hours. When significant extravasation occurs, the injection should be discontinued and conservative measures to treat damaged tissue and to relieve pain should be implemented. Do not mix or dilute with other solutions or drugs in syringe. Flush intravenous cannulas before

and after drugs are injected to avoid physical incompatibility reactions. Rare cases of death due to anaphylaxis have been reported (See PRECAUTIONS).
Precautions: General: Caution is to be exercised in patients with a history of allergy or bronchial asthma. An emergency tray including such items as 0.1% epinephrine for intravenous or intramuscular use; an antihistamine, soluble steroid, and aminophyllene for IV use; and oxygen should always be available in the event of possible reaction to fluorescein injection.[1] Use only if the container is undamaged.
Information for Patients: Skin will attain a temporary yellowish discoloration. Urine attains a bright yellow color. Discoloration of the skin fades in 6 to 12 hours; urine fluorescein in 24 to 36 hours.
Carcinogenesis, Mutagenesis, Impairment of Fertility: There have been no long-term studies done using fluorescein in animals to evaluate carcinogenic potential.
Use in Pregnancy: Avoid angiography on patients who are pregnant, especially those in first trimester. There have been no reports of fetal complications from fluorescein injection during pregnancy.
Nursing Mothers: Fluorescein has been demonstrated to be excreted in human milk. Caution should be exercised when fluorescein is administered to a nursing woman.
Geriatric Use: No overall differences in safety or effectiveness have been observed between elderly and younger patients.
Adverse Reactions: Nausea and headache, gastrointestinal distress, syncope, vomiting, hypotension, and other symptoms and signs of hypersensitivity have occurred. Cardiac arrest, basilar artery ischemia, severe shock, convulsions, thrombophlebitis at the injection site and rare cases of death have been reported. Extravasation of the solution at the injection site causes intense pain at the site and a dull aching pain in the injected arm. (See WARNING.) Generalized hives and itching, bronchospasm and anaphylaxis have been reported. A strong taste may develop after injection.
Dosage and Administration: Parenteral drug products should be inspected visually for particulate matter and discoloration prior to administration, whenever solution and container permit. Do not mix or dilute with other solutions or drugs. Flush intravenous cannulas before and after drugs are injected to avoid physical incompatibility reactions. Inject the contents of the ampule rapidly into the antecubital vein, *after taking precautions to avoid extravasation*. A syringe, filled with fluorescein, is attached to transparent tubing and a 25 gauge scalp vein needle for injection. Insert the needle and draw the patient's blood to the hub of the syringe so that a *small* air bubble separates the patient's blood in the tubing from the fluorescein. With the room lights on, slowly inject the blood back into the vein while watching the skin over the needle tip. If the needle has extravasated, the patient's blood will be seen to bulge the skin and the injection should be stopped before any fluorescein is injected. When assured that extravasation has not occurred, the room light may be turned off and the fluorescein injection completed. Luminescence appears in the retina and choroidal vessels in 9 to 14 seconds and can be observed by standard viewing equipment. If potential allergy is suspected, an intradermal skin test may be performed prior to intravenous administration, i.e., 0.05 mL injected intradermally to be evaluated 30 to 60 minutes following injection. For children, the dose is calculated on the basis of 35 mg for each ten pounds of body weight.

Continued on next page

Fluorescite—Cont.

How Supplied: 10% in 5 mL ampule and 25% in 2 mL ampule.
10% NDC 0065-0092-05
25% NDC 0065-0094-02
Storage: Store at 8°–27°C (46°–80°F).
℞ Only
REFERENCE:
1. Schatz, Burton, Yannuzzi, Rabb. Interpretation of Fundus Fluorescein Angiography, Page 38, C. V. Mosby Co., St. Louis, 1978.

NAPHCON A®   OTC
Eye Drops
Relieves Itching & Redness
EYE ALLERGY RELIEF

Temporary relief of the minor eye symptoms of itching and redness caused by ragweed, pollen, grass, animal dander and hair.
Description: Actives: Naphazoline Hydrochloride 0.025%, Pheniramine Maleate 0.3%.
Preservative: Benzalkonium Chloride 0.01%.
Inactives: Boric Acid, Edetate Disodium 0.01%, Purified Water, Sodium Borate, Sodium Chloride, Sodium Hydroxide and/or Hydrochloric Acid (to adjust pH). The sterile ophthalmic solution has a pH of about 6 and a tonicity of about 270 mOsm/Kg.
Directions: Put 1 or 2 drops in the affected eye(s) up to 4 times every day.
Warnings: To avoid contamination, do not touch tip of container to any surface. Replace cap after using.
If solution changes color or becomes cloudy, do not use.
Stop use and ask a doctor if you feel eye pain, changes in vision occur, redness or irritation of the eye(s) gets worse or lasts more than 72 hours.
Overuse may cause more redness of the eye(s). When using this product, pupils may become enlarged temporarily.
If you are sensitive to any ingredient in this product, do not use. Do not use this product if you have heart disease, high blood pressure, narrow angle glaucoma or trouble urinating unless directed by a physician.
Accidental swallowing by infants and children may lead to coma and marked reduction in body temperature. Before using in children under 6 years of age, consult your physician.
Keep this and all drugs out of the reach of children. If swallowed, get medical help or contact a Poison Control Center right away.
Remove contact lenses before using.
Store at 20°–25°C (68°–77°F).
Protect from light.
Use before the expiration date marked on the carton or bottle.

NATACYN®   ℞
(natamycin ophthalmic suspension)
5% Sterile

Description: NATACYN® (natamycin ophthalmic suspension) 5% is a sterile, antifungal drug for topical ophthalmic administration.
Established name: Natamycin
  Chemical name:
    Stereoisomer of 22-[(3-amino-3, 6-dideoxy-β-D- mannopyranosyl)oxy]-1,3,26-trihydroxy-12-methyl-10-oxo-6,11,28-trioxatricyclo[22.3.1.0^{5,7}]octacosa-8,14,16,18,20-pentaene-25-carboxylic acid.
  Other: Pimaricin

Each mL of the suspension contains: **Active:** Natamycin 5% (50mg). **Preservative:** Benzalkonium Chloride 0.02%. **Inactive:** Sodium Hydroxide and/or Hydrochloric Acid (neutralized to adjust the pH), Purified Water.   DM-00
Clinical Pharmacology: Natamycin is a tetraene polyene antibiotic derived from *Streptomyces natalensis*. It possesses *in vitro* activity against a variety of yeast and filamentous fungi, including *Candida, Aspergillus, Cephalosporium, Fusarium* and *Penicillium*. The mechanism of action appears to be through binding of the molecule to the sterol moiety of the fungal cell membrane. The polyenesterol complex alters the permeability of the membrane to produce depletion of essential cellular constituents. Although the activity against fungi is dose-related, natamycin is predominantly fungicidal.* Natamycin is not effective *in vitro* against gram-positive or gram-negative bacteria. Topical administration appears to produce effective concentrations of natamycin within the corneal stroma but not in intraocular fluid. Systemic absorption should not be expected following topical administration of NATACYN (natamycin ophthalmic suspension) 5%. As with other polyene antibiotics, absorption from the gastrointestinal tract is very poor. Studies in rabbits receiving topical natamycin revealed no measurable compound in the aqueous humor or sera, but the sensitivity of the measurement was no greater than 2 mg/mL.
Indications and Usage: NATACYN (natamycin ophthalmic suspension) 5% is indicated for the treatment of fungal blepharitis, conjunctivitis, and keratitis caused by susceptible organisms including *Fusarium solani* keratitis. As in other forms of suppurative keratitis, initial and sustained therapy of fungal keratitis should be determined by the clinical diagnosis, laboratory diagnosis by smear and culture of corneal scrapings and drug response. Whenever possible, the *in vitro* activity of natamycin against the responsible fungus should be determined. The effectiveness of natamycin as a single agent in fungal endophthalmitis has not been established.
Contraindications: NATACYN® (natamycin ophthalmic suspension) 5% is contraindicated in individuals with a history of hypersensitivity to any of its components.
Precautions: General. For topical eye use only—NOT FOR INJECTION. Failure of improvement of keratitis following 7–10 days of administration of the drug suggests that the infection may be caused by a microorganism not susceptible to natamycin.
Continuation of therapy should be based on clinical re-evaluation and additional laboratory studies.
Adherence of the suspension to areas of epithelial ulceration or retention of the suspension in the fornices occurs regularly. There have only been a limited number of cases in which natamycin has been used; therefore, it is possible that adverse reactions of which we have no knowledge at present may occur. For this reason, patients on this drug should be monitored at least twice weekly. Should suspicion of drug toxicity occur, the drug should be discontinued.
Information for Patients: Do not touch dropper tip to any surface, as this may contaminate the suspension.
Carcinogenesis, Mutagenesis, Impairment of Fertility: There have been no long term studies done using natamycin in animals to evaluate carcinogenesis, mutagenesis, or impairment of fertility.
Pregnancy: Pregnancy Category C. Animal reproduction studies have not been conducted with natamycin. It is also not known whether natamycin can cause fetal harm when administered to a pregnant woman or can affect reproduction capacity. NATACYN® (natamycin ophthalmic suspension) 5% should be given to a pregnant woman only if clearly needed.
Nursing Mothers: It is not known whether these drugs are excreted in human milk. Because many drugs are excreted in human milk, caution should be exercised when natamycin is administered to a nursing woman.
Pediatric Use: Safety and effectiveness in pediatric patients have not been established.
Adverse Reactions: One case of conjunctival chemosis and hyperemia, thought to be allergic in nature, has been reported.
Dosage and Administration: SHAKE WELL BEFORE USING. The preferred initial dosage in fungal keratitis is one drop of NATACYN (natamycin ophthalmic suspension) 5% instilled in the conjunctival sac at hourly or two-hourly intervals. The frequency of application can usually be reduced to one drop 6 to 8 times daily after the first 3 to 4 days. Therapy should generally be continued for 14 to 21 days or until there is resolution of active fungal keratitis. In many cases, it may be helpful to reduce the dosage gradually at 4 to 7 day intervals to assure that the replicating organism has been eliminated. Less frequent initial dosage (4 to 6 daily applications) may be sufficient in fungal blepharitis and conjunctivitis.
How Supplied: 15 mL in glass bottles with sterile dropper assembly.
NDC 0065-0645-15.
Storage: May be stored in refrigerator [(36°–46°F) (2°–8°C)] or at room temperature [(46°–75°F) (8°–24°C)]. *Do not freeze*. Avoid exposure to light and excessive heat.
℞ Only
* Laupen, J.O.; McLellan, W.L.; El Nakeeb, M.A.: "Antibiotics and Fungal Physiology," Antimicrobial Agents and Chemotherapy, 1965:1006, 1965.

References:
1. Barckhausen, B.: Die Behandlung der Probleminfektionen das vorderen Augenabschnittes in der Praxis. Landarzt 46:842, 1970.
2. Cuendet, J.F.; Nouri, A.: Traitement local en ophtalmologie par un nouvel antibiotique fungicide, la "pimaricine". Ophthalmologica 145:297, 1963.
3. Forster, R.K.; Rebell, G.: "The Diagnosis and Management of Keratomycoses", Arch. Ophth. 93:1134, 1975.
4. Francois, J.; de Vos, El: Traitement des mycoses oculaires par la pimaricine. Bull. Soc. Belge Ophthal. 131:382, 1962.
5. Jones, D.B.; Sexton, R.; Rebell, G.: "Mycotic keratitis in South Florida: A Review of Thirty-nine Cases." Transactions ophthal. Soc. U.K. 89:781, 1969.
6. Jones, D.B.; Forster, R.K.; Rebell, G.: "*Fusarium solani* keratitis treated with Natamycin (pimaricin), 18 consecutive cases." Arch. Ophth. 88:147, 1972.
7. L'Editeur: Traitement des mycoses oculaires. Presse med. 77:147, 1969.
8. Vozza, R.; Bagolini, B.: Su di un caso di grave ulcerazione bilaterale delle palpebra de Candida albicans. Bol. Oculist. 43:433, 1964.

PATANOL®   ℞
[pă'tə-nŏl]
(olopatadine hydrochloride ophthalmic solution 0.1%)

Description: PATANOL® (olopatadine hydrochloride ophthalmic solution) 0.1% is a sterile ophthalmic solution containing olopatadine, a relatively selective H_1- receptor antagonist and inhibitor of histamine release from the mast cell for topical administration to the eyes. Olopatadine hydrochloride is a white, crystalline, water-soluble powder with a molecular weight of 373.88. The chemical structure is presented below:

Chemical Name: 11-[(Z)-3-(Dimethylamino)propylidene]-6-11-dihydrodibenz[b,e] oxepin-2-acetic acid hydrochloride

Each mL of PATANOL contains: **Active:** 1.11 mg olopatadine hydrochloride equivalent to 1 mg olopatadine. **Preservative:** benzalkonium chloride 0.01%. **Inactives:** dibasic sodium phosphate; sodium chloride; hydrochloric acid/sodium hydroxide (adjust pH); and purified water. It has a pH of approximately 7 and an osmolality of approximately 300 mOsm/kg.
Clinical Pharmacology: Olopatadine is an inhibitor of the release of histamine from the mast cell and a relatively selective histamine H_1 –antagonist that inhibits the *in vivo* and *in vitro* type 1 immediate hypersensitivity reaction including inhibition of histamine induced effects on human conjunctival epithelial cells. Olopatadine is devoid of effects on alpha-adrenergic, dopamine and muscarinic type 1 and 2 receptors. Following topical ocular administration in man, olopatadine was shown to have low systemic exposure. Two studies in normal volunteers (totaling 24 subjects) dosed bilaterally with olopatadine 0.15% ophthalmic solution once every 12 hours for 2 weeks demonstrated plasma concentrations to be generally below the quantitation limit of the assay (<0.5 ng/mL). Samples in which olopatadine was quantifiable were typically found within 2 hours of dosing and ranged from 0.5 to 1.3 ng/mL. The half-life in plasma was approximately 3 hours, and elimination was predominantly through renal excretion. Approximately 60–70% of the dose was recovered in the urine as parent drug. Two metabolites, the mono-desmethyl and the N-oxide, were detected at low concentrations in the urine.
Results from an environmental study demonstrated that PATANOL was effective in the treatment of the signs and symptoms of allergic conjunctivitis when dosed twice daily for up to 6 weeks. Results from conjunctival antigen challenge studies demonstrated that PATANOL®, when subjects were challenged with antigen both initially and up to 8 hours after dosing, was significantly more effective than its vehicle in preventing ocular itching associated with allergic conjunctivitis.
Indications And Usage: PATANOL (olopatadine hydrochloride ophthalmic solution) 0.1% is indicated for the treatment of the signs and symptoms of allergic conjunctivitis.
Contraindications: PATANOL (olopatadine hydrochloride ophthalmic solution) 0.1% is contraindicated in persons with a known hypersensitivity to olopatadine hydrochloride or any components of PATANOL.
Warnings: PATANOL (olopatadine hydrochloride ophthalmic solution) 0.1% is for topical use only and not for injection or oral use.
Precautions:
Information for Patients: To prevent contaminating the dropper tip and solution, care should be taken not to touch the eyelids or surrounding areas with the dropper tip of the bottle. Keep bottle tightly closed when not in use. Patients should be advised not to wear a contact lens if their eye is red. PATANOL® (olopatadine hydrochloride ophthalmic solution) 0.1% should not be used to treat contact lens related irritation. The preservative in PATANOL, benzalkonium chloride, may be absorbed by soft contact lenses. Patients who wear soft contact lenses and **whose eyes are not red** should be instructed to wait at least ten minutes after instilling PATANOL (olopatadine hydrochloride ophthalmic solution) 0.1% before they insert their contact lenses.
Carcinogenesis, Mutagenesis, Impairment of Fertility: Olopatadine administered orally was not carcinogenic in mice and rats in doses up to 500 mg/kg/day and 200 mg/kg/day, respectively. Based on a 40 µL drop size, these doses were 78,125 and 31,250 times higher than the maximum recommended ocular human dose (MROHD). No mutagenic potential was observed when olopatadine was tested in an *in vitro* bacterial reverse mutation (Ames) test, an *in vitro* mammalian chromosome aberration assay or an *in vivo* mouse micronucleus test. Olopatadine administered to male and female rats at oral doses of 62,500 times MROHD level resulted in a slight decrease in the fertility index and reduced implantation rate; no effects on reproductive function were observed at doses of 7,800 times the maximum recommended ocular human use level.
Pregnancy: Pregnancy Category C. Olopatadine was found not to be teratogenic in rats and rabbits. However, rats treated at 600 mg/kg/day, or 93,750 times the MROHD and rabbits treated at 400 mg/kg/day, or 62,500 times the MROHD, during organogenesis showed a decrease in live fetuses. There are, however, no adequate and well controlled studies in pregnant women. Because animal studies are not always predictive of human responses, this drug should be used in pregnant women only if the potential benefit to the mother justifies the potential risk to the embryo or fetus.
Nursing Mothers: Olopatadine has been identified in the milk of nursing rats following oral administration. It is not known whether topical ocular administration could result in sufficient systemic absorption to produce detectable quantities in the human breast milk. Nevertheless, caution should be exercised when PATANOL® (olopatadine hydrochloride ophthalmic solution) 0.1% is administered to a nursing mother.
Pediatric Use: Safety and effectiveness in pediatric patients below the age of 3 years have not been established.
Geriatric Use: No overall differences in safety or effectiveness have been observed between elderly and younger patients.
Adverse Reactions: Headaches have been reported at an incidence of 7%. The following adverse experiences have been reported in less than 5% of patients: asthenia, blurred vision, burning or stinging, cold syndrome, dry eye, foreign body sensation, hyperemia, hypersensitivity, keratitis, lid edema, nausea, pharyngitis, pruritus, rhinitis, sinusitis, and taste perversion. Some of these events were similar to the underlying disease being studied.
Dosage And Administration: The recommended dose is one drop in each affected eye two times per day at an interval of 6 to 8 hours.
How Supplied: PATANOL (olopatadine hydrochloride ophthalmic solution) 0.1% is supplied as follows: 5 mL in plastic DROP-TAINER® dispenser.
    5 mL: NDC 0065-0271-05
Storage: Store at 39°F-77°F (4°C-25°C)
Rx Only
U.S. Patents Nos. 4,871,865; 4,923,892; 5,116,863; 5,641,805.
©2000, 2003 Alcon, Inc.
340337-0104   **Revised: December 2003**
ALCON LABORATORIES, INC.
Fort Worth, Texas 76134 USA
Printed in USA

SYSTANE® OTC
[sistan]
Lubricant Eye Drops

Description: SYSTANE® is scientifically formulated to shield eyes from dry eye discomfort so that eyes feel moist and refreshed longer. For the temporary relief of burning and irritation due to dryness of the eye.
Active Ingredients: Polyethylene Glycol 400 0.4% and Propylene Glycol 0.3% as lubricants.
Inactive Ingredients: boric acid, calcium chloride, hydroxypropyl guar, magnesium chloride, polyquaternium-1 as a preservative, potassium chloride, purified water, sodium chloride, zinc chloride.
Warnings: If you experience eye pain, changes in vision, continued redness or irritation of the eye, or if the condition worsens or persists for more than 72 hours, discontinue use and consult a doctor. Do not use if product changes color or becomes cloudy or if you are sensitive to any ingredient in this product. To avoid contamination, do not touch tip of container to any surface. Replace cap after each use. Keep this and all drugs out of the reach of children. In case of accidental ingestion, seek professional assistance or contact a Poison Control Center immediately.
How Supplied: SYSTANE® Lubricant Eye Drops are supplied in 15 mL and 30 mL bottles.

TEARS NATURALE® FORTE OTC
Lubricant Eye Drops
TEARS NATURALE FREE® OTC
Lubricant Eye Drops

Description: TEARS NATURALE® FORTE contains TriSorb™ Triple Demulcent Technology. This unique combination of ingredients works together to retain moisture on the eye and slow evaporation of the tear film. TEARS NATURALE® FORTE is preserved with POLYQUAD®, gentle enough for the most sensitive eyes. *In vitro* studies have shown that POLYQUAD substantially avoids the damaging effects of epithelial cell toxicity possible with other tear substitute preservatives and allows epithelial cell growth. POLYQUAD has been shown to be 99% reaction-free in normal subjects and 97% reaction-free in subjects known to be preservative sensitive. TEARS NATURALE® FORTE is designed to more closely mimic your natural tears. The unique formulation of TEARS NATURALE® FORTE Lubricant Eye Drops protects against the recurrence of dry eye symptoms.
TEARS NATURALE FREE® Lubricant Eye Drops provide lasting relief and are the most convenient preservative-free artificial tears. TEARS NATURALE FREE® is the only preservative-free lubricant eye drop with reclosable vials. Each vial of TEARS NATURALE FREE® contains up to 3 times as much volume as other products.
With their unique mucin like polymeric formulation, and with their natural pH, low viscosity, and isotonicity, TEARS NATURALE FORTE and TEARS NATURALE FREE provide dry eye patients with comfort and prompt relief of dry eye symptoms.
Sterile-For Topical Eye Use Only
Ingredients: TEARS NATURALE FORTE: Each mL contains: **Active Ingredients:** TriSorb™ lubricating and moisturizing demulcents containing Dextran 70 0.1%, Glycerin 0.2%, and Hypromellose 0.3%. **Preservative:** POLYQUAD® (Polyquaternium-1) 0.001%. **Inactive Ingredients:** Boric Acid, Calcium Chloride, Glycine, Hydrochloric Acid and/or Sodium Hydroxide (to adjust pH), Magnesium

Continued on next page

Tears Naturale—Cont.

Chloride, Polysorbate 80, Potassium Chloride, Purified Water, Sodium Chloride, Zinc Chloride.

TEARS NATURALE FREE: **Actives:** DUASORB® water soluble polymeric system containing Dextran 70 0.1% and Hypromellose 2910 0.3%. **Inactives:** Sodium Borate, Potassium Chloride, Sodium Chloride, Purified Water.

May contain Hydrochloric Acid and/or Sodium Hydroxide to adjust pH.

Indications: For the temporary relief of burning and irritation due to dryness of the eye and for use as a protectant against further irritation. For the temporary relief of discomfort due to minor irritations of the eye, or to exposure to wind or sun.

Warnings: If you experience eye pain, changes in vision, continued redness or irritation of the eye, or if the condition worsens or persists for more than 72 hours, discontinue use and consult a doctor.

If solution changes color or becomes cloudy, do not use.

To avoid contamination, do not touch tip of container to any surface. Replace cap after using. Keep this and all drugs out of the reach of children. In case of accidental ingestion, seek professional assistance or contact a Poison Control Center immediately.

Directions: TEARS NATURALE® FORTE: Instill 1 or 2 drops in the affected eye(s) as needed. TEARS NATURALE FREE®: Make sure container is intact before use. To open, completely TWIST off tab and set aside for reclosure. DO NOT pull off. Instill 1 or 2 drops in the affected eye(s) as needed. To close, press tab down over container tip and twist. Reclosed vial may leak under pressure. **DISCARD CONTAINER 12 HOURS AFTER OPENING.**

How Supplied: TEARS NATURALE FORTE Lubricant Eye Drops are supplied in 15 mL and 30 mL plastic DROP-TAINER® bottles.

15 mL NDC 0065-0426-15
30 mL NDC 0065-0426-30

TEARS NATURALE FREE Lubricant Eye Drops are supplied in boxes of 36 and 60 0.03 fl. oz. reclosable vials.

36s NDC 0065-0416-25
60s NDC 0065-0416-22

Storage: Store at room temperature.

TOBRADEX® ℞
(tobramycin and dexamethasone ophthalmic suspension)
Sterile

Description: TOBRADEX® (tobramycin and dexamethasone ophthalmic suspension) is a sterile, multiple dose antibiotic and steroid combination for topical ophthalmic use.

Each mL of TOBRADEX® Suspension contains:
Actives: Tobramycin 0.3% (3 mg) and Dexamethasone 0.1% (1 mg). **Preservative:** Benzalkonium Chloride 0.01%. **Inactives:** Tyloxapol, Edetate Disodium, Sodium Chloride, Hydroxyethyl Cellulose, Sodium Sulfate, Sulfuric Acid and/or Sodium Hydroxide (to adjust pH) and Purified Water. DM-00

Clinical Pharmacology: Corticoids suppress the inflammatory response to a variety of agents and they probably delay or slow healing. Since corticoids may inhibit the body's defense mechanism against infection, a concomitant antimicrobial drug may be used when this inhibition is considered to be clinically significant. Dexamethasone is a potent corticoid.

The antibiotic component in the combination (tobramycin) is included to provide action against susceptible organisms. *In vitro* studies have demonstrated that tobramycin is active against susceptible strains of the following microorganisms:

Staphylococci, including *S. aureus* and *S. epidermidis* (coagulase-positive and coagulase-negative), including penicillin-resistant strains.

Streptococci, including some of the Group A-beta-hemolytic species, some nonhemolytic species, and some *Streptococcus pneumoniae*.

Pseudomonas aeruginosa, Escherichia coli, Klebsiella pneumoniae, Enterobacter aerogenes, Proteus mirabilis, Morganella morganii, most *Proteus vulgaris* strains, *Haemophilus influenzae* and *H. aegyptius, Moraxella lacunata, Acinetobacter calcoaceticus* and some *Neisseria* species.

Bacterial susceptibility studies demonstrate that in some cases microorganisms resistant to gentamicin remain susceptible to tobramycin. No data are available on the extent of systemic absorption from TOBRADEX Ophthalmic Suspension; however, it is known that some systemic absorption can occur with ocularly applied drugs. If the maximum dose of TOBRADEX Ophthalmic Suspension is given for the first 48 hours (two drops in each eye every 2 hours) and complete systemic absorption occurs, which is highly unlikely, the daily dose of dexamethasone would be 2.4 mg. The usual physiologic replacement dose is 0.75 mg daily. If TOBRADEX Ophthalmic Suspension is given after the first 48 hours as two drops in each eye every 4 hours, the administered dose of dexamethasone would be 1.2 mg daily.

Indications And Usage: TOBRADEX Ophthalmic Suspension is indicated for steroid-responsive inflammatory ocular conditions for which a corticosteroid is indicated and where superficial bacterial ocular infection or a risk of bacterial ocular infection exists.

Ocular steroids are indicated in inflammatory conditions of the palpebral and bulbar conjunctiva, cornea and anterior segment of the globe where the inherent risk of steroid use in certain infective conjunctivities is accepted to obtain a diminution in edema and inflammation. They are also indicated in chronic anterior uveitis and corneal injury from chemical, radiation or thermal burns, or penetration of foreign bodies.

The use of a combination drug with an anti-infective component is indicated where the risk of superficial ocular infection is high or where there is an expectation that potentially dangerous numbers of bacteria will be present in the eye.

The particular anti-infective drug in this product is active against the following common bacterial eye pathogens:

Staphylococci, including *S. aureus* and *S. epidermidis* (coagulase-positive and coagulase-negative), including penicillin-resistant strains.

Streptococci, including some of the Group A-beta-hemolytic species, some nonhemolytic species, and some *Streptococcus pneumoniae*.

Pseudomonas aeruginosa, Escherichia coli, Klebsiella pneumoniae, Enterobacter aerogenes, Proteus mirabilis, Morganella morganii, most *Proteus vulgaris* strains, *Haemophilus influenzae* and *H. aegyptius, Moraxella lacunata, Acinetobacter calcoaceticus* and some *Neisseria* species.

Contraindications: Epithelial herpes simplex keratitis (dendritic keratitis), vaccinia, varicella, and many other viral diseases of the cornea and conjunctiva. Mycobacterial infection of the eye. Fungal diseases of ocular structures. Hypersensitivity to a component of the medication.

Warnings: NOT FOR INJECTION INTO THE EYE. Sensitivity to topically applied aminoglycosides may occur in some patients. If a sensitivity reaction does occur, discontinue use.

Prolonged use of steroids may result in glaucoma, with damage to the optic nerve, defects in visual acuity and fields of vision, and posterior subcapsular cataract formation. Intraocular pressure should be routinely monitored even though it may be difficult in pediatric patients and uncooperative patients. Prolonged use may suppress the host response and thus increase the hazard of secondary ocular infections. In those diseases causing thinning of the cornea or sclera, perforations have been known to occur with the use of topical steroids. In acute purulent conditions of the eye, steroids may mask infection or enhance existing infection.

Precautions:
General. The possibility of fungal infections of the cornea should be considered after long-term steroid dosing. As with other antibiotic preparations, prolonged use may result in overgrowth of nonsusceptible organisms, including fungi. If superinfection occurs, appropriate therapy should be initiated. When multiple prescriptions are required, or whenever clinical judgement dictates, the patient should be examined with the aid of magnification, such as slit lamp biomicroscopy and, where appropriate, fluorescein staining.

Cross-sensitivity to other aminoglycoside antibiotics may occur; if hypersensitivity develops with this product, discontinue use and institute appropriate therapy.

Information for Patients: Do not touch dropper tip to any surface, as this may contaminate the contents. Contact lenses should not be worn during the use of this product.

Carcinogenesis, Mutagenesis, Impairment of Fertility: No studies have been conducted to evaluate the carcinogenic or mutagenic potential. No impairment of fertility was noted in studies of subcutaneous tobramycin in rats at doses of 50 and 100 mg/kg/day.

Pregnancy Category C. Corticosteroids have been found to be teratogenic in animal studies. Ocular administration of 0.1% dexamethasone resulted in 15.6% and 32.3% incidence of fetal anomalies in two groups of pregnant rabbits. Fetal growth retardation and increased mortality rates have been observed in rats with chronic dexamethasone therapy. Reproduction studies have been performed in rats and rabbits with tobramycin at doses up to 100 mg/kg/day parenterally and have revealed no evidence of impaired fertility or harm to the fetus. There are no adequate and well controlled studies in pregnant women. TOBRADEX® Ophthalmic Suspension should be used during pregnancy only if the potential benefit justifies the potential risk to the fetus.

Nursing Mothers. Systemically administered corticosteroids appear in human milk and could suppress growth, interfere with endogenous corticosteroid production, or cause other untoward effects. It is not known whether topical administration of corticosteroids could result in sufficient systemic absorption to produce detectable quantities in human milk. Because many drugs are excreted in human milk, caution should be exercised when TOBRADEX® Ophthalmic Suspension is administered to a nursing woman.

Pediatric Use. Safety and effectiveness in pediatric patients below the age of 2 years have not been established.

Adverse Reactions: Adverse reactions have occurred with steroid/anti-infective combination drugs which can be attributed to the steroid component, the anti-infective component, or the combination. Exact incidence figures are not available. The most frequent adverse reactions to topical ocular tobramycin (TOBREX®) are hypersensitivity and localized ocular toxicity, including lid itching and swelling, and conjunctival erythema. These reactions occur in less than 4% of patients. Similar reactions may occur with the topical use of other aminoglycoside antibiotics. Other adverse reactions have not been reported, however, if topical ocular tobramycin is administered concomitantly with systemic aminoglycoside antibiotics, care should be taken to monitor the total serum concentration. The reactions due to the steroid component are: elevation of intraocular pressure (IOP) with possible development of glaucoma, and infrequent optic nerve damage; posterior subcapsular cataract formation; and delayed wound healing.

Secondary Infection. The development of secondary infection has occurred after use of combinations containing steroids and antimicrobials. Fungal infections of the cornea are particularly prone to develop coincidentally with long-term applications of steroids. The possibility of fungal invasion must be considered in any persistent corneal ulceration where steroid treatment has been used. Secondary bacterial ocular infection following suppression of host responses also occurs.

Overdosage: Clinically apparent signs and symptoms of an overdosage of TOBRADEX Ophthalmic Suspension (punctate keratitis, erythema, increased lacrimation, edema and lid itching) may be similar to adverse reaction effects seen in some patients.

Dosage and Administration: One or two drops instilled into the conjunctival sac(s) every four to six hours. During the initial 24 to 48 hours, the dosage may be increased to one or two drops every two (2) hours. Frequency should be decreased gradually as warranted by improvement in clinical signs. Care should be taken not to discontinue therapy prematurely. Not more than 20 mL should be prescribed initially and the prescription should not be refilled without further evaluation as outlined in PRECAUTIONS above.

How Supplied: Sterile ophthalmic suspension in 2.5 mL (**NDC** 0065-0647-25), 5 mL (**NDC** 0065-0647-05) and 10 mL (**NDC** 0065-0647-10) DROP-TAINER® dispensers.

Storage: Store at 8° to 27°C (46° to 80°F). Store suspension upright and shake well before using.

℞ Only

U.S. Patent No. 5,149,694

TOBRADEX® ℞
(tobramycin and dexamethasone ophthalmic ointment)
Sterile

Description: TOBRADEX® (tobramycin and dexamethasone ophthalmic ointment) is a sterile, multiple dose antibiotic and steroid combination for topical ophthalmic use.

Each gram of **TOBRADEX® Ointment contains:**
Actives: Tobramycin 0.3% (3mg) and Dexamethasone 0.1% (1mg). **Preservative:** Chlorobutanol 0.5%. **Inactives:** Mineral Oil and White Petrolatum. DM-00

Clinical Pharmacology: Corticoids suppress the inflammatory response to a variety of agents and they probably delay or slow healing. Since corticoids may inhibit the body's defense mechanism against infection, a concomitant antimicrobial drug may be used when this inhibition is considered to be clinically significant. Dexamethasone is a potent corticoid.

The antibiotic component in the combination (tobramycin) is included to provide action against susceptible organisms. *In vitro* studies have demonstrated that tobramycin is active against susceptible strains of the following microorganisms:

Staphylococci, including *S. aureus* and *S. epidermidis* (coagulase-positive and coagulase-negative), including penicillin-resistant strains.

Streptococci, including some of the Group A-beta-hemolytic species, some nonhemolytic species, and some *Streptococcus pneumoniae*. *Pseudomonas aeruginosa, Escherichia coli, Klebsiella pneumoniae, Enterobacter aerogenes, Proteus mirabilis, Morganella morganii*, most *Proteus vulgaris* strains, *Haemophilus influenzae* and *H. aegyptius, Moraxella lacunata, Acinetobacter calcoaceticus* and some *Neisseria* species.

Bacterial susceptibility studies demonstrate that in some cases microorganisms resistant to gentamicin remain susceptible to tobramycin.
No data are available on the extent of systemic absorption from TOBRADEX Ophthalmic Ointment; however, it is known that some systemic absorption can occur with ocularly applied drugs. The usual physiologic replacement dose is 0.75 mg daily. The administered dose for TOBRADEX® Ophthalmic Ointment in both eyes four times daily would be 0.4 mg of dexamethasone daily.

Indications and Usage: TOBRADEX Ophthalmic Ointment is indicated for steroid-responsive inflammatory ocular conditions for which a corticosteroid is indicated and where superficial bacterial ocular infection or a risk of bacterial ocular infection exists.

Ocular steroids are indicated in inflammatory conditions of the palpebral and bulbar conjunctiva, cornea and anterior segment of the globe where the inherent risk of steroid use in certain infective conjunctivitides is accepted to obtain a diminution in edema and inflammation. They are also indicated in chronic anterior uveitis and corneal injury from chemical, radiation or thermal burns, or penetration of foreign bodies.

The use of a combination drug with an anti-infective component is indicated where the risk of superficial ocular infection is high or where there is an expectation that potentially dangerous numbers of bacteria will be present in the eye.

The particular anti-infective drug in this product is active against the following common bacterial eye pathogens:

Staphylococci, including *S. aureus* and *S. epidermidis* (coagulase-positive and coagulase-negative), including penicillin-resistant strains.

Streptococci, including some of the Group A-beta-hemolytic species, some nonhemolytic species, and some *Streptococcus pneumoniae*. *Pseudomonas aeruginosa, Escherichia coli, Klebsiella pneumoniae, Enterobacter aerogenes, Proteus mirabilis, Morganella morganii*, most *Proteus vulgaris* strains, *Haemophilus influenzae* and *H. aegyptius, Moraxella lacunata, Acinetobacter calcoaceticus* and some *Neisseria* species.

Contraindications: Epithelial herpes simplex keratitis (dendritic keratitis), vaccinia, varicella, and many other viral diseases of the cornea and conjunctiva. Mycobacterial infection of the eye. Fungal diseases of ocular structures. Hypersensitivity to a component of the medication.

Warnings: NOT FOR INJECTION INTO THE EYE. Sensitivity to topically applied aminoglycosides may occur in some patients. If a sensitivity reaction does occur, discontinue use.

Prolonged use of steroids may result in glaucoma, with damage to the optic nerve, defects in visual acuity and fields of vision, and posterior subcapsular cataract formation. Intraocular pressure should be routinely monitored even though it may be difficult in pediatric patients and uncooperative patients. Prolonged use may suppress the host response and thus increase the hazard of secondary ocular infections. In those diseases causing thinning of the cornea or sclera, perforations have been known to occur with the use of topical steroids. In acute purulent conditions of the eye, steroids may mask infection or enhance existing infection.

Precautions:
General. The possibility of fungal infections of the cornea should be considered after long-term steroid dosing. As with other antibiotic preparations, prolonged use may result in overgrowth of nonsusceptible organisms, including fungi. If superinfection occurs, appropriate therapy should be initiated. When multiple prescriptions are required, or whenever clinical judgement dictates, the patient should be examined with the aid of magnification, such as slit lamp biomicroscopy and, where appropriate, fluorescein staining.

Cross-sensitivity to other aminoglycoside antibiotics may occur; if hypersensitivity develops with this product, discontinue use and institute appropriate therapy.

Ophthalmic ointment may retard corneal wound healing.

Information for Patients: Do not touch tube tip to any surface, as this may contaminate the contents. Contact lenses should not be worn during the use of this product.

Carcinogenesis, Mutagenesis, Impairment of Fertility. No studies have been conducted to evaluate the carcinogenic or mutagenic potential. No impairment of fertility was noted in studies of subcutaneous tobramycin in rats at doses of 50 and 100 mg/kg/day.

Pregnancy Category C. Corticosteroids have been found to be teratogenic in animal studies. Ocular administration of 0.1% dexamethasone resulted in 15.6% and 32.3% incidence of fetal anomalies in two groups of pregnant rabbits. Fetal growth retardation and increased mortality rates have been observed in rats with chronic dexamethasone therapy. Reproduction studies have been performed in rats and rabbits with tobramycin at doses up to 100 mg/kg/day parenterally and have revealed no evidence of impaired fertility or harm to the fetus. There are no adequate and well controlled studies in pregnant women. TOBRADEX® Ophthalmic Ointment should be used during pregnancy only if the potential benefit justifies the potential risk to the fetus.

Nursing Mothers. Systemically administered corticosteroids appear in human milk and could suppress growth, interfere with endogenous corticosteroid production, or cause other untoward effects. It is not known whether topical administration of corticosteroids could result in sufficient systemic absorption to produce detectable quantities in human milk. Because many drugs are excreted in human milk, caution should be exercised when TOBRADEX® Ophthalmic Ointment is administered to a nursing woman.

Pediatric Use. Safety and effectiveness in pediatric patients below the age of 2 years have not been established.

Adverse Reactions: Adverse reactions have occurred with steroid/anti-infective combination drugs which can be attributed to the steroid component, the anti-infective component, or the combination. Exact incidence figures are not available. The most frequent adverse reactions to topical ocular tobramycin (TOBREX®) are hypersensitivity and localized ocular toxicity, including lid itching and swelling, and conjunctival erythema. These reactions occur in less than 4% of patients. Similar reactions may occur with the topical use of other aminoglycoside antibiotics. Other adverse reactions have not been reported; however, if topical ocular tobramycin is administered concomitantly with systemic aminoglycoside antibiotics, care should be taken to monitor the total serum concentration. The reactions due to the steroid component are: elevation of intraocular pressure (IOP) with possible devel-

Continued on next page

TobraDex Ointment—Cont.

opment of glaucoma, and infrequent optic nerve damage; posterior subcapsular cataract formation; and delayed wound healing.

Secondary Infection. The development of secondary infection has occurred after use of combinations containing steroids and antimicrobials. Fungal infections of the cornea are particularly prone to develop coincidentally with long-term applications of steroids. The possibility of fungal invasion must be considered in any persistent corneal ulceration where steroid treatment has been used. Secondary bacterial ocular infection following suppression of host responses also occurs.

Overdosage: Clinically apparent signs and symptoms of an overdose of TOBRADEX Ophthalmic Ointment (punctate keratitis, erythema, increased lacrimation, edema and lid itching) may be similar to adverse reaction effects seen in some patients.

Dosage and Administration: Apply a small amount (approximately ½ inch ribbon) into the conjunctival sac(s) up to three or four times daily.

How to apply TOBRADEX Ophthalmic Ointment:
1. Tilt your head back.
2. Place a finger on your cheek just under your eye and gently pull down until a "V" pocket is formed between your eyeball and your lower lid.
3. Place a small amount (about ½ inch) of TOBRADEX® Ophthalmic Ointment in the "V" pocket. Do not let the tip of the tube touch your eye.
4. Look downward before closing your eye.

Not more than 8 g should be prescribed initially and the prescription should not be refilled without further evaluation as outlined in PRECAUTIONS above.

How Supplied: Sterile ophthalmic ointment in 3.5 g ophthalmic tube (NDC 0065-0648-35).

Storage: Store at 8° to 27°C (46° to 80°F).

℞ Only

U.S. Patent No. 5,149,694

TRAVATAN® ℞
[tra-va-tan]
(travoprost ophthalmic solution) 0.004%
Sterile

Description: Travoprost is a synthetic prostaglandin $F_{2\alpha}$ analogue. Its chemical name is isopropyl (Z)-7-[(1R,2R,3R,5S)-3,5-dihydroxy-2-[(1E,3R)-3-hydroxy-4-[(α,α,α-trifluoro-m-tolyl)oxy]-1-butenyl]cyclopentyl]-5-heptenoate. It has a molecular formula of $C_{26}H_{35}F_3O_6$ and a molecular weight of 500.56. The chemical structure of travoprost is:

Travoprost is a clear, colorless to slightly yellow oil that is very soluble in acetonitrile, methanol, octanol, and chloroform. It is practically insoluble in water.

TRAVATAN® Ophthalmic Solution 0.004% is supplied as sterile, buffered aqueous solution of travoprost with a pH of approximately 6.0 and an osmolality of approximately 290 mOsmol/kg.

Each mL of TRAVATAN® 0.004% contains 40 μg travoprost. Benzalkonium chloride 0.015% is added as a preservative. Inactive ingredients are: polyoxyl 40 hydrogenated castor oil, tromethamine, boric acid, mannitol, edetate disodium, sodium hydroxide and/or hydrochloric acid (to adjust pH) and purified water.

Clinical Pharmacology:
Mechanism of Action
Travoprost free acid is a selective FP prostanoid receptor agonist which is believed to reduce intraocular pressure by increasing uveoscleral outflow. The exact mechanism of action is unknown at this time.

Pharmacokinetics/Pharmacodynamics
Absorption: Travoprost is absorbed through the cornea and is hydrolyzed to the active free acid. Data from four multiple dose pharmacokinetic studies (totaling 107 subjects) have shown that plasma concentrations of the free acid are below 0.01 ng/mL (the quantitation limit of the assay) in two-thirds of the subjects. In those individuals with quantifiable plasma concentrations (N=38), the mean plasma C_{max} was 0.018 ± 007 ng/mL (ranged 0.01 to 0.052 ng/mL) and was reached within 30 minutes. From these studies, travoprost is estimated to have a plasma half-life of 45 minutes. There was no difference in plasma concentrations between Days 1 and 7, indicating steady-state was reached early and that there was no significant accumulation.

Metabolism: Travoprost, an isopropyl ester prodrug, is hydrolyzed by esterases in the cornea to its biologically active free acid. Systemically, travoprost free acid is metabolized to inactive metabolites via beta-oxidation of the α(carboxylic acid) chain to give the 1,2-dinor and 1,2,3,4-tetranor analogs, via oxidation of the 15-hydroxyl moiety, as well as via reduction of the 13,14 double bond.

Elimination: The elimination of travoprost free acid from plasma was rapid and levels were generally below the limit of quantification within one hour after dosing. The terminal elimination half-life of travoprost free acid was estimated from fourteen subjects and ranged from 17 minutes to 86 minutes with the mean half-life of 45 minutes. Less than 2% of the topical ocular dose of travoprost was excreted in the urine within 4 hours as the travoprost free acid.

Clinical Studies
In clinical studies, patients with open-angle glaucoma or ocular hypertension and baseline pressure of 25–27 mm Hg who were treated with TRAVATAN® Ophthalmic Solution 0.004% dosed once-daily in the evening demonstrated 7–8 mm Hg reductions in intraocular pressure. In subgroup analyses of these studies, mean IOP reduction in black patients was up to 1.8 mm Hg greater than in non-black patients. It is not known at this time whether this difference is attributed to race or to heavily pigmented irides.

In a multi-center, randomized, controlled trial, patients with mean baseline intraocular pressure of 24–26 mm Hg on TIMOPTIC* 0.5% BID who were treated with TRAVATAN® 0.004% dosed QD adjunctively to TIMOPTIC* 0.5% BID demonstrated 6–7 mm Hg reductions in intraocular pressure.

TRAVATAN® has been studied in patients with hepatic impairment and also in patients with renal impairment. No clinically relevant changes in hematology, blood chemistry, or urinalysis laboratory data were observed in these patients.

Indications and Usage: TRAVATAN® Ophthalmic Solution is indicated for the reduction of elevated intraocular pressure in patients with open-angle glaucoma or ocular hypertension who are intolerant of other intraocular pressure lowering medications or insufficiently responsive (failed to achieve target IOP determined after multiple measurements over time) to another intraocular pressure lowering medication.

Contraindications: Known hypersensitivity to travoprost, benzalkonium chloride or any other ingredients in this product.

Warnings: **TRAVATAN® has been reported to cause changes to pigmented tissues. The most frequently reported changes have been increased pigmentation of the iris and periorbital tissue (eyelid) and increased pigmentation and growth of eyelashes. These changes may be permanent.**

TRAVATAN® may gradually change eye color, increasing the amount of brown pigmentation in the iris by increasing the number of melanosomes (pigment granules) in melanocytes. The long term effects on the melanocytes and the consequences of potential injury to the melanocytes and/or deposition of pigment granules to other areas of the eye are currently unknown. The change in iris color occurs slowly and may not be noticeable for months to years. Patients should be informed of the possibility of iris color change.

Eyelid skin darkening has been reported in association with the use of TRAVATAN®.

TRAVATAN® Ophthalmic Solution may gradually change eyelashes in the treated eye; these changes include increased length, thickness, pigmentation, and/or number of lashes. Patients who are expected to receive treatment in only one eye should be informed about the potential for increased brown pigmentation of the iris, periorbital and/or eyelid tissue, and eyelashes in the treated eye and thus heterochromia between the eyes. They should also be advised of the potential for a disparity between the eyes in length, thickness, and/or number of eyelashes.

Precautions:
General
There have been reports of bacterial keratitis associated with the use of multiple-dose containers of topical ophthalmic products. These containers had been inadvertently contaminated by patients who, in most cases, had a concurrent corneal disease or a disruption of the epithelial surface (see Information for Patients).

Patients may slowly develop increased brown pigmentation of the iris. This change may not be noticeable for months to years (see Warnings). Iris pigmentation changes may be more noticeable in patients with mixed colored irides, i.e., blue-brown, grey-brown, yellow-brown, and green-brown; however, it has also been observed in patients with brown eyes. The color change is believed to be due to increased melanin content in the stromal melanocytes of the iris. The exact mechanism of action is unknown at this time. Typically the brown pigmentation around the pupil spreads concentrically towards the periphery in affected eyes, but the entire iris or parts of it may become more brownish. Until more information about increased brown pigmentation is available, patients should be examined regularly and, depending on the situation, treatment may be stopped if increased pigmentation ensues.

TRAVATAN® should be used with caution in patients with a history of intraocular inflammation (iritis/uveitis) and should generally not be used in patients with active intraocular inflammation.

Macular edema, including cystoid macular edema, has been reported during treatment with prostaglandin $F_{2\alpha}$ analogues. These reports have mainly occurred in aphakic patients, pseudophakic patients with a torn posterior lens capsule, or in patients with known risk factors for macular edema. TRAVATAN® Ophthalmic Solution should be used with caution in these patients.

TRAVATAN® has not been evaluated for the treatment of angle closure, inflammatory or neovascular glaucoma.

TRAVATAN® Ophthalmic Solution should not be administered while wearing contact lenses. Patients should be advised that TRAVATAN® contains benzalkonium chloride which may be absorbed by contact lenses. Contact lenses should be removed prior to the administration of the solution. Lenses may be reinserted 15 minutes following administration of TRAVATAN®.

Information for Patients
Patients should be advised concerning all the information contained in the Warnings and Precautions sections.

Patients should also be instructed to avoid allowing the tip of the dispensing container to contact the eye or surrounding structures because this could cause the tip to become contaminated by common bacteria known to cause ocular infections. Serious damage to the eye and subsequent loss of vision may result from using contaminated solutions.

Patients also should be advised that if they develop an intercurrent ocular condition (e.g., trauma, or infection) or have ocular surgery, they should immediately seek their physician's advice concerning the continued use of the multi-dose container.

Patients should be advised that if they develop any ocular reactions, particularly conjunctivitis and lid reactions, they should immediately seek their physician's advice.

If more than one topical ophthalmic drug is being used, the drugs should be administered at least five (5) minutes apart.

Carcinogenesis, Mutagenesis, Impairment of Fertility
Two-year carcinogenicity studies in mice and rats at subcutaneous doses of 10, 30, or 100 µg/kg/day did not show any evidence of carcinogenic potential. However, at 100 µg/kg/day, male rats were only treated for 82 weeks, and the maximum tolerated dose (MTD) was not reached in the mouse study. The high dose (100 µg/kg) corresponds to exposure levels over 400 times the human exposure at the maximum recommended human ocular dose (MRHOD) of 0.04 µg/kg, based on plasma active drug levels.

Travoprost was not mutagenic in the Ames test, mouse micronucleus test or rat chromosome aberration assay. A slight increase in the mutant frequency was observed in one of two mouse lymphoma assays in the presence of rat S-9 activation enzymes.

Travoprost did not affect mating or fertility indices in male or female rats at subcutaneous doses up to 10 µg/kg/day [250 times the maximum recommended human ocular dose of 0.04 µg/kg/day on a µg/kg basis (MRHOD)]. At 10 µg/kg/day, the mean number of corpora lutea was reduced, and the post-implantation losses were increased. These effects were not observed at 3 µg/kg/day (75 times the MRHOD).

Pregnancy: Teratogenic Effects
Pregnancy Category: C
Travoprost was teratogenic in rats, at an intravenous (IV) dose up to 10 µg/kg/day (250 times the MRHOD), evidenced by an increase in the incidence of skeletal malformations as well as external and visceral malformations, such as fused sternebrae, domed head and hydrocephaly. Travoprost was not teratogenic in rats at IV doses up to 3 µg/kg/day (75 times the MRHOD), or in mice at subcutaneous doses up to 1.0 µg/kg/day (25 times the MRHOD). Travoprost produced an increase in post-implantation losses and a decrease in fetal viability in rats at IV doses > 3 µg/kg/day (75 times the MRHOD) and in mice at subcutaneous doses > 0.3 µg/kg/day (7.5 times the MRHOD).

In the offspring of female rats that received travoprost subcutaneously from Day 7 of pregnancy to lactation Day 21 at the doses of ≥ 0.12 µg/kg/day (3 times the MRHOD), the incidence of postnatal mortality was increased, and neonatal body weight gain was decreased. Neonatal development was also affected, evidenced by delayed eye opening, pinna detachment and preputial separation, and by decreased motor activity.

There are no adequate and well-controlled studies in pregnant women. TRAVATAN® should be used during pregnancy only if the potential benefit justifies the potential risk to the fetus.

Nursing Mothers
A study in lactating rats demonstrated that radiolabeled travoprost and/or its metabolites were excreted in milk. It is not known whether this drug or its metabolites are excreted in human milk. Because many drugs are excreted in human milk, caution should be exercised when TRAVATAN® is administered to a nursing woman.

Pediatric Use
Safety and effectiveness in pediatric patients have not been established.

Geriatric Use
No overall differences in safety or effectiveness have been observed between elderly and other adult patients.

Adverse Reactions: The most common ocular adverse event observed in controlled clinical studies with TRAVATAN® 0.004% was ocular hyperemia which was reported in 35 to 50% of patients. Approximately 3% of patients discontinued therapy due to conjunctival hyperemia.

Ocular adverse events reported at an incidence of 5 to 10% included decreased visual acuity, eye discomfort, foreign body sensation, pain, and pruritus.

Ocular adverse events reported at an incidence of 1 to 4% included abnormal vision, blepharitis, blurred vision, cataract, cells, conjunctivitis, dry eye, eye disorder, flare, iris discoloration, keratitis, lid margin crusting, photophobia, subconjunctival hemorrhage, and tearing.

Nonocular adverse events reported at a rate of 1 to 5% were accidental injury, angina pectoris, anxiety, arthritis, back pain, bradycardia, bronchitis, chest pain, cold syndrome, depression, dyspepsia, gastrointestinal disorder, headache, hypercholesterolemia, hypertension, hypotension, infection, pain, prostate disorder, sinusitis, urinary incontinence, and urinary tract infection.

Dosage and Administration: The recommended dosage is one drop in the affected eye(s) once-daily in the evening. The dosage of TRAVATAN® should not exceed once-daily since it has been shown that more frequent administration may decrease the intraocular pressure lowering effect.

Reduction of intraocular pressure starts approximately 2 hours after administration and the maximum effect is reached after 12 hours. TRAVATAN® may be used concomitantly with other topical ophthalmic drug products to lower intraocular pressure. If more than one topical ophthalmic drug is being used, the drugs should be administered at least five (5) minutes apart.

How Supplied: TRAVATAN® (travoprost ophthalmic solution) 0.004% is a sterile, isotonic, buffered, preserved, aqueous solution of travoprost (0.04 mg/mL) supplied in Alcon's oval DROP-TAINER® package system.

TRAVATAN® is supplied as a 2.5 mL solution in a 4 mL and a 5 mL solution in a 7.5 mL natural polypropylene dispenser bottle with a natural polypropylene dropper tip and a turquoise polypropylene overcap. Tamper evidence is provided with a shrink band around the closure and neck area of the package.

NDC 0065-0266-25, 2.5 mL fill
NDC 0065-0266-17, 2 units, 2.5 mL fill each
NDC 0065-0266-34, 5 mL fill

Storage
Store at 2°-25°C (36°-77°F).
Rx Only

U.S. Patent Nos. 5,631,287; 5,849,792; 5,889,052; 6,011,062 and 6,235,781.

*TIMOPTIC is a registered trademark of Merck & Co., Inc.
Alcon®
ALCON LABORATORIES, INC.
Fort Worth, Texas 76134 USA
© 2004 Alcon, Inc.

VIGAMOX™ ℞
[Vi-ga-mox]
(moxifloxacin hydrochloride ophthalmic solution)
0.5% as base

Description: VIGAMOX™ (moxifloxacin HCl ophthalmic solution) 0.5% is a sterile ophthalmic solution. It is an 8-methoxy fluoroquinolone anti-infective for topical ophthalmic use.

$C_{21}H_{24}FN_3O_4 \cdot HCl$ Mol. Wt 437.9

Chemical Name: 1-Cyclopropyl-6-fluoro-1,4-dihydro-8-methoxy-7-[(4aS,7aS)-octahydro-6H-pyrrolol[3,4-b]pyridin-6-yl]-4-oxo-3-quinolinecarboxylic acid, monohydrochloride.

Moxifloxacin hydrochloride is a slightly yellow to yellow crystalline powder. Each mL of VIGAMOX™ contains 5.45 mg moxifloxacin hydrochloride equivalent to 5 mg moxifloxacin base.

Contains:
Active: Moxifloxacin 0.5% (5 mg/mL); **Inactives:** Boric acid, sodium chloride, and purified water. May also contain hydrochloric acid/sodium hydroxide to adjust pH to approximately 6.8.

VIGAMOX™ is an isotonic solution with an osmolality of approximately 290 mOsm/kg.

Clinical Pharmacology:
Pharmacokinetics: Plasma concentrations of moxifloxacin were measured in healthy adult male and female subjects who received bilateral topical ocular doses of VIGAMOX™ 3 times a day. The mean steady-state C_{max} (2.7 ng/mL) and estimated daily exposure AUC (45 ng·hr/mL) values were 1,600 and 1,000 times lower than the mean C_{max} and AUC reported after therapeutic 400 mg oral doses of moxifloxacin. The plasma half-life of moxifloxacin was estimated to be 13 hours.

Microbiology
Moxifloxacin is an 8-methoxy fluoroquinolone with a diazabicyclononyl ring at the C7 position. The antibacterial action of moxifloxacin results from inhibition of the topoisomerase II (DNA gyrase) and topoisomerase IV. DNA gyrase is an essential enzyme that is involved in the replication, transcription and repair of bacterial DNA. Topoisomerase IV is an enzyme known to play a key role in the partitioning of the chromosomal DNA during bacterial cell division.

The mechanism of action for quinolones, including moxifloxacin, is different from that of macrolides, aminoglycosides, or tetracyclines. Therefore, moxifloxacin may be active against pathogens that are resistant to these antibiotics and these antibiotics may be active against pathogens that are resistant to moxifloxacin. There is no cross-resistance between moxifloxacin and the aforementioned classes of an-

Continued on next page

Vigamox—Cont.

tibiotics. Cross resistance has been observed between systemic moxifloxacin and some other quinolones.

In vitro resistance to moxifloxacin develops via multiple-step mutations. Resistance to moxifloxacin occurs *in vitro* at a general frequency of between 1.8×10^{-9} to $< 1 \times 10^{-11}$ for Gram-positive bacteria.

Moxifloxacin has been shown to be active against most strains of the following microorganisms, both *in vitro* and in clinical infections as described in the INDICATIONS AND USAGE section:

Aerobic Gram-positive microorganisms:
Corynebacterium species*
Micrococcus luteus
Staphylococcus aureus
Staphylococcus epidermidis
Staphylococcus haemolyticus
Staphylococcus hominis
Staphylococcus warneri
Streptococcus pneumoniae
Streptococcus viridans group
Aerobic Gram-negative microorganisms:
Acinetobacter lwoffii
Haemophilus influenzae
Haemophilus parainfluenzae
Other microorganisms:
Chlamydia trachomatis

---

*Efficacy for this organism was studied in fewer than 10 infections.
The following *in vitro* data are also available, **but their clinical significance in ophthalmic infections is unknown.** The safety and effectiveness of VIGAMOX™ in treating ophthalmological infections due to these microorganisms have not been established in adequate and well-controlled trials.
The following organisms are considered susceptible when evaluated using systemic breakpoints. However, a correlation between the *in vitro* systemic breakpoint and ophthalmological efficacy has not been established. The list of organisms is provided as guidance only in assessing the potential treatment of conjunctival infections. Moxifloxacin exhibits *in vitro* minimal inhibitory concentrations (MICs) of 2 µg/ml or less (systemic susceptible breakpoint) against most ($\geq 90\%$) of strains of the following ocular pathogens.
Aerobic Gram-positive microorganisms:
Streptococcus pyogenes
Aerobic Gram-negative microorganisms:
Escherichia coli
Klebsiella oxytoca
Klebsiella pneumoniae
Moraxella catarrhalis
Proteus mirabilis
Anaerobic microorganisms:
Fusobacterium species
Prevotella species
Clinical Studies:
In two randomized, double-masked, multicenter, controlled clinical trials in which patients were dosed 3 times a day for 4 days, VIGAMOX™ solution produced clinical cures on day 5–6 in 66% to 69% of patients treated for bacterial conjunctivitis. Microbiological success rates for the eradication of the baseline pathogens ranged from 84% to 94%. Please note that microbiologic eradication does not always correlate with clinical outcome in anti-infective trials.
Indications And Usage: VIGAMOX™ solution is indicated for the treatment of bacterial conjunctivitis caused by susceptible strains of the following organisms:
Aerobic Gram-positive microorganisms:
Corynebacterium species*
Micrococcus luteus
Staphylococcus aureus
Staphylococcus epidermidis
Staphylococcus haemolyticus
Staphylococcus hominis
Staphylococcus warneri
Streptococcus pneumoniae
Streptococcus viridans group
Aerobic Gram-negative microorganisms:
Acinetobacter lwoffii
Haemophilus influenzae
Haemophilus parainfluenzae
Other microorganisms:
Chlamydia trachomatis

---

*Efficacy for this organism was studied in fewer than 10 infections.
Contraindications: VIGAMOX™ (moxifloxacin HCl ophthalmic solution) is contraindicated in patients with a history of hypersensitivity to moxifloxacin, to other quinolones, or to any of the components in this medication.
Warnings: NOT FOR INJECTION.
VIGAMOX™ solution should not be injected subconjunctivally, nor should it be introduced directly into the anterior chamber of the eye. In patients receiving systemically administered quinolones, including moxifloxacin, serious and occasionally fatal hypersensitivity (anaphylactic) reactions have been reported, some following the first dose. Some reactions were accompanied by cardiovascular collapse, loss of consciousness, angioedema (including laryngeal, pharyngeal or facial edema), airway obstruction, dyspnea, urticaria, and itching. If an allergic reaction to moxifloxacin occurs, discontinue use of the drug. Serious acute hypersensitivity reactions may require immediate emergency treatment. Oxygen and airway management should be administered as clinically indicated.
Precautions:
General: As with other anti-infectives, prolonged use may result in overgrowth of non-susceptible organisms, including fungi. If superinfection occurs, discontinue use and institute alternative therapy. Whenever clinical judgment dictates, the patient should be examined with the aid of magnification, such as slit-lamp biomicroscopy, and, where appropriate, fluorescein staining. Patients should be advised not to wear contact lenses if they have signs and symptoms of bacterial conjunctivitis.
Information for Patients: Avoid contaminating the applicator tip with material from the eye, fingers or other source. Systemically administered quinolones including moxifloxacin have been associated with hypersensitivity reactions, even following a single dose. Discontinue use immediately and contact your physician at the first sign of a rash or allergic reaction.
Drug Interactions: Drug-drug interaction studies have not been conducted with VIGAMOX™ solution. *In vitro* studies indicate that moxifloxacin does not inhibit CYP3A4, CYP2D6, CYP2C9, CYP2C19, or CYP1A2 indicating that moxifloxacin is unlikely to alter the pharmacokinetics of drugs metabolized by these cytochrome P450 isozymes.
Carcinogenesis, Mutagenesis, Impairment of Fertility: Long-term studies in animals to determine the carcinogenic potential of moxifloxacin have not been performed. However, in an accelerated study with initiators and promoters, moxifloxacin was not carcinogenic in rats following up to 38 weeks of oral dosing at 500 mg/kg/day (approximately 21,700 times the highest recommended total daily human ophthalmic dose for a 50 kg person, on a mg/kg basis).
Moxifloxacin was not mutagenic in four bacterial strains used in the Ames *Salmonella* reversion assay. As with other quinolones, the positive response observed with moxifloxacin in strain TA 102 using the same assay may be due to the inhibition of DNA gyrase. Moxifloxacin was not mutagenic in the CHO/HGPRT mammalian cell gene mutation assay. An equivocal result was obtained in the same assay when v79 cells were used. Moxifloxacin was clastogenic in the v79 chromosome aberration assay, but it did not induce unscheduled DNA synthesis in cultured rat hepatocytes. There was no evidence of genotoxicity *in vivo* in a micronucleus test or a dominant lethal test in mice.
Moxifloxacin had no effect on fertility in male and female rats at oral doses as high as 500 mg/kg/day, approximately 21,700 times the highest recommended total daily human ophthalmic dose. At 500 mg/kg orally there were slight effects on sperm morphology (head-tail separation) in male rats and on the estrous cycle in female rats.
Pregnancy: Teratogenic Effects.
Pregnancy Category C: Moxifloxacin was not teratogenic when administered to pregnant rats during organogenesis at oral doses as high as 500 mg/kg/day (approximately 21,700 times the highest recommended total daily human ophthalmic dose); however, decreased fetal body weights and slightly delayed fetal skeletal development were observed. There was no evidence of teratogenicity when pregnant Cynomolgus monkeys were given oral doses as high as 100 mg/kg/day (approximately 4,300 times the highest recommended total daily human ophthalmic dose). An increased incidence of smaller fetuses was observed at 100 mg/kg/day.
Since there are no adequate and well-controlled studies in pregnant women, VIGAMOX™ solution should be used during pregnancy only if the potential benefit justifies the potential risk to the fetus.
Nursing Mothers: Moxifloxacin has not been measured in human milk, although it can be presumed to be excreted in human milk. Caution should be exercised when VIGAMOX™ solution is administered to a nursing mother.
Pediatric Use: The safety and effectiveness of VIGAMOX™ solution in infants below 1 year of age have not been established. There is no evidence that the ophthalmic administration of VIGAMOX™ has any effect on weight bearing joints, even though oral administration of some quinolones has been shown to cause arthropathy in immature animals.
Geriatric Use: No overall differences in safety and effectiveness have been observed between elderly and younger patients.
Adverse Reactions: The most frequently reported ocular adverse events were conjunctivitis, decreased visual acuity, dry eye, keratitis, ocular discomfort, ocular hyperemia, ocular pain, ocular pruritus, subconjunctival hemorrhage, and tearing. These events occurred in approximately 1-6% of patients.
Nonocular adverse events reported at a rate of 1-4% were fever, increased cough, infection, otitis media, pharyngitis, rash, and rhinitis.
Dosage and Administration: Instill one drop in the affected eye 3 times a day for 7 days.
How Supplied: VIGAMOX™ (moxifloxacin hydrochloride ophthalmic solution) 0.5% is supplied as a sterile ophthalmic solution in Alcon's DROP-TAINER® dispensing system consisting of a natural low density polyethylene bottle and dispensing plug and tan polypropylene closure. Tamper evidence is provided with a shrink band around the closure and neck area of the package.
3 mL in 6 mL bottle - **NDC** 0065-4013-03
Storage: Store at 2°C-25°C (36°F-77°F).
Rx Only
Manufactured by
Alcon Laboratories, Inc.
Fort Worth, Texas 76134 USA
Licensed from Bayer AG to Alcon, Inc.
U.S. PAT. NO. 4,990,517; 5,607,942; 5,849,752
© 2003 Alcon, Inc.

Allergan, Inc.
2525 DUPONT DRIVE
P.O. BOX 19534
IRVINE, CA 92623-9534

Direct Inquiries to:
(714) 246-4500

ACULAR® ℞
(ketorolac tromethamine ophthalmic solution)
0.5%
Sterile

Description: ACULAR® (ketorolac tromethamine ophthalmic solution) is a member of the pyrrolo-pyrrole group of nonsteroidal anti-inflammatory drugs (NSAIDs) for ophthalmic use. Its chemical name is (±)-5-Benzoyl-2,3-dihydro-1H-pyrrolizine-1-carboxylic acid, compound with 2-amino-2-(hydroxymethyl)-1,3-propanediol (1:1)
ACULAR® ophthalmic solution is supplied as a sterile isotonic aqueous 0.5% solution, with a pH of 7.4. ACULAR® ophthalmic solution is a racemic mixture of R-(+)- and S-(−)- ketorolac tromethamine. Ketorolac tromethamine may exist in three crystal forms. All forms are equally soluble in water. The pKa of ketorolac is 3.5. This white to off-white crystalline substance discolors on prolonged exposure to light. The molecular weight of ketorolac tromethamine is 376.41. The osmolality of ACULAR® ophthalmic solution is 290 mOsm/kg. Each mL of ACULAR® ophthalmic solution contains: **Active:** ketorolac tromethamine 0.5%. **Preservative:** benzalkonium chloride 0.01%. **Inactives:** edetate disodium 0.1%; octoxynol 40; purified water; sodium chloride; and hydrochloric acid and/or sodium hydroxide to adjust the pH.

Clinical Pharmacology: Ketorolac tromethamine is a nonsteroidal anti-inflammatory drug which, when administered systemically, has demonstrated analgesic, anti-inflammatory, and anti-pyretic activity. The mechanism of its action is thought to be due to its ability to inhibit prostaglandin biosynthesis. Ketorolac tromethamine given systemically does not cause pupil constriction.
Prostaglandins have been shown in many animal models to be mediators of certain kinds of intraocular inflammation. In studies performed in animal eyes, prostaglandins have been shown to produce disruption of the blood-aqueous humor barrier, vasodilation, increased vascular permeability, leukocytosis, and increased intraocular pressure. Prostaglandins also appear to play a role in the miotic response produced during ocular surgery by constricting the iris sphincter independently of cholinergic mechanisms.
Two drops (0.1 mL) of 0.5% ACULAR® ophthalmic solution instilled into the eyes of patients 12 hours and 1 hour prior to cataract extraction achieved measurable levels in 8 of 9 patients' eyes (mean ketorolac concentration 95 ng/mL aqueous humor, range 40 to 170 ng/mL). Ocular administration of ketorolac tromethamine reduces prostaglandin E_2 (PGE_2) levels in aqueous humor. The mean concentration of PGE_2 was 80 pg/mL in the aqueous humor of eyes receiving vehicle and 28 pg/mL in the eyes receiving ACULAR® 0.5% ophthalmic solution.
One drop (0.05 mL) of 0.5% ACULAR® ophthalmic solution was instilled into one eye and one drop of vehicle into the other eye TID in 26 normal subjects. Only 5 of 26 subjects had a detectable amount of ketorolac in their plasma (range 10.7 to 22.5 ng/mL) at Day 10 during topical ocular treatment. When ketorolac tromethamine 10 mg is administered systemically every 6 hours, peak plasma levels at steady state are around 960 ng/mL.
Two controlled clinical studies showed that ACULAR® ophthalmic solution was significantly more effective than its vehicle in relieving ocular itching caused by seasonal allergic conjunctivitis.
Two controlled clinical studies showed that patients treated for two weeks with ACULAR® ophthalmic solution were less likely to have measurable signs of inflammation (cell and flare) than patients treated with its vehicle.
Results from clinical studies indicated that ketorolac tromethamine has no significant effect upon intraocular pressure; however, changes in intraocular pressure may occur following cataract surgery.

Indications and Usage: ACULAR® ophthalmic solution is indicated for the temporary relief of ocular itching due to seasonal allergic conjunctivitis. ACULAR® ophthalmic solution is also indicated for the treatment of postoperative inflammation in patients who have undergone cataract extraction.

Contraindications: ACULAR® ophthalmic solution is contraindicated in patients with previously demonstrated hypersensitivity to any of the ingredients in the formulation.

Warnings: There is the potential for cross-sensitivity to acetylsalicylic acid, phenylacetic acid derivatives, and other nonsteroidal anti-inflammatory agents. Therefore, caution should be used when treating individuals who have previously exhibited sensitivities to these drugs.
With some nonsteroidal anti-inflammatory drugs, there exists the potential for increased bleeding time due to interference with thrombocyte aggregation. There have been reports that ocularly applied nonsteroidal anti-inflammatory drugs may cause increased bleeding of ocular tissues (including hyphemas) in conjunction with ocular surgery.

Precautions:
General: All topical nonsteroidal anti-inflammatory drugs (NSAIDs) may slow or delay healing. Topical corticosteroids are also known to slow or delay healing. Concomitant use of topical NSAIDs and topical steroids may increase the potential for healing problems.
Use of topical NSAIDs may result in keratitis. In some susceptible patients, continued use of topical NSAIDs may result in epithelial breakdown, corneal thinning, corneal erosion, corneal ulceration or corneal perforation. These events may be sight threatening. Patients with evidence of corneal epithelial breakdown should immediately discontinue use of topical NSAIDs and should be closely monitored for corneal health.
Postmarketing experience with topical NSAIDs suggests that patients with complicated ocular surgeries, corneal denervation, corneal epithelial defects, diabetes mellitus, ocular surface diseases (e.g., dry eye syndrome), rheumatoid arthritis, or repeat ocular surgeries within a short period of time may be at increased risk for corneal adverse events which may become sight threatening. Topical NSAIDs should be used with caution in these patients.
Postmarketing experience with topical NSAIDs also suggests that use more than 24 hours prior to surgery or use beyond 14 days post-surgery may increase patient risk for the occurrence and severity of corneal adverse events.
It is recommended that ACULAR® ophthalmic solution be used with caution in patients with known bleeding tendencies or who are receiving medications which may prolong bleeding time.

Information for Patients: ACULAR® ophthalmic solution should not be administered while wearing contact lenses.

Carcinogenesis, Mutagenesis, and Impairment of Fertility: Ketorolac tromethamine was not carcinogenic in rats given up to 5 mg/kg/day orally for 24 months (151 times the maximum recommended human topical ophthalmic dose, on a mg/kg basis, assuming 100% absorption in humans and animals) nor in mice given 2 mg/kg/day orally for 18 months (60 times the maximum recommended human topical ophthalmic dose, on a mg/kg basis, assuming 100% absorption in humans and animals).
Ketorolac tromethamine was not mutagenic *in vitro* in the Ames assay or in forward mutation assays. Similarly, it did not result in an *in vitro* increase in unscheduled DNA synthesis or an *in vivo* increase in chromosome breakage in mice. However, ketorolac tromethamine did result in an increased incidence in chromosomal aberrations in Chinese hamster ovary cells.
Ketorolac tromethamine did not impair fertility when administered orally to male and female rats at doses up to 272 and 484 times the maximum recommended human topical ophthalmic dose, respectively, on a mg/kg basis, assuming 100% absorption in humans and animals.

Pregnancy: Teratogenic Effects: Pregnancy Category C. Ketorolac tromethamine, administered during organogenesis, was not teratogenic in rabbits or rats at oral doses up to 109 times and 303 times the maximum recommended human topical ophthalmic dose, respectively, on a mg/kg basis assuming 100% absorption in humans and animals. When administered to rats after Day 17 of gestation at oral doses up to 45 times the maximum recommended human topical ophthalmic dose, respectively, on a mg/kg basis, assuming 100% absorption in humans and animals, ketorolac tromethamine resulted in dystocia and increased pup mortality. There are no adequate and well-controlled studies in pregnant women. ACULAR® ophthalmic solution should be used during pregnancy only if the potential benefit justifies the potential risk to the fetus.

Nonteratogenic Effects: Because of the known effects of prostaglandin-inhibiting drugs on the fetal cardiovascular system (closure of the ductus arteriosus), the use of ACULAR® ophthalmic solution during late pregnancy should be avoided.

Nursing Mothers: Caution should be exercised when ACULAR® ophthalmic solution is administered to a nursing woman.

Pediatric Use: Safety and efficacy in pediatric patients below the age of 3 have not been established.

Geriatric Use: No overall differences in safety or effectiveness have been observed between elderly and younger patients.

Adverse Reactions: The most frequent adverse events reported with the use of ketorolac tromethamine ophthalmic solutions have been transient stinging and burning on instillation. These events were reported by up to 40% of patients participating in clinical trials.
Other adverse events occurring approximately 1 to 10% of the time during treatment with ketorolac tromethamine ophthalmic solutions included allergic reactions, corneal edema, iritis, ocular inflammation, ocular irritation, superficial keratitis and superficial ocular infections.
Other adverse events reported rarely with the use of ketorolac tromethamine ophthalmic solutions included: corneal infiltrates, corneal ulcer, eye dryness, headaches, and visual disturbance (blurry vision).
Clinical Practice: The following events have been identified during postmarketing use of ketorolac tromethamine ophthalmic solution 0.5% in clinical practice. Because they are reported voluntarily from a population of unknown size, estimates of frequency cannot be made. The events, which have been chosen for inclusion due to either their seriousness, fre-

Continued on next page

Acular—Cont.

quency of reporting, possible causal connection to topical ketorolac tromethamine ophthalmic solution 0.5%, or a combination of these factors, include corneal erosion, corneal perforation, corneal thinning and epithelial breakdown (see **Precautions, General**).

Dosage and Administration: The recommended dose of ACULAR® ophthalmic solution is one drop (0.25 mg) four times a day for relief of ocular itching due to seasonal allergic conjunctivitis.

For the treatment of postoperative inflammation in patients who have undergone cataract extraction, one drop of ACULAR® ophthalmic solution should be applied to the affected eye(s) four times daily beginning 24 hours after cataract surgery and continuing through the first 2 weeks of the postoperative period.

ACULAR® ophthalmic solution has been safely administered in conjunction with other ophthalmic medications such as antibiotics, beta blockers, carbonic anhydrase inhibitors, cycloplegics, and mydriatics.

How Supplied: ACULAR® (ketorolac tromethamine ophthalmic solution) is supplied sterile in opaque white LDPE plastic bottles with droppers with gray high impact polystyrene (HIPS) caps as follows:

3 mL in 5 mL bottle **NDC** 0023-2181-03
5 mL in 10 mL bottle **NDC** 0023-2181-05
10 mL in 10 mL bottle **NDC** 0023-2181-10

Store at 15–25°C (59–77°F) with protection from light.

℞ only

U.S. Pat.: 5,110,493.
©2004 Allergan, Inc., Irvine, CA 92612, U.S.A.
ACULAR®, a registered trademark of Roche Palo Alto LLC, is manufactured and distributed by Allergan, Inc. under license from its developer, Roche Palo Alto LLC, Palo Alto, California, U.S.A.

ALLERGAN
Irvine, CA 92612

Shown in Product Identification Guide, page 103

ACULAR LS™ ℞
[ă-kew-lar]
(ketorolac tromethamine ophthalmic solution) 0.4%
Sterile

Description: ACULAR LS™ (ketorolac tromethamine ophthalmic solution) 0.4% is a member of the pyrrolo-pyrrole group of nonsteroidal anti-inflammatory drugs (NSAIDs) for ophthalmic use.

Structural and Molecular Formula:

$C_{19}H_{24}N_2O_6$ Mol Wt 376.41

Chemical Name: (±)-5-Benzoyl-2,3-dihydro-1H-pyrrolizine-1-carboxylic acid, compound with 2-amino-2-(hydroxymethyl)-1,3-propanediol (1:1)

Contains: Active: ketorolac tromethamine 0.4%. **Preservative:** benzalkonium chloride 0.006%. **Inactives:** sodium chloride; edetate disodium 0.015%; octoxynol 40; purified water; and hydrochloric acid and/or sodium hydroxide to adjust the pH.

ACULAR LS™ ophthalmic solution is supplied as a sterile isotonic aqueous 0.4% solution, with a pH of approximately 7.4. ACULAR LS™ ophthalmic solution is a racemic mixture of R-(+) and S-(−)- ketorolac tromethamine. Ketorolac tromethamine may exist in three crystal forms. All forms are equally soluble in water. The pKa of ketorolac is 3.5. This white to off-white crystalline substance discolors on prolonged exposure to light. The osmolality of ACULAR LS™ ophthalmic solution is approximately 290 mOsml/kg.

Clinical Pharmacology:
Mechanism of Action
Ketorolac tromethamine is a nonsteroidal anti-inflammatory drug which, when administered systemically, has demonstrated analgesic, anti-inflammatory, and anti-pyretic activity. The mechanism of its action is thought to be due to its ability to inhibit prostaglandin biosynthesis. Ketorolac tromethamine given systemically does not cause pupil constriction.

Pharmacokinetics
One drop (0.05 mL) of 0.5% ketorolac tromethamine ophthalmic solution was instilled into one eye and one drop of vehicle into the other eye TID in 26 normal subjects. Only 5 of 26 subjects had a detectable amount of ketorolac in their plasma (range 10.7 to 22.5 ng/mL) at day 10 during topical ocular treatment. When ketorolac tromethamine 10 mg is administered systemically every 6 hours, peak plasma levels at steady state are around 960 ng/mL.

Clinical Studies: In two double-masked, multi-centered, parallel-group studies, 313 patients who had undergone photorefractive keratectomy received ACULAR LS™ 0.4% or its vehicle QID for up to 4 days. Significant differences favored ACULAR LS™ for the reduction of ocular pain and burning/stinging following photorefractive keratectomy surgery.

Results from clinical studies indicate that ketorolac tromethamine has no significant effect upon intraocular pressure.

Indications and Usage: ACULAR LS™ ophthalmic solution is indicated for the reduction of ocular pain and burning/stinging following corneal refractive surgery.

Contraindications: ACULAR LS™ ophthalmic solution is contraindicated in patients with previously demonstrated hypersensitivity to any of the ingredients in the formulation.

Warnings: There is the potential for cross-sensitivity to acetylsalicylic acid, phenylacetic acid derivatives, and other nonsteroidal anti-inflammatory agents. Therefore, caution should be used when treating individuals who have previously exhibited sensitivities to these drugs.

With some nonsteroidal anti-inflammatory drugs there exists the potential for increased bleeding time due to interference with thrombocyte aggregation. There have been reports that ocularly applied nonsteroidal anti-inflammatory drugs may cause increased bleeding of ocular tissues (including hyphemas) in conjunction with ocular surgery.

Precautions:
General: All topical nonsteroidal anti-inflammatory drugs (NSAIDs), including ketorolac tromethamine ophthalmic solution, may slow or delay healing. Topical corticosteroids are also known to slow or delay healing. Concomitant use of topical NSAIDS and topical steroids may increase the potential for healing problems.

Use of topical NSAIDs may result in keratitis. In some susceptible patients, continued use of topical NSAIDs may result in epithelial breakdown, corneal thinning, corneal erosion, corneal ulceration or corneal perforation. These events may be sight threatening. Patients with evidence of corneal epithelial breakdown should immediately discontinue use of topical NSAIDs and should be closely monitored for corneal health.

Postmarketing experience with topical NSAIDs suggests that patients with complicated ocular surgeries, corneal denervation, corneal epithelial defects, diabetes mellitus, ocular surface diseases (e.g., dry eye syndrome), rheumatoid arthritis, or repeat ocular surgeries within a short period of time may be at increased risk for corneal adverse events which may become sight threatening. Topical NSAIDs should be used with caution in these patients.

Postmarketing experience with topical NSAIDs also suggests that use more than 24 hours prior to surgery or use beyond 14 days post-surgery may increase patient risk for the occurrence and severity of corneal adverse events.

It is recommended that ACULAR LS™ ophthalmic solution be used with caution in patients with known bleeding tendencies or who are receiving other medications, which may prolong bleeding time.

Information for Patients: ACULAR LS™ ophthalmic solution should not be administered while wearing contact lenses.

Carcinogenesis, Mutagenesis, Impairment of Fertility:
Ketorolac tromethamine was neither carcinogenic in rats given up to 5 mg/kg/day orally for 24 months (156 times the maximum recommended human topical ophthalmic dose, on a mg/kg basis, assuming 100% absorption in humans and animals) nor in mice given 2 mg/kg/day orally for 18 months (62.5 times the maximum recommended human topical ophthalmic dose, on a mg/kg basis, assuming 100% absorption in humans and animals).

Ketorolac tromethamine was not mutagenic *in vitro* in the Ames assay or in forward mutation assays. Similarly, it did not result in an *in vitro* increase in unscheduled DNA synthesis or an *in vivo* increase in chromosome breakage in mice. However, ketorolac tromethamine did result in an increased incidence in chromosomal aberrations in Chinese hamster ovary cells.

Ketorolac tromethamine did not impair fertility when administered orally to male and female rats at doses up to 280 and 499 times the maximum recommended human topical ophthalmic dose, respectively, on a mg/kg basis, assuming 100% absorption in humans and animals.

Pregnancy:
Teratogenic Effects: Pregnancy Category C:
Ketorolac tromethamine, administered during organogenesis, was not teratogenic in rabbits or rats at oral doses up to 112 times and 312 times the maximum recommended human topical ophthalmic dose, respectively, on a mg/kg basis assuming 100% absorption in humans and animals. When administered to rats after Day 17 of gestation at oral doses up to 46 times the maximum recommended human topical ophthalmic dose on a mg/kg basis, assuming 100% absorption in humans and animals, ketorolac tromethamine resulted in dystocia and increased pup mortality. There are no adequate and well-controlled studies in pregnant women. ACULAR LS™ ophthalmic solution should be used during pregnancy only if the potential benefit justifies the potential risk to the fetus.

Nonteratogenic Effects:
Because of the known effects of prostaglandin-inhibiting drugs on the fetal cardiovascular system (closure of the ductus arteriosus), the use of ACULAR LS™ ophthalmic solution during late pregnancy should be avoided.

Nursing Mothers: Caution should be exercised when ACULAR LS™ ophthalmic solution is administered to a nursing woman.

Pediatric Use: Safety and effectiveness of ketorolac tromethamine in pediatric patients below the age of 3 have not been established.

Geriatric use: No overall differences in safety or effectiveness have been observed between elderly and younger patients.

Adverse Reactions: The most frequently reported adverse reactions for ACULAR LS™

ophthalmic solution occurring in approximately 1 to 5% of the overall study population were conjunctival hyperemia, corneal infiltrates, headache, ocular edema and ocular pain.

The most frequent adverse events reported with the use of ketorolac tromethamine ophthalmic solutions have been transient stinging and burning on instillation. These events were reported by 20%-40% of patients participating in these other clinical trials.

Other adverse events occurring approximately 1%-10% of the time during treatment with ketorolac tromethamine ophthalmic solutions included allergic reactions, corneal edema, iritis, ocular inflammation, ocular irritation, ocular pain, superficial keratitis, and superficial ocular infections.

Clinical Practice: The following events have been identified during postmarketing use of ketorolac tromethamine ophthalmic solutions in clinical practice. Because they are reported voluntarily from a population of unknown size, estimates of frequency cannot be made. The events, which have been chosen for inclusion due to either their seriousness, frequency of reporting, possible causal connection to topical ketorolac tromethamine ophthalmic solutions, or a combination of these factors, include corneal erosion, corneal perforation, corneal thinning and epithelial breakdown (see **Precautions, General**).

Dosage and Administration: The recommended dose of ACULAR LS™ ophthalmic solution is one drop four times a day in the operated eye as needed for pain and burning/stinging for up to 4 days following corneal refractive surgery.

Ketorolac tromethamine ophthalmic solution has been safely administered in conjunction with other ophthalmic medications such as antibiotics, beta blockers, carbonic anhydrase inhibitors, cycloplegics, and mydriatics.

How Supplied: ACULAR LS™ (ketorolac tromethamine ophthalmic solution) 0.4% is supplied sterile in an opaque white LDPE plastic bottle with a white dropper with a gray high impact polystyrene (HIPS) cap as follows:
5 mL in 10 mL bottle- NDC 0023-9277-05
Note: Store at 15°C-25°C (59°F-77°F).

℞ only

U.S. Pat. 5,110,493
©2003 Allergan, Inc., Irvine, CA 92612, U.S.A.
This product is manufactured and distributed by Allergan, Inc. under license from its developer, Roche Palo Alto LLC, Palo Alto, California, U.S.A.
May 2003
9437X

Shown in Product Identification Guide, page 103

ACULAR® PF ℞
(ketorolac tromethamine ophthalmic solution) 0.5%
Preservative-Free

Description: ACULAR® PF (ketorolac tromethamine ophthalmic solution) Preservative-Free is a member of the pyrrolo-pyrrole group of nonsteroidal anti-inflammatory drugs (NSAIDs) for ophthalmic use. Its chemical name is (±)-5-Benzoyl-2,3-dihydro-1H-pyrrolizine-1-carboxylic acid, compound with 2-amino-2-(hydroxymethyl)-1,3-propanediol (1:1)

ACULAR® PF is a racemic mixture of R-(+) and S-(-)-ketorolac tromethamine. Ketorolac tromethamine may exist in three crystal forms. All forms are equally soluble in water. The pKa of ketorolac is 3.5. This white to off-white crystalline substance discolors on prolonged exposure to light. The molecular weight of ketorolac tromethamine is 376.41. The osmolality of ACULAR® PF is 290 mOsmol/kg. Each ml of ACULAR® PF contains: **Active:** ketorolac tromethamine 0.5%. **Inactives:** purified water; sodium chloride; and hydrochloric acid and/or sodium hydroxide to adjust the pH to 7.4.

Clinical Pharmacology: Ketorolac tromethamine is a nonsteroidal anti-inflammatory drug which, when administered systemically, has demonstrated analgesic, anti-inflammatory, and anti-pyretic activity. The mechanism of its action is thought to be due to its ability to inhibit prostaglandin biosynthesis. Ketorolac tromethamine given systemically does not cause pupil constriction.

One drop (0.05 mL) of ketorolac tromethamine (preserved) was instilled into one eye and one drop of vehicle into the other eye TID in 26 normal subjects. Only 5 of 26 subjects had a detectable amount of ketorolac in their plasma (range 10.7 to 22.5 ng/mL) at day 10 during topical ocular treatment. When ketorolac tromethamine 10 mg is administered systemically every 6 hours, peak plasma levels at steady state are around 960 ng/mL.

In two double-masked, multi-centered, parallel-group studies, 340 patients who had undergone incisional refractive surgery received ACULAR® PF or its vehicle QID for up to 3 days. Significant differences favored ACULAR® PF for the treatment of ocular pain and photophobia.

Results from clinical studies indicate that ketorolac tromethamine has no significant effect upon intraocular pressure.

Indications and Usage: ACULAR® PF ophthalmic solution is indicated for the reduction of ocular pain and photophobia following incisional refractive surgery.

Contraindications: ACULAR® PF ophthalmic solution is contraindicated in patients with previously demonstrated hypersensitivity to any of the ingredients in the formulation.

Warnings: There is the potential for cross-sensitivity to acetylsalicylic acid, phenylacetic acid derivatives, and other nonsteroidal anti-inflammatory agents. Therefore, caution should be used when treating individuals who have previously exhibited sensitivities to these drugs.

With some nonsteroidal anti-inflammatory drugs, there exists the potential for increased bleeding time due to interference with thrombocyte aggregation. There have been reports that ocularly applied nonsteroidal anti-inflammatory drugs may cause increased bleeding of ocular tissues (including hyphemas) in conjunction with ocular surgery.

Precautions
General: All topical nonsteroidal anti-inflammatory drugs (NSAIDs) may slow or delay healing. Topical corticosteroids are also known to slow or delay healing. Concomitant use of topical NSAIDs and topical steroids may increase the potential for healing problems.

Use of topical NSAIDs may result in keratitis. In some susceptible patients, continued use of topical NSAIDs may result in epithelial breakdown, corneal thinning, corneal erosion, corneal ulceration or corneal perforation. These events may be sight threatening. Patients with evidence of corneal epithelial breakdown should immediately discontinue use of topical NSAIDs and should be closely monitored for corneal health.

Postmarketing experience with topical NSAIDs suggests that patients with complicated ocular surgeries, corneal denervation, corneal epithelial defects, diabetes mellitus, ocular surface diseases (e.g., dry eye syndrome), rheumatoid arthritis, or repeat ocular surgeries within a short period of time may be at increased risk for corneal adverse events which may become sight threatening. Topical NSAIDs should be used with caution in these patients.

Postmarketing experience with topical NSAIDs also suggests that use more than 24 hours prior to surgery or use beyond 14 days post-surgery may increase patient risk for the occurrence and severity of corneal adverse events.

It is recommended that ACULAR® PF ophthalmic solution be used with caution in patients with known bleeding tendencies or who are receiving other medications which may prolong bleeding time.

Information for Patients: ACULAR® PF should not be administered while wearing contact lenses.

The solution from one individual single-use vial is to be used immediately after opening for administration to one or both eyes, and the remaining contents should be discarded immediately after administration. To avoid contamination, do not touch tip of unit-dose vial to eye or any other surface.

Carcinogenesis, Mutagenesis, and Impairment of Fertility: Ketorolac tromethamine was not carcinogenic in rats given up to 5 mg/kg/day orally for 24 months (151 times the maximum recommended human topical ophthalmic dose, on a mg/kg basis, assuming 100% absorption in humans and animals) nor in mice given 2 mg/kg/day orally for 18 months (60 times the maximum recommended human topical ophthalmic dose, on a mg/kg basis, assuming 100% absorption in humans and animals).

Ketorolac tromethamine was not mutagenic *in vitro* in the Ames assay or in forward mutation assays. Similarly, it did not result in an *in vitro* increase in unscheduled DNA synthesis or an *in vivo* increase in chromosome breakage in mice. However, ketorolac tromethamine did result in an increased incidence in chromosomal aberrations in Chinese hamster ovary cells.

Ketorolac tromethamine did not impair fertility when administered orally to male and female rats at doses up to 272 and 484 times the maximum recommended human topical ophthalmic dose, respectively, on a mg/kg basis, assuming 100% absorption in humans and animals.

Pregnancy:
Teratogenic Effects: Pregnancy Category C. Ketorolac tromethamine, administered during organogenesis, was not teratogenic in rabbits or rats at oral doses up to 109 times and 303 times the maximum recommended human topical ophthalmic dose, respectively, on a mg/kg basis assuming 100% absorption in humans and animals. When administered to rats after Day 17 of gestation at oral doses up to 45 times the maximum recommended human topical ophthalmic dose, respectively, on a mg/kg basis, assuming 100% absorption in humans and animals, ketorolac tromethamine resulted in dystocia and increased pup mortality. There are no adequate and well-controlled studies in pregnant women. ACULAR® PF ophthalmic solution should be used during pregnancy only if the potential benefit justifies the potential risk to the fetus.

Nonteratogenic Effects: Because of the known effects of prostaglandin-inhibiting drugs on the fetal cardiovascular system (closure of the ductus arteriosus), the use of ACULAR® PF during late pregnancy should be avoided.

Nursing Mothers: Caution should be exercised when ACULAR® PF is administered to a nursing woman.

Pediatric Use: Safety and efficacy in pediatric patients below the age of 3 years have not been established.

Geriatric Use: No overall differences in safety or effectiveness have been observed between elderly and younger patients.

Continued on next page

Acular PF—Cont.

Adverse Reactions: The most frequent adverse events reported with the use of ketorolac tromethamine ophthalmic solutions have been transient stinging and burning on instillation. These events were reported by approximately 20% of patients participating in clinical trials.
Other adverse events occurring approximately 1%–10% of the time during treatment with ketorolac tromethamine ophthalmic solutions included allergic reactions, corneal edema, iritis, ocular inflammation, ocular irritation, superficial keratitis, and superficial ocular infections. Other adverse events reported rarely with the use of ketorolac tromethamine ophthalmic solutions include: corneal infiltrates, corneal ulcer, eye dryness, headaches, and visual disturbance (blurry vision).
Clinical Practice: The following events have been identified during postmarketing use of ketorolac tromethamine ophthalmic solution 0.5% in clinical practice. Because they are reported voluntarily from a population of unknown size, estimates of frequency cannot be made. The events, which have been chosen for inclusion due to either their seriousness, frequency of reporting, possible causal connection to topical ketorolac tromethamine ophthalmic solution 0.5%, or a combination of these factors, include corneal erosion, corneal perforation, corneal thinning and epithelial breakdown (see **PRECAUTIONS, General**).
Dosage And Administration: The recommended dose of ACULAR® PF is one drop (0.25 mg) four times a day in the operated eye as needed for pain and photophobia for up to 3 days after incisional refractive surgery.
How Supplied: ACULAR® PF (ketorolac tromethamine ophthalmic solution) 0.5% Preservative-Free is available as a sterile solution supplied in clear, LDPE single-use vials as follows: ACULAR® PF 12 Single-Use Vials 0.4 mL each - NDC 0023-9055-04. Store ACULAR® PF at 15°C–30°C (59°F–86°F) with protection from light.
℞ only
U.S. Pat.: 5,110,493
ALLERGAN ©2002 Allergan, Irvine, CA 92612, U.S.A.
ACULAR® is a registered trademark of Roche Palo Alto LLC. ACULAR® PF is manufactured and distributed by ALLERGAN under license from its developer, Roche Palo Alto LLC, Palo Alto, California, U.S.A.
Revised February 2002
Shown in Product Identification Guide, page 103

ALBALON®
(naphazoline hydrochloride ophthalmic solution, USP) 0.1%
Sterile

Description: Naphazoline hydrochloride, an ocular vasoconstrictor, is an imidazoline derivative sympathomimetic amine. It occurs as a white, odorless crystalline powder having a bitter taste and is freely soluble in water and in alcohol.
Chemical Name: 2-(1-Naphthylmethyl)-2-imidazoline monohydrochloride
Contains:
Active: naphazoline HCl 0.1%. **Preservative:** benzalkonium chloride 0.004%.
Inactives: citric acid, monohydrate; edetate disodium; polyvinyl alcohol 1.4%; purified water; sodium chloride; sodium citrate, dihydrate; and sodium hydroxide to adjust the pH. It has a shelf life pH range of 5.5 to 6.5.
Clinical Pharmacology: Naphazoline constricts the vascular system of the conjunctiva. It is presumed that this effect is due to direct stimulation action of the drug upon the alpha-adrenergic receptors in the arterioles of the conjunctiva, resulting in decreased conjunctival congestion. Naphazoline belongs to the imidazoline class of sympathomimetics.
Indications and Usage: ALBALON® (naphazoline hydrochloride ophthalmic solution, USP) 0.1% is indicated for use as a topical ocular vasoconstrictor.
Contraindications: ALBALON® ophthalmic solution is contraindicated in the presence of an anatomically narrow angle or in narrow-angle glaucoma or in persons who have shown hypersensitivity to any component of this preparation.
Warnings: Patients under therapy with MAO inhibitors may experience a severe hypertensive crisis if given a sympathomimetic drug. Use in children, especially infants, may result in CNS depression leading to coma and marked reduction in body temperature.
Precautions:
General: Use with caution in the presence of hypertension, cardiovascular abnormalities, hyperglycemia (diabetes), hyperthyroidism, infection or injury.
Patient Information: Patients should be advised to discontinue the drug and consult a physician if relief is not obtained within 48 hours of therapy, if irritation, blurring or redness persists or increases, or if symptoms of systemic absorption occur, i.e., dizziness, headache, nausea, decrease in body temperature, or drowsiness.
To prevent contaminating the dropper tip and solution, do not touch the eyelids or the surrounding area with the dropper tip of the bottle. If solution changes color or becomes cloudy, do not use.
Drug Interactions: Concurrent use of maprotiline or tricyclic antidepressants and naphazoline may potentiate the pressor effect of naphazoline. Patients under therapy with MAO inhibitors may experience a severe hypertensive crisis if given a sympathomimetic drug. (See **Warnings**).
Pregnancy: Pregnancy Category C: Animal reproduction studies have not been conducted with naphazoline. It is also not known whether naphazoline can cause fetal harm when administered to a pregnant woman or can affect reproduction capacity. Naphazoline should be given to a pregnant woman only if clearly needed.
Nursing Mothers: It is not known whether naphazoline is excreted in human milk. Because many drugs are excreted in human milk, caution should be exercised when naphazoline is administered to a nursing woman.
Pediatric Use: Safety and effectiveness in pediatric patients have not been established. See "**Warnings**" AND "**Contraindications**."
Adverse Reactions:
Ocular: Mydriasis, increased redness, irritation, discomfort, blurring, punctate keratitis, lacrimation, increased intraocular pressure.
Systemic: Dizziness, headache, nausea, sweating, nervousness, drowsiness, weakness, hypertension, cardiac irregularities, and hyperglycemia.
Dosage and Administration: Instill one or two drops in the conjunctival sac(s) every three to four hours as needed.
How Supplied: ALBALON® (naphazoline hydrochloride ophthalmic solution, USP) 0.1% is supplied sterile in opaque white LDPE plastic bottles with dropper tips and white high impact polystyrene (HIPS) caps as follows:
15 mL in 15 mL bottle – **NDC** 11980-154-15
Note: Store between 15° to 25°C (59° to 77°F).
℞ only
Revised January 2003

ALPHAGAN® P
(brimonidine tartrate ophthalmic solution) 0.15%
STERILE

Description: ALPHAGAN® P (brimonidine tartrate ophthalmic solution) 0.15% is a relatively selective alpha-2 adrenergic agonist for ophthalmic use. The chemical name of brimonidine tartrate is 5-bromo-6- (2-imidazolidinylideneamino) quinoxaline L-tartrate. It is an off-white to pale yellow powder. It has a molecular weight of 442.24 as the tartrate salt, and is both soluble in water (1.5 mg/mL) and in the product vehicle (3.0 mg/mL) at pH 7.2. The structural formula is:

Formula: $C_{11}H_{10}BrN_5 \bullet C_4H_6O_6$
CAS Number: 70359-46-5
In solution, ALPHAGAN® P (brimonidine tartrate ophthalmic solution) 0.15% has a clear, greenish-yellow color. It has an osmolality of 250–350 mOsmol/kg and a pH of 6.6–7.4.
Each mL of ALPHAGAN® P contains:
Active Ingredient: brimonidine tartrate 0.15% (1.5 mg/mL)
Preservative: *Purite*® 0.005% (0.05 mg/mL)
Inactives: boric acid; calcium chloride; magnesium chloride; potassium chloride; purified water; sodium borate; sodium carboxymethylcellulose; sodium chloride; with hydrochloric acid and/or sodium hydroxide to adjust pH.
Clinical Pharmacology:
Mechanism of Action: ALPHAGAN® P ophthalmic solution is an alpha adrenergic receptor agonist. It has a peak ocular hypotensive effect occurring at two hours post-dosing. Fluorophotometric studies in animals and humans suggest that brimonidine tartrate has a dual mechanism of action by reducing aqueous humor production and increasing uveoscleral outflow.
Pharmacokinetics: After ocular administration of either a 0.1% or 0.2% solution, plasma concentrations peaked within 0.5 to 2.5 hours and declined with a systemic half-life of approximately 2 hours. In humans, systemic metabolism of brimonidine is extensive. It is metabolized primarily by the liver. Urinary excretion is the major route of elimination of the drug and its metabolites. Approximately 87% of an orally-administered radioactive dose was eliminated within 120 hours, with 74% found in the urine.
Clinical Evaluations: Elevated IOP presents a major risk factor in glaucomatous field loss. The higher the level of IOP, the greater the likelihood of optic nerve damage and visual field loss. Brimonidine tartrate has the action of lowering intraocular pressure with minimal effect on cardiovascular and pulmonary parameters.
Two clinical studies were conducted to evaluate the safety, efficacy, and acceptability of ALPHAGAN® P (brimonidine tartrate ophthalmic solution) 0.15% compared with ALPHAGAN®, administered three-times-daily in patients with open-angle glaucoma or ocular hypertension. Those results indicated that ALPHAGAN® P (brimonidine tartrate ophthalmic solution) 0.15% is comparable in IOP lowering effect to ALPHAGAN® (brimonidine tartrate ophthalmic solution) 0.2%, and effectively lowers IOP in patients with open-angle glaucoma or ocular hypertension by approximately 2–5 mmHg.

Indications and Usage: ALPHAGAN® P is indicated for the lowering of intraocular pressure in patients with open-angle glaucoma or ocular hypertension.

Contraindications: ALPHAGAN® P is contraindicated in patients with hypersensitivity to brimonidine tartrate or any component of this medication. It is also contraindicated in patients receiving monoamine oxidase (MAO) inhibitor therapy.

Precautions:

General: Although ALPHAGAN® P ophthalmic solution had minimal effect on the blood pressure of patients in clinical studies, caution should be exercised in treating patients with severe cardiovascular disease.

ALPHAGAN® P has not been studied in patients with hepatic or renal impairment; caution should be used in treating such patients. ALPHAGAN® P should be used with caution in patients with depression, cerebral or coronary insufficiency, Raynaud's phenomenon, orthostatic hypotension, or thromboangiitis obliterans. Patients prescribed IOP-lowering medication should be routinely monitored for IOP.

Information for Patients: As with other drugs in this class, ALPHAGAN® P ophthalmic solution may cause fatigue and/or drowsiness in some patients. Patients who engage in hazardous activities should be cautioned of the potential for a decrease in mental alertness.

Drug Interactions: Although specific drug interaction studies have not been conducted with ALPHAGAN® P, the possibility of an additive or potentiating effect with CNS depressants (alcohol, barbiturates, opiates, sedatives, or anesthetics) should be considered. Alpha-agonists, as a class, may reduce pulse and blood pressure. Caution in using concomitant drugs such as beta-blockers (ophthalmic and systemic), anti-hypertensives and/or cardiac glycosides is advised.

Tricyclic antidepressants have been reported to blunt the hypotensive effect of systemic clonidine. It is not known whether the concurrent use of these agents with ALPHAGAN® P ophthalmic solution in humans can lead to resulting interference with the IOP lowering effect. No data on the level of circulating catecholamines after ALPHAGAN® P administration are available. Caution, however, is advised in patients taking tricyclic antidepressants which can affect the metabolism and uptake of circulating amines.

Carcinogenesis, Mutagenesis, and Impairment of Fertility: No compound-related carcinogenic effects were observed in either mice or rats following a 21-month and 24-month study, respectively. In these studies, dietary administration of brimonidine tartrate at doses up to 2.5 mg/kg/day in mice and 1.0 mg/kg/day in rats achieved 86 and 55 times, respectively, the plasma drug concentration estimated in humans treated with one drop of ALPHAGAN® P ophthalmic solution into both eyes 3 times per day.

Brimonidine tartrate was not mutagenic or cytogenic in a series of *in vitro* and *in vivo* studies including the Ames test, chromosomal aberration assay in Chinese Hamster Ovary (CHO) cells, a host-mediated assay and cytogenic studies in mice, and dominant lethal assay.

Reproductive studies performed in rats with oral doses of 0.66 mg base/kg revealed no evidence of impaired fertility due to ALPHAGAN® P.

Pregnancy: Teratogenic Effects: Pregnancy Category B. Reproductive studies performed in rats with oral doses of 0.66 mg base/kg revealed no evidence of harm to the fetus due to ALPHAGAN® P ophthalmic solution. Dosing at this level produced an exposure that is 189 times higher than the exposure seen in humans following multiple ophthalmic doses.

There are no adequate and well-controlled studies in pregnant women. In animal studies, brimonidine crossed the placenta and entered into the fetal circulation to a limited extent. ALPHAGAN® P should be used during pregnancy only if the potential benefit to the mother justifies the potential risk to the fetus.

Nursing Mothers: It is not known whether this drug is excreted in human milk; in animal studies brimonidine tartrate was excreted in breast milk. A decision should be made whether to discontinue nursing or to discontinue the drug, taking into account the importance of the drug to the mother.

Pediatric Use: In a well-controlled clinical study conducted in pediatric glaucoma patients (ages 2 to 7 years) the most commonly observed adverse events with brimonidine tartrate ophthalmic solution 0.2% dosed three times daily were somnolence (50%–83% in patients ages 2 to 6 years) and decreased alertness. In pediatric patients 7 years of age or older (>20kg), somnolence appears to occur less frequently (25%). Approximately 16% of patients on brimonidine tartrate ophthalmic solution discontinued from the study due to somnolence.

The safety and effectiveness of brimonidine tartrate ophthalmic solution have not been studied in pediatric patients below the age of 2 years. Brimonidine tartrate ophthalmic solution is not recommended for use in pediatric patients under the age of 2 years. (Also refer to Adverse Reactions section.)

Geriatric Use: No overall differences in safety or effectiveness have been observed between elderly and other adult patients.

Adverse Reactions: Adverse events occurring in approximately 10–20% of the subjects included: allergic conjunctivitis, conjunctival hyperemia, and eye pruritus.

Adverse events occurring in approximately 5–9% of the subjects included: burning sensation, conjunctival folliculosis, hypertension, oral dryness, and visual disturbance.

Events occurring in approximately 1–4% of subjects included: allergic reaction, asthenia, blepharitis, bronchitis, conjunctival edema, conjunctival hemorrhage, conjunctivitis, cough, dizziness, dyspepsia, dyspnea, epiphora, eye discharge, eye dryness, eye irritation, eye pain, eyelid edema, eyelid erythema, flu syndrome, follicular conjunctivitis, foreign body sensation, headache, pharyngitis, photophobia, rash, rhinitis, sinus infection, sinusitis, stinging, superficial punctate keratopathy, visual field defect, vitreous floaters, and worsened visual acuity.

The following events were reported in less than 1% of subjects: corneal erosion, insomnia, nasal dryness, somnolence, and taste perversion.

The following events have been identified during post-marketing use of ALPHAGAN® ophthalmic solution in clinical practice. Because they are reported voluntarily from a population of unknown size, estimates of frequency cannot be made. The events, which have been chosen for inclusion due to either their seriousness, frequency of reporting, possible causal connection to ALPHAGAN®, or a combination of these factors, include: bradycardia; hypotension; iritis; miosis; skin reactions (including erythema, eyelid pruritus, rash, and vasodilation) and tachycardia. Apnea, bradycardia, hypotension, hypothermia, hypotonia, and somnolence have been reported in infants receiving ALPHAGAN® ophthalmic solution.

Overdosage: No information is available on overdosage in humans. Treatment of an oral overdose includes supportive and symptomatic therapy; a patent airway should be maintained.

Dosage and Administration: The recommended dose is one drop of ALPHAGAN® P in the affected eye(s) three times daily, approximately 8 hours apart.

ALPHAGAN® P ophthalmic solution may be used concomitantly with other topical ophthalmic drug products to lower intraocular pressure. If more than one topical ophthalmic product is being used, the products should be administered at least 5 minutes apart.

How Supplied: ALPHAGAN® P (brimonidine tartrate ophthalmic solution) 0.15% is supplied sterile in opaque teal LDPE plastic bottles and tips with purple high impact polystyrene (HIPS) caps as follows:

5 mL in 10 mL bottle   NDC 0023-9177-05
10 mL in 10 mL bottle   NDC 0023-9177-10
15 mL in 15 mL bottle   NDC 0023-9177-15

NOTE: Store at 15°–25°C (59°–77°F).

℞ Only

® Marks owned by Allergan, Inc.

U.S. Pat. 5,424,078; 5,736,165; 6,194,415; 6,248,741; 6,465,464; 6,562,873; 6,627,210; 6,641,834; 6,673,337

ALLERGAN
©2003 Allergan, Inc
Irvine, CA 92612, U.S.A.

Shown in Product Identification Guide, page 103

BETAGAN® ℞
(levobunolol hydrochloride ophthalmic solution, USP)
sterile

Description: BETAGAN® (levobunolol hydrochloride ophthalmic solution, USP) sterile is a noncardioselective beta-adrenoceptor blocking agent for ophthalmic use. The solution is colorless to slightly light yellow in appearance with an osmolality range of 250–360 mOsm/kg. The shelf life pH range is 5.5 to 7.5.

Chemical Name: (-)-5-[3-(tert-Butylamino)-2-hydroxypropoxy]-3,4-dihydro-1(2H)-naphthalenone hydrochloride.

Contains: Active: levobunolol HCl 0.25% or 0.5%. **Preservative:** benzalkonium chloride 0.004% **Inactives:** edetate disodium; polyvinyl alcohol 1.4%; potassium phosphate, monobasic; purified water; sodium chloride; sodium metabisulfite, sodium phosphate, dibasic; and hydrochloric acid or sodium hydroxide to adjust pH.

Clinical Pharmacology: Levobunolol HCl is a noncardioselective beta-adrenoceptor blocking agent, equipotent at both beta$_1$ and beta$_2$ receptors. Levobunolol HCl is greater than 60 times more potent than its dextro isomer in its beta-blocking activity, yet equipotent in its potential for direct myocardial depression. Accordingly, the levo isomer, levobunolol HCl, is used. Levobunolol HCl does not have significant local anesthetic (membrane-stabilizing) or intrinsic sympathomimetic activity.

Beta-adrenergic receptor blockade reduces cardiac output in both healthy subjects and patients with heart disease. In patients with severe impairment of myocardial function, beta-adrenergic receptor blockade may inhibit the stimulatory effect of the sympathetic nervous system necessary to maintain adequate cardiac function.

Beta-adrenergic receptor blockade in the bronchi and bronchioles results in increased airway resistance from unopposed para-sympathetic activity. Such an effect in patients with asthma or other bronchospastic conditions is potentially dangerous.

BETAGAN® (levobunolol hydrochloride ophthalmic solution, USP) has been shown to be an active agent in lowering elevated as well as

Continued on next page

Betagan—Cont.

normal intraocular pressure (IOP) whether or not accompanied by glaucoma. Elevated IOP presents a major risk factor in glaucomatous field loss. The higher the level of IOP, the greater the likelihood of optic nerve damage and visual field loss.

The onset of action with one drop of BETAGAN® can be detected within one hour after treatment, with maximum effect seen between 2 and 6 hours.

A significant decrease in IOP can be maintained for up to 24 hours following a single dose.

In two separate, controlled studies (one three month and one up to 12 months duration) BETAGAN® ophthalmic solution 0.25% b.i.d. controlled the IOP of approximately 64% and 70% of the subjects.

The overall mean decrease from baseline was 5.4 mm Hg and 5.1 mm Hg respectively. In an open-label study, BETAGAN® ophthalmic solution 0.25% q.d. controlled the IOP of 72% of the subjects while achieving an overall mean decrease of 5.9 mm Hg.

In controlled clinical studies of approximately two years duration, intraocular pressure was well-controlled in approximately 80% of subjects treated with BETAGAN® ophthalmic solution 0.5% b.i.d. The mean IOP decrease from baseline was between 6.87 mm Hg and 7.81 mm Hg. No significant effects on pupil size, tear production or corneal sensitivity were observed. BETAGAN® at the concentrations tested, when applied topically, decreased heart rate and blood pressure in some patients. The IOP-lowering effect of BETAGAN® was well maintained over the course of these studies.

In a three month clinical study, a single daily application of 0.5% BETAGAN® ophthalmic solution controlled the IOP of 72% of subjects achieving an overall mean decrease in IOP of 7.0 mm Hg.

The primary mechanism of the ocular hypotensive action of levobunolol HCl in reducing IOP is most likely a decrease in aqueous humor production. BETAGAN® reduces IOP with little or no effect on pupil size or accommodation in contrast to the miosis which cholinergic agents are known to produce. The blurred vision and night blindness often associated with miotics would not be expected and have not been reported with the use of BETAGAN® ophthalmic solution. This is particularly important in cataract patients with central lens opacities who would experience decreased visual acuity with pupillary constriction.

Indications and Usage: BETAGAN® ophthalmic solution has been shown to be effective in lowering intraocular pressure and may be used in patients with chronic open-angle glaucoma or ocular hypertension.

Contraindications: BETAGAN® ophthalmic solution is contraindicated in those individuals with bronchial asthma or with a history of bronchial asthma, or severe chronic obstructive pulmonary disease (see WARNINGS); sinus bradycardia; second and third degree atrioventricular block; overt cardiac failure (see WARNINGS); cardiogenic shock; or hypersensitivity to any component of these products.

Warnings: As with other topically applied ophthalmic drugs, BETAGAN® may be absorbed systemically. The same adverse reactions found with systemic administration of beta-adrenergic blocking agents may occur with topical administration. For example, severe respiratory reactions and cardiac reactions, including death due to bronchospasm in patients with asthma, and rarely death in association with cardiac failure, have been reported with topical application of beta-adrenergic blocking agents (see CONTRAINDICATIONS).

Cardiac Failure: Sympathetic stimulation may be essential for support of the circulation in individuals with diminished myocardial contractility, and its inhibition by beta-adrenergic receptor blockade may precipitate more severe failure.

In Patients Without a History of Cardiac Failure: Continued depression of the myocardium with beta-blocking agents over a period of time can, in some cases, lead to cardiac failure. At the first sign or symptom of cardiac failure, BETAGAN® ophthalmic solution should be discontinued.

Obstructive Pulmonary Disease:
PATIENTS WITH CHRONIC OBSTRUCTIVE PULMONARY DISEASE (e.g., CHRONIC BRONCHITIS, EMPHYSEMA) OF MILD OR MODERATE SEVERITY, BRONCHOSPASTIC DISEASE OR A HISTORY OF BRONCHOSPASTIC DISEASE (OTHER THAN BRONCHIAL ASTHMA OR A HISTORY OF BRONCHIAL ASTHMA, IN WHICH BETAGAN® IS CONTRAINDICATED, See CONTRAINDICATIONS), SHOULD IN GENERAL NOT RECEIVE BETA BLOCKERS, INCLUDING BETAGAN®. However, if BETAGAN® is deemed necessary in such patients, then it should be administered cautiously since it may block bronchodilation produced by endogenous and exogenous catecholamine stimulation of $beta_2$ receptors.

Major Surgery: The necessity or desirability of withdrawal of beta-adrenergic blocking agents prior to major surgery is controversial. Beta-adrenergic receptor blockade impairs the ability of the heart to respond to beta-adrenergically mediated reflex stimuli. This may augment the risk of general anesthesia in surgical procedures. Some patients receiving beta-adrenergic receptor blocking agents have been subject to protracted severe hypotension during anesthesia. Difficulty in restarting and maintaining the heartbeat has also been reported. For these reasons, in patients undergoing elective surgery, gradual withdrawal of beta-adrenergic receptor blocking agents may be appropriate.

If necessary during surgery, the effects of beta-adrenergic blocking agents may be reversed by sufficient doses of such agonists as isoproterenol, dopamine, dobutamine or levarterenol (See OVERDOSAGE).

Diabetes Mellitus: Beta-adrenergic blocking agents should be administered with caution in patients subject to spontaneous hypoglycemia or to diabetic patients (especially those with labile diabetes) who are receiving insulin or oral hypoglycemic agents. Beta-adrenergic receptor blocking agents may mask the signs and symptoms of acute hypoglycemia.

Thyrotoxicosis: Beta-adrenergic blocking agents may mask certain clinical signs (e.g., tachycardia) of hyperthyroidism. Patients suspected of developing thyrotoxicosis should be managed carefully to avoid abrupt withdrawal of beta-adrenergic blocking agents, which might precipitate a thyroid storm.

These products contain sodium metabisulfite, a sulfite that may cause allergic-type reactions including anaphylactic symptoms and life-threatening or less severe asthmatic episodes in certain susceptible people. The overall prevalence of sulfite sensitivity in the general population is unknown and probably low. Sulfite sensitivity is seen more frequently in asthmatic than in nonasthmatic people.

Precautions:
General: BETAGAN® (levobunolol hydrochloride ophthalmic solution, USP) sterile should be used with caution in patients with known hypersensitivity to other beta-adrenoceptor blocking agents.

Use with caution in patients with known diminished pulmonary function.

BETAGAN® should be used with caution in patients who are receiving a beta-adrenergic blocking agent orally, because of the potential for additive effects on systemic beta-blockade or on intraocular pressure. Patients should not typically use two or more topical ophthalmic beta-adrenergic blocking agents simultaneously.

Because of the potential effects of beta-adrenergic blocking agents on blood pressure and pulse rates, these medications must be used cautiously in patients with cerebrovascular insufficiency. Should signs or symptoms develop that suggest reduced cerebral blood flow while using BETAGAN® ophthalmic solution, alternative therapy should be considered. In patients with angle-closure glaucoma, the immediate objective of treatment is to reopen the angle. This requires, in most cases, constricting the pupil with a miotic. BETAGAN® ophthalmic solution has little or no effect on the pupil. When BETAGAN® is used to reduce elevated intraocular pressure in angle-closure glaucoma, it should be followed with a miotic and not alone.

Muscle Weakness: Beta-adrenergic blockade has been reported to potentiate muscle weakness consistent with certain myasthenic symptoms (e.g., diplopia, ptosis and generalized weakness).

Drug Interactions: Although BETAGAN® ophthalmic solution used alone has little or no effect on pupil size, mydriasis resulting from concomitant therapy with BETAGAN® and epinephrine may occur.

Close observation of the patient is recommended when a beta-blocker is administered to patients receiving catecholamine-depleting drugs such as reserpine, because of possible additive effects and the production of hypotension and/or marked bradycardia, which may produce vertigo, syncope, or postural hypotension.

Patients receiving beta-adrenergic blocking agents along with either oral or intravenous calcium antagonists should be monitored for possible atrioventricular conduction disturbances, left ventricular failure and hypotension. In patients with impaired cardiac function, simultaneous use should be avoided altogether.

The concomitant use of beta-adrenergic blocking agents with digitalis and calcium antagonists may have additive effects on prolonging atrioventricular conduction time.

Phenothiazine-related compounds and beta-adrenergic blocking agents may have additive hypotensive effects due to the inhibition of each other's metabolism.

Risk of anaphylactic reaction: While taking beta-blockers, patients with a history of severe anaphylactic reaction to a variety of allergens may be more reactive to repeated challenge, either accidental, diagnostic, or therapeutic. Such patients may be unresponsive to the usual doses of epinephrine used to treat allergic reaction.

Animal Studies: No adverse ocular effects were observed in rabbits administered BETAGAN® ophthalmic solution topically in studies lasting one year in concentrations up to 10 times the human dose concentration.

Carcinogenesis, mutagenesis, impairment of fertility: In a lifetime oral study in mice, there were statistically significant ($p \leq 0.05$) increases in the incidence of benign leiomyomas in female mice at 200 mg/kg/day (14,000 times the recommended human dose for glaucoma), but not at 12 or 50 mg/kg/day (850 and 3,500 times the human dose). In a two-year oral study of levobunolol HCl in rats, there was a statistically significant ($p \leq 0.05$) increase in the incidence of benign hepatomas in male rats administered 12,800 times the recommended human dose for glaucoma. Similar differences were not observed in rats administered oral doses equivalent to 350 times to 2,000 times the recommended human dose for glaucoma.

Levobunolol did not show evidence of mutagenic activity in a battery of microbiological and mammalian *in vitro* and *in vivo* assays. Reproduction and fertility studies in rats showed no adverse effect on male or female fertility at doses up to 1,800 times the recommended human dose for glaucoma.

Pregnancy Category C: Fetotoxicity (as evidenced by a greater number of resorption sites) has been observed in rabbits when doses of levobunolol HCl equivalent to 200 and 700 times the recommended dose for the treatment of glaucoma were given. No fetotoxic effects have been observed in similar studies with rats at up to 1,800 times the human dose for glaucoma. Teratogenic studies with levobunolol in rats at doses up to 25 mg/kg/day (1,800 times the recommended human dose for glaucoma) showed no evidence of fetal malformations. There were no adverse effects on postnatal development of offspring. It appears when results from studies using rats and studies with other beta-adrenergic blockers are examined, that the rabbit may be a particularly sensitive species. There are no adequate and well controlled studies in pregnant women. BETAGAN® ophthalmic solution should be used during pregnancy only if the potential benefit justifies the potential risk to the fetus.

Nursing Mothers: It is not known whether this drug is excreted in human milk. Systemic beta-blockers and topical timolol maleate are known to be excreted in human milk. Caution should be exercised when BETAGAN® is administered to a nursing woman.

Pediatric Use: Safety and effectiveness in pediatric patients have not been established.

Geriatric Use: No overall differences in safety or effectiveness have been observed between elderly and younger patients.

Adverse Reactions: In clinical trials, the use of BETAGAN® ophthalmic solution has been associated with transient ocular burning and stinging in up to 1 in 3 patients, and with blepharoconjunctivitis in up to 1 in 20 patients. Decreases in heart rate and blood pressure have been reported (see CONTRAINDICATIONS and WARNINGS).

The following adverse effects have been reported rarely with the use of BETAGAN®: iridocyclitis, headache, transient ataxia, dizziness, lethargy, urticaria and pruritus.

Decreased corneal sensitivity has been noted in a small number of patients. Although levobunolol has minimal membrane-stabilizing activity, there remains a possibility of decreased corneal sensitivity after prolonged use.

The following additional adverse reactions have been reported either with BETAGAN® ophthalmic solution or ophthalmic use of other beta-adrenergic receptor blocking agents:
BODY AS A WHOLE: Headache, asthenia, chest pain. **CARDIOVASCULAR:** Bradycardia, arrhythmia, hypotension, syncope, heart block, cerebral vascular accident, cerebral ischemia, congestive heart failure, palpitation, cardiac arrest. **DIGESTIVE:** Nausea, diarrhea. **PSYCHIATRIC:** Depression, confusion, increase in signs and symptoms of myasthenia gravis, paresthesia. **SKIN:** Hypersensitivity, including localized and generalized rash, alopecia, Stevens-Johnson Syndrome. **RESPIRATORY:** Bronchospasm (predominantly in patients with pre-existing bronchospastic disease), respiratory failure, dyspnea, nasal congestion. **UROGENITAL:** Impotence. **ENDOCRINE:** Masked symptoms of hypoglycemia in insulin-dependent diabetics (see WARNINGS). **SPECIAL SENSES:** Signs and symptoms of keratitis, blepharoptosis, visual disturbances including refractive changes (due to withdrawal of miotic therapy in some cases), diplopia, ptosis.

Other reactions associated with the oral use of non-selective adrenergic receptor blocking agents should be considered potential effects with ophthalmic use of these agents.

Overdosage: No data are available regarding overdosage in humans. Should accidental ocular overdosage occur, flush eye(s) with water or normal saline. If accidentally ingested, efforts to decrease further absorption may be appropriate (gastric lavage). The most common signs and symptoms to be expected with overdosage with administration of a systemic beta-adrenergic blocking agent are symptomatic bradycardia, hypotension, bronchospasm, and acute cardiac failure. Should these symptoms occur, discontinue BETAGAN® therapy and initiate appropriate supportive therapy. The following supportive measures should be considered:

1. Symptomatic bradycardia: Use atropine sulfate intravenously in a dosage of 0.25 mg to 2 mg to induce vagal blockade. If bradycardia persists, intravenous isoproterenol hydrochloride should be administered cautiously. In refractory cases, the use of a transvenous cardiac pacemaker should be considered.
2. Hypotension: Use sympathomimetic pressor drug therapy, such as dopamine, dobutamine or levarterenol. In refractory cases, the use of glucagon hydrochloride may be useful.
3. Bronchospasm: Use isoproterenol hydrochloride. Additional therapy with aminophylline may be considered.
4. Acute cardiac failure: Conventional therapy with digitalis, diuretics and oxygen should be instituted immediately. In refractory cases, the use of intravenous aminophylline is suggested. This may be followed, if necessary, by glucagon hydrochloride, which may be useful.
5. Heart block (second or third degree): Use isoproterenol hydrochloride or a transvenous cardiac pacemaker.

Dosage and Administration: The recommended starting dose is one to two drops of BETAGAN® ophthalmic solution 0.5% in the affected eye(s) once a day. Typical dosing with BETAGAN® 0.25% ophthalmic solution is one to two drops twice daily. In patients with more severe or uncontrolled glaucoma, BETAGAN® 0.5% can be administered b.i.d. As with any new medication, careful monitoring of patients is advised. Dosages above one drop of BETAGAN® 0.5% b.i.d. are not generally more effective. If the patient's IOP is not at a satisfactory level on this regimen, concomitant therapy with dipivefrin and/or epinephrine, and/or pilocarpine and other miotics, and/or systemically administered carbonic anhydrase inhibitors, such as acetazolamide, can be instituted. Patients should not typically use two or more topical ophthalmic beta-adrenergic blocking agents simultaneously.

How Supplied: BETAGAN® (levobunolol hydrochloride ophthalmic solution, USP) is supplied sterile in white low density polyethylene ophthalmic dispenser bottles and tips.
BETAGAN® 0.25% strength units include a light blue high intensity polystyrene cap.
BETAGAN® 0.5% strength units include a yellow high intensity polystyrene cap.
BETAGAN 0.25%:
  5 mL in 10 mL bottle—NDC 0023-4526-05
  10 mL in 15 mL bottle—NDC 0023-4526-10
BETAGAN 0.5%:
  2 mL in 5 mL bottle—NDC 0023-4385-02
  5 mL in 10 mL bottle—NDC 0023-4385-05
  10 mL in 15 mL bottle—NDC 0023-4385-10
  15 mL in 15 mL bottle—NDC 0023-4385-15
NOTE: Protect from light. Store at 15°–25°C (59°–77°F).
℞ only

BLEPH®-10 ℞
(sulfacetamide sodium
ophthalmic solution, USP) 10%

Description: BLEPH®-10 (sulfacetamide sodium ophthalmic solution USP) 10% is a sterile topical antibacterial agent for ophthalmic use.
Chemical Name: N-Sulfanilylacetamide monosodium salt monohydrate.
Contains:
BLEPH®-10 solution: Active: Sulfacetamide sodium 10% (100 mg/mL). **Preservative:** benzalkonium chloride (0.005%). **Inactives:** polyvinyl alcohol 1.4%; sodium thiosulfate; sodium phosphate dibasic; sodium phosphate monobasic; edetate disodium; polysorbate 80; hydrochloric acid and/or sodium hydroxide to adjust the pH; and purified water.
Clinical Pharmacology:
Microbiology: The sulfonamides are bacteriostatic agents and the spectrum of activity is similar for all. Sulfonamides inhibit bacterial synthesis of dihydrofolic acid by preventing the condensation of the pteridine with aminobenzoic acid through competitive inhibition of the enzyme dihydropteroate synthetase. Resistant strains have altered dihydropteroate synthetase with reduced affinity for sulfonamides or produce increased quantities of aminobenzoic acid.
Topically applied sulfonamides are considered active against susceptible strains of the following common bacterial eye pathogens: *Escherichia coli, Staphylococcus aureus, Streptococcus pneumoniae, Streptococcus* (viridans group), *Haemophilus influenzae, Klebsiella* species, and *Enterobacter* species.
Topically applied sulfonamides do not provide adequate coverage against *Neisseria* species, *Serratia marcescens* and *Pseudomonas aeruginosa*. A significant percentage of staphylococcal isolates are completely resistant to sulfa drugs.
Indications and Usage: BLEPH®-10 solution is indicated for the treatment of conjunctivitis and other superficial ocular infections due to the following susceptible microorganisms. BLEPH®-10 solution is also indicated as an adjunctive in systemic sulfonamide therapy of trachoma:
Escherichia coli, Staphylococcus aureus, Streptococcus pneumoniae, Streptococcus (viridans group), *Haemophilus influenzae, Klebsiella* species, and *Enterobacter* species.
Topically applied sulfonamides do not provide adequate coverage against *Neisseria* species, *Serratia marcescens* and *Pseudomonas aeruginosa*. A significant percentage of staphylococcal isolates are completely resistant to sulfa drugs.
Contraindications: BLEPH®-10 solution is contraindicated in individuals who have a hypersensitivity to sulfonamides or to any ingredient of the preparations.
Warnings: FOR TOPICAL EYE USE ONLY—NOT FOR INJECTION.
FATALITIES HAVE OCCURRED, ALTHOUGH RARELY, DUE TO SEVERE REACTIONS TO SULFONAMIDES INCLUDING STEVENS-JOHNSON SYNDROME, TOXIC EPIDERMAL NECROLYSIS, FULMINANT HEPATIC NECROSIS, AGRANULOCYTOSIS, APLASTIC ANEMIA AND OTHER BLOOD DYSCRASIAS. Sensitizations may recur when a sulfonamide is readministered, irrespective of the route of administration. Sen-

Continued on next page

Bleph-10—Cont.

sitivity reactions have been reported in individuals with no prior history of sulfonamide hypersensitivity. At the first sign of hypersensitivity, skin rash or other serious reaction, discontinue use of these preparations.

Precautions:
General: Prolonged use of topical antibacterial agents may give rise to overgrowth of nonsusceptible organisms including fungi. Bacterial resistance to sulfonamides may also develop.
The effectiveness of sulfonamides may be reduced by the para-aminobenzoic acid present in purulent exudates.
Sensitization may recur when a sulfonamide is readministered irrespective of the route of administration, and cross-sensitivity between different sulfonamides may occur.
At the first sign of hypersensitivity, increase in purulent discharge, or aggravation of inflammation or pain, the patient should discontinue use of the medication and consult a physician (see **Warnings**).
Information for patients: To avoid contamination, do not touch tip of container to the eye, eyelid or any surface.
Drug interactions: Sulfacetamide preparations are incompatible with silver preparations.
Carcinogenesis, Mutagenesis, Impairment of Fertility: No studies have been conducted in animals or in humans to evaluate the possibility of these effects with ocularly administered sulfacetamide. Rats appear to be especially susceptible to the goitrogenic effects of sulfonamides, and long-term oral administration of sulfonamides has resulted in thyroid malignancies in these animals.
Pregnancy: Pregnancy Category C. Animal reproduction studies have not been conducted with sulfonamide ophthalmic preparations. Kernicterus may occur in the newborn as a result of treatment of a pregnant woman at term with orally administered sulfonamides. There are no adequate and well controlled studies of sulfonamide ophthalmic preparations in pregnant women and it is not known whether topically applied sulfonamides can cause fetal harm when administered to a pregnant woman. This product should be used in pregnancy only if the potential benefit justifies the potential risk to the fetus.
Nursing mothers: Systematically administered sulfonamides are capable of producing kernicterus in infants of lactating women. Because of the potential for the development of kernicterus in neonates, a decision should be made whether to discontinue nursing or discontinue the drug taking into account the importance of the drug to the mother.
Pediatric Use: Safety and effectiveness in children below the age of two months have not been established.
Adverse Reactions: Bacterial and fungal corneal ulcers have developed during treatment with sulfonamide ophthalmic preparations.
The most frequently reported reactions are local irritation, stinging and burning. Less commonly reported reactions include non-specific conjunctivitis, conjunctival hyperemia, secondary infections and allergic reactions.
Fatalities have occurred, although rarely, due to severe reactions to sulfonamides including Stevens-Johnson syndrome, toxic epidermal necrolysis, fulminant hepatic necrosis, agranulocytosis, aplastic anemia, and other blood dyscrasias (see **Warnings**).
Dosage and Administration: For conjunctivitis and other superficial ocular infections:
BLEPH®-10 solution:
Instill one or two drops into the conjunctival sac(s) of the affected eye(s) every two to three hours initially. Dosages may be tapered by increasing the time interval between doses as the condition responds. The usual duration of treatment is seven to ten days.
For trachoma:
Instill two drops into the conjunctival sac(s) of the affected eye(s) every two hours. Topical administration must be accompanied by systemic administration.
How Supplied: BLEPH®-10 (sulfacetamide sodium ophthalmic solution, USP) 10% is supplied sterile in plastic bottles in the following sizes:
  5 mL—NDC 11980-011-05
  15 mL—NDC 11980-011-15
Note: Store between 8°–25°C (46°–77°F). Protect from light. Sulfonamide solutions, on long standing, will darken in color and should be discarded.
℞ only
®Marks owned by Allergan, Inc.

BLEPHAMIDE® ℞
(sulfacetamide sodium—prednisolone acetate ophthalmic suspension)
sterile

Description: BLEPHAMIDE® ophthalmic suspension is a topical anti-inflammatory/anti-infective combination product for ophthalmic use.
Chemical Names: Sulfacetamide sodium: N-sulfanilylacetamide monosodium salt monohydrate.
Prednisolone acetate: 11β, 17, 21-trihydroxypregna-1, 4-diene-3, 20-dione 21-acetate.
Contains: Actives: sulfacetamide sodium 10%, prednisolone acetate (microfine suspension) 0.2%. Preservative: benzalkonium chloride (0.004%). Inactives: polyvinyl alcohol 1.4%; polysorbate 80; edetate disodium; sodium phosphate, dibasic; potassium phosphate, monobasic; sodium thiosulfate; hydrochloric acid and/or sodium hydroxide to adjust the pH; and purified water.
Clinical Pharmacology: Corticosteroids suppress the inflammatory response to a variety of agents and they probably delay or slow healing. Since corticosteroids may inhibit the body's defense mechanism against infection, a concomitant antibacterial drug may be used when this inhibition is considered to be clinically significant in a particular case.
When a decision to administer both a corticosteroid and an antibacterial is made, the administration of such drugs in combination has the advantage of greater patient compliance and convenience, with the added assurance that the appropriate dosage of both drugs is administered. When both types of drugs are in the same formulation, compatibility of ingredients is assured and the correct volume of drug is delivered and retained. The relative potency of corticosteroids depends on the molecular structure, concentration and release from the vehicle.
Microbiology: Sulfacetamide sodium exerts a bacteriostatic effect against susceptible bacteria by restricting the synthesis of folic acid required for growth through competition with p-aminobenzoic acid.
Some strains of these bacteria may be resistant to sulfacetamide or resistant strains may emerge *in vivo*.
The anti-infective component in these products is included to provide action against specific organisms susceptible to it. Sulfacetamide sodium is active *in vitro* against susceptible strains of the following microorganisms: *Escherichia coli, Staphylococcus aureus, Streptococcus pneumoniae, Streptococcus* (*viridans* group), *Haemophilus influenzae, Klebsiella* species, and *Enterobacter* species. This product does not provide adequate coverage against: *Neisseria* species, *Pseudomonas* species, and *Serratia marcescens* (see **Indications and Usage**).
Indications and Usage: A steroid/anti-infective combination is indicated for steroid-responsive inflammatory ocular conditions for which a corticosteroid is indicated and where superficial bacterial ocular infection or a risk of bacterial ocular infection exists.
Ocular corticosteroids are indicated in inflammatory conditions of the palpebral and bulbar conjunctiva, cornea, and anterior segment of the globe where the inherent risk of corticosteroid use in certain infective conjunctivitides is accepted to obtain diminution in edema and inflammation. They are also indicated in chronic anterior uveitis and corneal injury from chemical, radiation, or thermal burns or penetration of foreign bodies.
The use of a combination drug with an anti-infective component is indicated where the risk of superficial ocular infection is high or where there is an expectation that potentially dangerous numbers of bacteria will be present in the eye.
The particular anti-bacterial drug in this product is active against the following common bacterial eye pathogens: *Escherichia coli, Staphylococcus aureus, Streptococcus pneumoniae, Streptococcus* (*viridans* group), *Haemophilus influenzae, Klebsiella* species, and *Enterobacter* species. This product does not provide adequate coverage against *Neisseria* species, *Pseudomonas* species, and *Serratia marcescens*.
A significant percentage of staphylococcal isolates are completely resistant to sulfa drugs.
Contraindications: BLEPHAMIDE® ophthalmic suspension is contraindicated in most viral diseases of the cornea and conjunctiva including epithelial herpes simplex keratitis (dendritic keratitis), vaccinia, and varicella, and also in mycobacterial infection of the eye and fungal diseases of ocular structures.
This product is also contraindicated in individuals with known or suspected hypersensitivity to any of the ingredients of this preparation, to other sulfonamides and to other corticosteroids. See **Warnings**. (Hypersensitivity to the antimicrobial component occurs at a higher rate than for other components.)
Warnings:
NOT FOR INJECTION INTO THE EYE.
Prolonged use of corticosteroids may result in ocular hypertension/glaucoma with damage to the optic nerve, defects in visual acuity and fields of vision, and in posterior subcapsular cataract formation.
Acute anterior uveitis may occur in susceptible individuals, primarily Blacks.
Prolonged use of BLEPHAMIDE® ophthalmic suspension may suppress the host response and thus increase the hazard of secondary ocular infections. In those diseases causing thinning of the cornea or sclera, perforation has been known to occur with the use of topical corticosteroids. In acute purulent conditions of the eye, corticosteroids may mask infection or enhance existing infection.
If the product is used for 10 days or longer, intraocular pressure should be routinely monitored even though it may be difficult in children and uncooperative patients. Corticosteroids should be used with caution in the presence of glaucoma. Intraocular pressure should be checked frequently.
A significant percentage of staphylococcal isolates are completely resistant to sulfonamides. The use of steroids after cataract surgery may delay healing and increase the incidence of filtering blebs.
The use of ocular corticosteroids may prolong the course and may exacerbate the severity of many viral infections of the eye (including her-

pes simplex). Employment of corticosteroid medication in the treatment of herpes simplex requires great caution.

Topical steroids are not effective in mustard gas keratitis and Sjögren's keratoconjunctivitis.

Fatalities have occurred, although rarely, due to severe reactions to sulfonamides including Stevens-Johnson syndrome, toxic epidermal necrolysis, fulminant hepatic necrosis, agranulocytosis, aplastic anemia and other blood dyscrasias. Sensitization may recur when a sulfonamide is readministered, irrespective of the route of administration.

If signs of hypersensitivity or other serious reactions occur, discontinue use of this preparation. Cross-sensitivity among corticosteroids has been demonstrated (see **Adverse Reactions**).

Precautions:
General: The initial prescription and renewal of the medication order beyond 20 milliliters of the suspension should be made by a physician only after examination of the patient with the aid of magnification, such as slit lamp biomicroscopy and, where appropriate, fluorescein staining. If signs and symptoms fail to improve after two days, the patient should be re-evaluated.

The possibility of fungal infections of the cornea should be considered after prolonged corticosteroid dosing. Use with caution in patients with severe dry eye. Fungal cultures should be taken when appropriate.

The p-amino benzoic acid present in purulent exudates competes with sulfonamides and can reduce their effectiveness.

Information for Patients: If inflammation or pain persists longer than 48 hours or becomes aggravated, the patient should be advised to discontinue use of the medication and consult a physician (see **Warnings**).

Contact lenses should not be worn during the use of this product.

This product is sterile when packaged. To prevent contamination, care should be taken to avoid touching the applicator tip to eyelids or to any other surface. The use of this bottle by more than one person may spread infection. Keep bottle tightly closed when not in use. Protect from light. Sulfonamide solutions darken on prolonged standing and exposure to heat and light. Do not use if solution has darkened. Yellowing does not affect activity. Keep out of the reach of children.

Laboratory Tests: Eyelid cultures and tests to determine the susceptibility of organisms to sulfacetamide may be indicated if signs and symptoms persist or recur in spite of the recommended course of treatment with BLEPHAMIDE® ophthalmic suspension.

Drug Interactions: BLEPHAMIDE® ophthalmic suspension is incompatible with silver preparations. Local anesthetics related to p-amino benzoic acid may antagonize the action of the sulfonamides.

Carcinogenesis, Mutagenesis, Impairment of Fertility: Prednisolone has been reported to be noncarcinogenic. Long-term animal studies for carcinogenic potential have not been performed with sulfacetamide.

One author detected chromosomal nondisjunction in the yeast *Saccharomyces cerevisiae* following application of sulfacetamide sodium. The significance of this finding to topical ophthalmic use of sulfacetamide sodium in the human is unknown.

Mutagenic studies with prednisolone have been negative. Studies on reproduction and fertility have not been performed with sulfacetamide. A long-term chronic toxicity study in dogs showed that high oral doses of prednisolone prevented estrus. A decrease in fertility was seen in male and female rats that were mated following oral dosing with another glucocorticosteroid.

Pregnancy: Teratogenic Effects: Pregnancy Category C. Animal reproduction studies have not been conducted with sulfacetamide sodium. Prednisolone has been shown to be teratogenic in rabbits, hamsters, and mice. In mice, prednisolone has been shown to be teratogenic when given in doses 1 to 10 times the human ocular dose. Dexamethasone, hydrocortisone and prednisolone were ocularly applied to both eyes of pregnant mice five times per day on days 10 through 13 of gestation. A significant increase in the incidence of cleft palate was observed in the fetuses of the treated mice. There are no adequate well-controlled studies in pregnant women dosed with corticosteroids.

Kernicterus may be precipitated in infants by sulfonamides being given systemically during the third trimester of pregnancy. It is not known whether sulfacetamide sodium can cause fetal harm when administered to a pregnant woman or whether it can affect reproductive capacity.

BLEPHAMIDE® ophthalmic suspension should be used during pregnancy only if the potential benefit justifies the potential risk to the fetus.

Nursing Mothers: It is not known whether topical administration of corticosteroids could result in sufficient systemic absorption to produce detectable quantities in human milk. Systemically administered corticosteroids appear in human milk and could suppress growth, interfere with endogenous corticosteroid production, or cause other untoward effects. Systemically administered sulfonamides are capable of producing kernicterus in infants of lactating women. Because of the potential for serious adverse reactions in nursing infants from sulfacetamide sodium and prednisolone acetate ophthalmic suspensions, a decision should be made whether to discontinue nursing or to discontinue the medication.

Pediatric Use: Safety and effectiveness in pediatric patients below the age of six have not been established.

Adverse Reactions: Adverse reactions have occurred with corticosteroid/antibacterial combination drugs which can be attributed to the corticosteroid component, the antibacterial component, or the combination. Exact incidence figures are not available since no denominator of treated patients is available.

Reactions occurring most often from the presence of the antibacterial ingredient are allergic sensitizations. Fatalities have occurred, although rarely, due to severe reactions to sulfonamides including Stevens-Johnson syndrome, toxic epidermal necrolysis, fulminant hepatic necrosis, agranulocytosis, aplastic anemia and other blood dyscrasias (See **Warnings**).

Sulfacetamide sodium may cause local irritation.

The reactions due to the corticosteroid component in decreasing order of frequency are: elevation of intraocular pressure (IOP) with possible development of glaucoma and infrequent optic nerve damage, posterior subcapsular cataract formation, and delayed wound healing.

Although systemic effects are extremely uncommon, there have been rare occurrences of systemic hypercorticoidism after use of topical corticosteroids.

Corticosteroid-containing preparations can also cause acute anterior uveitis or perforation of the globe. Mydriasis, loss of accommodation and ptosis have occasionally been reported following local use of corticosteroids.

Secondary Infection: The development of secondary infection has occurred after use of combinations containing corticosteroids and antibacterials. Fungal and viral infections of the cornea are particularly prone to develop coincidentally with long-term applications of corticosteroid. The possibility of fungal invasion must be considered in any persistent corneal ulceration where corticosteroid treatment has been used.

Secondary bacterial ocular infection following suppression of host responses also occurs.

Dosage and Administration: SHAKE WELL BEFORE USING. Two drops should be instilled into the conjunctival sac every four hours during the day and at bedtime.

Not more than 20 milliliters should be prescribed initially, and the prescription should not be refilled without further evaluation as outlined in **Precautions** above.

BLEPHAMIDE® dosage may be reduced, but care should be taken not to discontinue therapy prematurely. In chronic conditions, withdrawal of treatment should be carried out by gradually decreasing the frequency of application.

If signs and symptoms fail to improve after two days, the patient should be re-evaluated (see **Precautions**).

How Supplied: BLEPHAMIDE® ophthalmic suspension is supplied in plastic dropper bottles in the following sizes:

     5 mL—NDC 11980-022-05
    10 mL—NDC 11980-022-10

Note: Protect from freezing. **Shake well before using.**

Storage: Store BLEPHAMIDE® at 8°–24°C (46°–75°F) in an upright position.

PROTECT FROM LIGHT

Sulfonamide solutions darken on prolonged standing and exposure to heat and light. Do not use if solution has darkened.

Yellowing does not affect activity.

KEEP OUT OF REACH OF CHILDREN

Rx only.

®Marks owned by Allergan, Inc.

BLEPHAMIDE® ℞
(sulfacetamide sodium and prednisolone acetate ophthalmic ointment, USP)
10%/0.2% sterile

Description: BLEPHAMIDE® (sulfacetamide sodium and prednisolone acetate ophthalmic ointment, USP) is a sterile topical ophthalmic ointment combining an antibacterial and a corticosteroid.

Chemical Names: Sulfacetamide sodium: N-sulfanilylacetamide monosodium salt monohydrate.

Prednisolone acetate: 11β, 17, 21-trihydroxy-pregna-1,4-diene-3, 20-dione, 21-acetate.

Contains: Actives: sulfacetamide sodium 10% and prednisolone acetate 0.2%. Preservative: phenylmercuric acetate (0.0008%). Inactives: mineral oil; white petrolatum; and petrolatum (and) lanolin alcohol.

Clinical Pharmacology: Corticosteroids suppress the inflammatory response to a variety of agents and they probably delay or slow healing. Since corticosteroids may inhibit the body's defense mechanism against infection, a concomitant antibacterial drug may be used when this inhibition is considered to be clinically significant in a particular case.

When a decision to administer both a corticosteroid and an antibacterial is made, the administration of such drugs in combination has the advantage of greater patient compliance and convenience, with the added assurance that the appropriate dosage of both drugs is administered, plus assured compatibility of ingredients when both types of drugs are in the same formulation and, particularly, that the correct volume of drug is delivered and retained.

Continued on next page

Blephamide Ointment—Cont.

The relative potency of corticosteroids depends on the molecular structure, concentration and release from the vehicle.

Microbiology: Sulfacetamide exerts a bacteriostatic effect against susceptible bacteria by restricting the synthesis of folic acid required for growth through competition with p-amino benzoic acid.

Some strains of these bacteria may be resistant to sulfacetamide or resistant strains may emerge *in vivo*.

The anti-infective component in BLEPHAMIDE® ointment is included to provide action against specific organisms susceptible to it. Sulfacetamide sodium is active *in vitro* against susceptible strains of the following microorganisms: *Escherichia coli, Staphylococcus aureus, Streptococcus pneumoniae, Streptococcus* (*viridans* group), *Haemophilus influenzae, Klebsiella* species, and *Enterobacter* species. This product does not provide adequate coverage against: *Neisseria* species, *Pseudomonas* species, and *Serratia marcescens* (see **Indications and Usage**).

Indications and Usage: BLEPHAMIDE® ophthalmic ointment is indicated for steroid-responsive inflammatory ocular conditions for which a corticosteroid is indicated and where superficial bacterial ocular infection or a risk of bacterial ocular infection exists.

Ocular corticosteroids are indicated in inflammatory conditions of the palpebral and bulbar conjunctiva, cornea, and anterior segment of the globe where the inherent risk of corticosteroid use in certain infective conjunctivitides is accepted to obtain diminution in edema and inflammation. They are also indicated in chronic anterior uveitis and corneal injury from chemical, radiation or thermal burns or penetration of foreign bodies.

The use of a combination drug with an anti-infective component is indicated where the risk of superficial ocular infection is high or where there is an expectation that potentially dangerous numbers of bacteria will be present in the eye.

The particular antibacterial drug in this product is active against the following common bacterial eye pathogens: *Escherichia coli, Staphylococcus aureus, Streptococcus pneumoniae, Streptococcus* (*viridans* group), *Haemophilus influenzae, Klebsiella* species, and *Enterobacter* species.

The product does not provide adequate coverage against: *Neisseria* species, *Pseudomonas* species, and *Serratia marcescens*.

A significant percentage of staphylococcal isolates are completely resistant to sulfa drugs.

Contraindications: BLEPHAMIDE® ophthalmic ointment is contraindicated in most viral diseases of the cornea and conjunctiva including epithelial herpes simplex keratitis (dendritic keratitis), vaccinia, and varicella, and also in mycobacterial infection of the eye and fungal diseases of ocular structures.
This product is also contraindicated in individuals with known or suspected hypersensitivity to any of the ingredients of this preparation, to other sulfonamides and to other corticosteroids. See **Warnings**. (Hypersensitivity to the antimicrobial component occurs at a higher rate than for other components).

Warnings:
NOT FOR INJECTION INTO THE EYE.
Prolonged use of corticosteroids may result in ocular hypertension/glaucoma with damage to the optic nerve, defects in visual acuity and fields of vision, and in posterior subcapsular cataract formation.
Acute anterior uveitis may occur in susceptible individuals, primarily Blacks.

Prolonged use of BLEPHAMIDE® ophthalmic ointment may suppress the host response and thus increase the hazard of secondary ocular infections. In those diseases causing thinning of the cornea or sclera, perforation has been known to occur with the use of topical corticosteroids. In acute purulent conditions of the eye, corticosteroids may mask infection or enhance existing infection.

If the product is used for 10 days or longer, intraocular pressure should be routinely monitored even though it may be difficult in children and uncooperative patients. Corticosteroids should be used with caution in the presence of glaucoma. Intraocular pressure should be checked frequently.

A significant percentage of staphylococcal isolates are completely resistant to sulfonamides. The use of steroids after cataract surgery may delay healing and increase the incidence of filtering blebs.

The use of ocular corticosteroids may prolong the course and may exacerbate the severity of many viral infections of the eye (including herpes simplex). Employment of corticosteroid medication in the treatment of herpes simplex requires great caution.

Topical steroids are not effective in mustard gas keratitis and Sjogren's keratoconjunctivitis.

Fatalities have occurred, although rarely, due to severe reactions to sulfonamides including Stevens-Johnson syndrome, toxic epidermal necrolysis, fulminant hepatic necrosis, agranulocytosis, aplastic anemia and other blood dyscrasias. Sensitization may recur when a sulfonamide is readministered, irrespective of the route of administration.

If signs of hypersensitivity or other serious reactions occur, discontinue use of this preparation. Cross-sensitivity among corticosteroids has been demonstrated (see **Adverse Reactions**).

Precautions:
General: The initial prescription and renewal of the medication order beyond 8 g of ointment should be made by a physician only after examination of the patient with the aid of magnification, such as slit lamp biomicroscopy and, where appropriate, fluorescein staining. If signs and symptoms fail to improve after two days, the patient should be re-evaluated. The possibility of fungal infections of the cornea should be considered after prolonged corticosteroid dosing. Use with caution in patients with severe dry eye. Fungal cultures should be taken when appropriate.

The p-amino benzoic acid present in purulent exudates competes with sulfonamides and can reduce their effectiveness. Ophthalmic ointments may retard corneal healing.

Information for Patients: If inflammation or pain persists longer than 48 hours or becomes aggravated, the patient should be advised to discontinue use of the medication and consult a physician (see **Warnings**).

This product is sterile when packaged. To prevent contamination, care should be taken to avoid touching the tube tip to eyelids or to any other surface. The use of this tube by more than one person may spread infection. Keep tube tightly closed when not in use. Keep out of the reach of children.

Laboratory Tests: Eyelid cultures and tests to determine the susceptibility of organisms to sulfacetamide may be indicated if signs and symptoms persist or recur in spite of the recommended course of treatment with BLEPHAMIDE® ophthalmic ointment.

Drug Interactions: BLEPHAMIDE® ophthalmic ointment is incompatible with silver preparations. Local anesthetics related to p-amino benzoic acid may antagonize the action of the sulfonamides.

Carcinogenesis, Mutagenesis, Impairment of Fertility: Prednisolone has been reported to be noncarcinogenic. Long-term animal studies for carcinogenic potential have not been performed with sulfacetamide.

One author detected chromosomal nondisjunction in the yeast *Saccharomyces cerevisiae* following application of sulfacetamide sodium. The significance of this finding to topical ophthalmic use of sulfacetamide sodium in the human is unknown.

Mutagenic studies with prednisolone have been negative. Studies on reproduction and fertility have not been performed with sulfacetamide. A long-term chronic toxicity study in dogs showed that high oral doses of prednisolone prevented estrus. A decrease in fertility was seen in male and female rats that were mated following oral dosing with another glucocorticosteroid.

Pregnancy: Teratogenic Effects: Pregnancy Category C. Animal reproduction studies have not been conducted with sulfacetamide sodium. Prednisolone has been shown to be teratogenic in rabbits, hamsters, and mice. In mice, prednisolone has been shown to be teratogenic when given in doses 1 to 10 times the human ocular dose. Dexamethasone, hydrocortisone and prednisolone were ocularly applied to both eyes of pregnant mice five times per day on days 10 through 13 of gestation. A significant increase in the incidence of cleft palate was observed in the fetuses of the treated mice. There are no adequate well-controlled studies in pregnant women dosed with corticosteroids.

Kernicterus may be precipitated in infants by sulfonamides being given systemically during the third trimester of pregnancy. It is not known whether sulfacetamide sodium can cause fetal harm when administered to a pregnant woman or whether it can affect reproductive capacity.

BLEPHAMIDE® ophthalmic ointment should be used during pregnancy only if the potential benefit justifies the potential risk to the fetus.

Nursing Mothers: It is not known whether topical administration of corticosteroids could result in sufficient systemic absorption to produce detectable quantities in human milk. Systemically administered corticosteroids appear in human milk and could suppress growth, interfere with endogenous corticosteroid production, or cause other untoward effects. Systemically administered sulfonamides are capable of producing kernicterus in infants of lactating women. Because of the potential for serious adverse reactions in nursing infants from sulfacetamide sodium and prednisolone acetate ophthalmic ointments, a decision should be made whether to discontinue nursing or to discontinue the medication.

Pediatric Use: Safety and effectiveness in children below the age of six have not been established.

Adverse Reactions: Adverse reactions have occurred with corticosteroid/antibacterial combination drugs which can be attributed to the corticosteroid component, the antibacterial component, or the combination. Exact incidence figures are not available since no denominator of treated patients is available.

Reactions occurring most often from the presence of the antibacterial ingredient are allergic sensitizations. Fatalities have occurred, although rarely, due to severe reactions to sulfonamides including Stevens-Johnson syndrome, toxic epidermal necrolysis, fulminant hepatic necrosis, agranulocytosis, aplastic anemia, and other blood dyscrasias (See **Warnings**).

Sulfacetamide sodium may cause local irritation.

The reactions due to the corticosteroid component in decreasing order of frequency are: elevation of intraocular pressure (IOP) with possible development of glaucoma and infrequent optic nerve damage, posterior subcapsular cataract formation, and delayed wound healing. Although systemic effects are extremely uncommon, there have been rare occurrences of systemic hypercorticoidism after use of topical steroids.

Corticosteroid-containing preparations can also cause acute anterior uveitis or perforation of the globe. Mydriasis, loss of accommodation and ptosis have occasionally been reported following local use of corticosteroids.

Secondary Infection: The development of secondary infection has occurred after use of combinations containing corticosteroids and antibacterials. Fungal and viral infections of the cornea are particularly prone to develop coincidentally with long-term applications of corticosteroid. The possibility of fungal invasion must be considered in any persistent corneal ulceration where corticosteroid treatment has been used.

Secondary bacterial ocular infection following suppression of host responses also occurs.

Dosage and Administration: A small amount, approximately $1/2$ inch ribbon of ointment, should be applied in the conjunctival sac three or four times daily and once or twice at night.

Not more than 8 g should be prescribed initially.

The dosing of BLEPHAMIDE® ophthalmic ointment may be reduced, but care should be taken not to discontinue therapy prematurely. In chronic conditions, withdrawal of treatment should be carried out by gradually decreasing the frequency of application.

If signs and symptoms fail to improve after two days, the patient should be re-evaluated (see **Precautions**).

How Supplied: BLEPHAMIDE® (sulfacetamide sodium and prednisolone acetate ophthalmic ointment, USP) 10%/0.2% is supplied sterile in ointment tubes of the following size:
3.5 g—NDC 0023-0313-04.

Note: Store between 15–25°C (59–77°F).
® Marks owned by Allergan, Inc.

Rx only

© 2000 Allergan, Inc. Irvine, California 92612, U.S.A.

Shown in Product Identification Guide, page 103

ELESTAT™   ℞
[ĕl-ĕ-stăt]
(epinastine HCl ophthalmic solution) 0.05%
Sterile

Description: ELESTAT™ (epinastine HCl ophthalmic solution) 0.05% is a clear, colorless, sterile isotonic solution containing epinastine HCl, an antihistamine and an inhibitor of histamine release from the mast cell for topical administration to the eyes.

Epinastine HCl is represented by the following structural formula:

$C_{16}H_{15}N_3$ • HCl Mol. Wt. 285.78

Chemical Name: 3-Amino-9, 13b-dihydro-1H-dibenz[c,f]imidazo[1,5-a]azepine hydrochloride

Each mL contains: Active: Epinastine HCl 0.05% (0.5mg/mL) equivalent to epinastine 0.044% (0.44mg/mL); **Preservative:** Benzalkonium chloride 0.01%; **Inactives:** Edetate disodium; purified water; sodium chloride; sodium phosphate, monobasic; and sodium hydroxide and/or hydrochloric acid (to adjust the pH).

ELESTAT™ has a pH of approximately 7 and an osmolality range of 250 to 310 mOsm/kg.

Clinical Pharmacology: Epinastine is a topically active, direct H_1-receptor antagonist and an inhibitor of the release of histamine from the mast cell. Epinastine is selective for the histamine H_1-receptor and has affinity for the histamine H_2-receptor. Epinastine also possesses affinity for the α_1-, α_2-, and 5-HT$_2$-receptors. Epinastine does not penetrate the blood/brain barrier and, therefore, is not expected to induce side effects of the central nervous system.

Fourteen subjects, with allergic conjunctivitis, received one drop of ELESTAT™ ophthalmic solution in each eye twice daily for seven days. On day seven average maximum epinastine plasma concentrations of 0.04 ± 0.014 ng/ml were reached after about two hours indicating low systemic exposure. While these concentrations represented an increase over those seen following a single dose, the day 1 and day 7 Area Under the Curve (AUC) values were unchanged indicating that there is no increase in systemic absorption with multiple dosing. Epinastine is 64% bound to plasma proteins. The total systemic clearance is approximately 56 L/hr and the terminal plasma elimination half-life is about 12 hours. Epinastine is mainly excreted unchanged. About 55% of an intravenous dose is recovered unchanged in the urine with about 30% in feces. Less than 10% is metabolized. The renal elimination is mainly via active tubular secretion.

Clinical studies: Epinastine HCl 0.05% has been shown to be significantly superior to vehicle for improving ocular itching in patients with allergic conjunctivitis in clinical studies using two different models: (1) conjunctival antigen challenge (CAC) where patients were dosed and then received antigen instilled into the inferior conjunctival fornix; and (2) environmental field studies where patients were dosed and evaluated during allergy season in their natural habitat. Results demonstrated a rapid onset of action for epinastine HCl 0.05% within 3 to 5 minutes after conjunctival antigen challenge. Duration of effect was shown to be 8 hours, making a twice daily regimen suitable. This dosing regimen was shown to be safe and effective for up to 8 weeks, without evidence of tachyphylaxis.

Indications and Usage: ELESTAT™ ophthalmic solution is indicated for the prevention of itching associated with allergic conjunctivitis.

Contraindications: ELESTAT™ ophthalmic solution is contraindicated in those patients who have shown hypersensitivity to epinastine or to any of the other ingredients.

Warnings: ELESTAT™ is for topical ophthalmic use only and not for injection or oral use.

Precautions:
Information for Patients: Patients should be advised not to wear a contact lens if their eye is red. ELESTAT™ ophthalmic solution should not be used to treat contact lens related irritation. The preservative in ELESTAT™, benzalkonium chloride, may be absorbed by soft contact lenses. Contact lenses should be removed prior to instillation of ELESTAT™ ophthalmic solution and may be reinserted after 10 minutes following its administration.
Patients should be instructed to avoid allowing the tip of the dispensing container to contact the eye, surrounding structures, fingers, or any other surface in order to avoid contamination of the solution by common bacteria known to cause ocular infections. Serious damage to the eye and subsequent loss of vision may result from using contaminated solutions.
Bottle should be kept tightly closed when not in use.

Carcinogenesis, Mutagenesis, Impairment of Fertility: In 18-month or 2-year dietary carcinogenicity studies in mice or rats, respectively, epinastine was not carcinogenic at doses up to 40 mg/kg [approximately 30,000 times higher than the maximum recommended ocular human dose of 0.0014 mg/kg/day (MROHD) on a mg/kg basis, assuming 100% absorption in humans and animals].

Epinastine in newly synthesized batches was negative for mutagenicity in the Ames/*Salmonella* assay and *in vitro* chromosome aberration assay using human lymphocytes. Positive results were seen with early batches of epinastine in two *in vitro* chromosomal aberration studies conducted in 1980s with human peripheral lymphocytes and with V79 cells, respectively. Epinastine was negative in the *in vivo* clastogenicity studies, including the mouse micronucleus assay and chromosome aberration assay in Chinese hamsters. Epinastine was also negative in the cell transformation assay using Syrian hamster embryo cells, V79/HGPRT mammalian cell point mutation assay, and *in vivo/in vitro* unscheduled DNA synthesis assay using rat primary hepatocytes.

Epinastine had no effect on fertility of male rats. Decreased fertility in female rats was observed at an oral dose up to approximately 90,000 times the MROHD.

Pregnancy: Teratogenic Effects: Pregnancy Category C In an embryofetal developmental study in pregnant rats, maternal toxicity with no embryofetal effects was observed at an oral dose that was approximately 150,000 times the MROHD. Total resorptions and abortion were observed in an embryofetal study in pregnant rabbits at an oral dose that was approximately 55,000 times the MROHD. In both studies, no drug-induced teratogenic effects were noted.

Epinastine reduced pup body weight gain following an oral dose to pregnant rats that was approximately 90,000 times the MROHD.

There are, however, no adequate and well-controlled studies in pregnant women. Because animal reproduction studies are not always predictive of human response, ELESTAT™ ophthalmic solution should be used during pregnancy only if the potential benefit justifies the potential risk to the fetus.

Nursing Mothers: A study in lactating rats revealed excretion of epinastine in the breast milk. It is not known whether this drug is excreted in human milk. Because many drugs are excreted in human milk, caution should be exercised when ELESTAT™ ophthalmic solution is administered to a nursing woman.

Pediatric Use: Safety and effectiveness in pediatric patients below the age of 3 years have not been established.

Geriatric Use: No overall differences in safety or effectiveness have been observed between elderly and younger patients.

Adverse Reactions: The most frequently reported ocular adverse events occurring in approximately 1-10% of patients were burning sensation in the eye, folliculosis, hyperemia, and pruritus.

The most frequently reported non-ocular adverse events were infection (cold symptoms and upper respiratory infections) seen in approximately 10% of patients, and headache, rhinitis, sinusitis, increased cough, and pharyngitis seen in approximately 1-3% of patients. Some of these events were similar to the underlying disease being studied.

Dosage and Administration: The recommended dosage is one drop in each eye twice a day.

Treatment should be continued throughout the period of exposure (i.e., until the pollen season is over or until exposure to the offending allergen is terminated), even when symptoms are absent.

Continued on next page

Elestat—Cont.

How Supplied: ELESTAT™ (epinastine HCl ophthalmic solution) 0.05% is supplied sterile in opaque white LDPE plastic bottles with dropper tips and white high impact polystyrene (HIPS) caps as follows:
5 mL in 8 mL bottle   NDC 0023-9201-05
Storage: Store at 15-25°C (59-77°F). Keep bottle tightly closed and out of the reach of children.
Rx Only   October 2003
© 2003 Allergan, Inc.
Irvine, CA 92612 U.S.A.
® and ™ Marks owned by Allergan, Inc.
9343X
Licensed from Boehringer Ingelheim Int. GmbH   71634US10M
Inspire and the Inspire logo are registered trademarks of Inspire Pharmaceuticals Inc.

EPIFRIN® ℞
(epinephrine, USP)
sterile ophthalmic solution

Description: EPIFRIN® (epinephrine, USP) sterile ophthalmic solution is a topical sympathomimetic agent for ophthalmic use.
Chemical Name: 1,2-Benzenediol,4-[1-hydroxy-2-(methylamino)ethyl]-, (R)-.
Contains:
Active: epinephrine, USP 0.5%, 1%, or 2%
Preservative: benzalkonium chloride
Inactives: sodium metabisulfite; edetate disodium; hydrochloric acid; and purified water.
Clinical Pharmacology: Epinephrine is an adrenergic agonist that stimulates α- and β-adrenergic receptors. The capacity of EPIFRIN® (epinephrine, USP) to decrease the aqueous inflow in open-angle glaucoma has been well documented. Studies have also shown that prolonged topical epinephrine therapy offers significant improvement in the coefficient of aqueous outflow.
EPIFRIN® ophthalmic solution is effective alone in reducing intraocular pressure and is particularly useful in combination with miotics or beta-adrenergic blocking agents for the difficult-to-control patients. The addition of EPIFRIN® to the patient's regimen often provides better control of intraocular pressure than the original agent alone.
Indications and Usage: EPIFRIN® ophthalmic solution is indicated for the treatment of chronic simple glaucoma.
Contraindications: EPIFRIN® ophthalmic solution should not be used in patients who have had an attack of narrow-angle glaucoma, since dilation of the pupil may trigger an acute attack. Do not use if hypersensitive to any ingredient.
Warnings:
1. EPIFRIN® ophthalmic solution should be used with caution in patients with a narrow angle, since dilation of the pupil may trigger an acute attack of narrow-angle glaucoma.
2. Use with caution in patients with hypertensive cardiovascular disease or coronary artery disease.
3. Epinephrine has been reported to produce reversible macular edema in some aphakic patients and should be used with caution in these patients.

Contains sodium metabisulfite, a sulfite that may cause allergic-type reactions, including anaphylactic symptoms and life-threatening or less severe asthmatic episodes in certain susceptible people. The overall prevalence of sulfite sensitivity in the general population is unknown and probably low. Sulfite sensitivity is seen more frequently in asthmatic than in nonasthmatic people.

Precautions:
General: Epinephrine in any form is relatively uncomfortable upon instillation. However, discomfort lessens as the concentration of epinephrine decreases. EPIFRIN® is not for injection.
Carcinogenesis, mutagenesis and impairment of fertility: No studies have been conducted in animals or in humans to evaluate the potential of these effects.
Pregnancy Category C: Animal reproduction studies have not been conducted with epinephrine. It is also not known whether epinephrine can cause fetal harm when administered to a pregnant woman or if it can affect reproduction capacity. Epinephrine should be given to a pregnant woman only if clearly needed.
Pediatric Use: Safety and effectiveness in pediatric patients have not been established.
Adverse Reactions: Undesirable reactions to topical epinephrine include eye pain or ache, browache, headache, conjunctival hyperemia and allergic lid reactions.
Adrenochrome deposits in the conjunctiva and cornea after prolonged epinephrine therapy have been reported. Topical epinephrine has been reported to produce reversible macular edema in some aphakic patients.
Overdosage: Accidental ingestion will not cause problems because pharmacologically active concentrations of epinephrine cannot be achieved orally in man. Should accidental overdosage in the eye(s) occur, flush eye(s) with water or normal saline.
Dosage and Administration: The usual dosage is 1 drop in the affected eye(s) once or twice daily. However, the dosage should be adjusted to meet the needs of the individual patients. This is made easier with EPIFRIN® (epinephrine, USP) sterile ophthalmic solution available in three strengths.
How Supplied: EPIFRIN® is available in plastic dropper bottles in the following concentrations and sizes:
0.5%   15 mL—NDC 11980-119-15
1%   15 mL—NDC 11980-122-15
2%   15 mL—NDC 11980-058-15
Note: Protect from light and excessive heat. If the solution discolors or a precipitate forms, it should be discarded.
Rx Only
May 2002
®Registered marks of Allergan, Inc.
Allergan, Inc.
Irvine, CA 92612, U.S.A.

FML FORTE® ℞
(fluorometholone ophthalmic suspension, USP) 0.25%
sterile

Description: FML FORTE® sterile ophthalmic suspension is a topical anti-inflammatory product for ophthalmic use.
Chemical Name: Fluorometholone: 9-Fluoro-11β, 17-dihydroxy-6α-methylpregna-1,4-diene-3,20-dione.
Contains: Active: fluorometholone 0.25%. **Preservative:** benzalkonium chloride 0.005%. **Inactives:** edetate disodium; polysorbate 80; polyvinyl alcohol 1.4%; purified water; sodium chloride; sodium phosphate, dibasic; sodium phosphate, monobasic; and sodium hydroxide to adjust the pH. FML Forte® suspension is formulated with a pH from 6.2 to 7.5
Clinical Pharmacology: Corticosteroids inhibit the inflammatory response to a variety of inciting agents and probably delay or slow healing. They inhibit the edema, fibrin deposition, capillary dilation, leukocyte migration, capillary proliferation, fibroblast proliferation, deposition of collagen, and scar formation associated with inflammation.
There is no generally accepted explanation for the mechanism of action of ocular corticosteroids. However, corticosteroids are thought to act by the induction of phospholipase A_2 inhibitory proteins, collectively called lipocortins. It is postulated that these proteins control the biosynthesis of potent mediators of inflammation such as prostaglandins and leukotrienes by inhibiting the release of their common precursor, arachidonic acid. Arachidonic acid is released from membrane phospholipids by phospholipase A_2.
Corticosteroids are capable of producing a rise in intraocular pressure. In clinical studies of documented steroid-responders, fluorometholone demonstrated a significantly longer average time to produce a rise in intraocular pressure than dexamethasone phosphate; however, in a small percentage of individuals a significant rise in intraocular pressure occurred within one week. The ultimate magnitude of the rise was equivalent for both drugs.
Indications and Usage: FML FORTE® suspension is indicated for the treatment of corticosteroid-responsive inflammation of the palpebral and bulbar conjunctiva, cornea and anterior segment of the globe.
Contraindications: FML FORTE® suspension is contraindicated in most viral diseases of the cornea and conjunctiva, including epithelial herpes simplex keratitis (dendritic keratitis), vaccinia, and varicella, and also in mycobacterial infection of the eye and fungal diseases of ocular structures. FML FORTE® suspension is also contraindicated in individuals with known or suspected hypersensitivity to any of the ingredients of this preparation and to other corticosteroids.
Warnings: Prolonged use of corticosteroids may result in glaucoma, with damage to the optic nerve, defects in visual acuity and fields of vision, and in posterior subcapsular cataract formation. Prolonged use may also suppress the host immune response and thus increase the hazard of secondary ocular infections.
Various ocular diseases and long-term use of topical corticosteroids have been known to cause corneal and scleral thinning. Use of topical corticosteroids in the presence of thin corneal or scleral tissue may lead to perforation. Acute purulent infections of the eye may be masked or activity enhanced by the presence of corticosteroid medication.
If this product is used for 10 days or longer, intraocular pressure should be routinely monitored even though it may be difficult in children and uncooperative patients. Steroids should be used with caution in the presence of glaucoma. Intraocular pressure should be checked frequently.
The use of steroids after cataract surgery may delay healing and increase the incidence of bleb formation.
Use of ocular steroids may prolong the course and may exacerbate the severity of many viral infections of the eye (including herpes simplex). Employment of a corticosteroid medication in the treatment of patients with a history of herpes simplex requires great caution; frequent slit lamp microscopy is recommended.
Corticosteroids are not effective in mustard gas keratitis and Sjögren's keratoconjunctivitis.
Precautions:
General: The initial prescription and renewal of the medication order beyond 20 milliliters of FML FORTE® suspension should be made by a physician only after examination of the patient with the aid of magnification, such as slit lamp biomicroscopy and, where appropriate, fluorescein staining. If signs and symptoms fail to improve after two days, the patient should be re-evaluated.
As fungal infections of the cornea are particularly prone to develop coincidentally with long-term local corticosteroid applications, fungal invasion should be suspected in any persistent

corneal ulceration where a corticosteroid has been used or is in use. Fungal cultures should be taken when appropriate.
If this product is used for 10 days or longer, intraocular pressure should be monitored (see **Warnings**).
Information for Patients: If inflammation or pain persists longer than 48 hours or becomes aggravated, the patient should be advised to discontinue use of the medication and consult a physician.
This product is sterile when packaged. To prevent contamination, care should be taken to avoid touching the bottle tip to eyelids or to any other surface. The use of this bottle by more than one person may spread infection. Keep bottle tightly closed when not in use. Keep out of reach of children.
Carcinogenesis, mutagenesis, impairment of fertility: No studies have been conducted in animals or in humans to evaluate the possibility of these effects with fluorometholone.
Pregnancy: Teratogenic effects. Pregnancy Category C: Fluorometholone has been shown to be embryocidal and teratogenic in rabbits when administered at low multiples of the human ocular dose. Fluorometholone was applied ocularly to rabbits daily on days 6–18 of gestation, and dose-related fetal loss and fetal abnormalities including cleft palate, deformed rib cage, anomalous limbs and neural abnormalities such as encephalocele, craniorachischisis, and spina bifida were observed. There are no adequate and well-controlled studies of fluorometholone in pregnant women, and it is not known whether fluorometholone can cause fetal harm when administered to a pregnant woman. Fluorometholone should be used during pregnancy only if the potential benefit justifies the potential risk to the fetus.
Nursing Mothers: It is not known whether topical ophthalmic administration of corticosteroids could result in sufficient systemic absorption to produce detectable quantities in human milk. Systemically administered corticosteroids appear in human milk and could suppress growth, interfere with endogenous corticosteroid production, or cause other untoward effects. Because of the potential for serious adverse reactions in nursing infants from fluorometholone, a decision should be made whether to discontinue nursing or to discontinue the drug, taking into account the importance of the drug to the mother.
Pediatric Use: Safety and effectiveness in infants below the age of two years have not been established.
Geriatric Use: No overall differences in safety or effectiveness have been observed between elderly and younger patients.
Adverse Reactions: Adverse reactions include, in decreasing order of frequency, elevation of intraocular pressure (IOP) with possible development of glaucoma and infrequent optic nerve damage, posterior subcapsular cataract formation, and delayed wound healing.
Although systemic effects are extremely uncommon, there have been rare occurrences of systemic hypercorticoidism after use of topical steroids.
Corticosteroid-containing preparations have also been reported to cause acute anterior uveitis and perforation of the globe. Keratitis, conjunctivitis, corneal ulcers, mydriasis, conjunctival hyperemia, loss of accommodation and ptosis have occasionally been reported following local use of corticosteroids.
The development of secondary ocular infection (bacterial, fungal and viral) has occurred. Fungal and viral infections of the cornea are particularly prone to develop coincidentally with long-term applications of steroids. The possibility of fungal invasion should be considered in any persistent corneal ulceration where steroid treatment has been used (see **Warnings**).

Other adverse events reported with the use of FML FORTE® include transient burning and stinging upon instillation, ocular irritation, taste perversion, and visual disturbance (blurry vision).
Dosage and Administration: Instill one drop into the conjunctival sac two to four times daily. Care should be taken not to discontinue therapy prematurely. If signs and symptoms fail to improve after two days, the patient should be re-evaluated (see **Precautions**).
The dosing of FML FORTE® suspension may be reduced, but care should be taken not to discontinue therapy prematurely. In chronic conditions, withdrawal of treatment should be carried out by gradually decreasing the frequency of applications.
How Supplied: FML FORTE® (fluorometholone ophthalmic suspension, USP) 0.25% is supplied sterile in opaque white LDPE plastic bottles with droppers with white high impact polystyrene (HIPS) caps as follows:
  2 mL in 6 mL bottle—NDC 11980-228-02
  5 mL in 10 mL bottle—NDC 11980-228-05
  10 mL in 15 mL bottle—NDC 11980-228-10
  15 mL in 15 mL bottle—NDC 11980-228-15
Note: Store at or below 25°C (77°F); protect from freezing. **Shake well before using.**
℞ only
©2001 Allergan, Inc.
Irvine, CA 92612 U.S.A.
® Marks owned by Allergan, Inc.

FML® ℞
(fluorometholone ophthalmic suspension, USP) 0.1%
Sterile

Description: FML® (fluorometholone ophthalmic suspension, USP) 0.1% is a sterile, topical anti-inflammatory agent for ophthalmic use.
Chemical Name: Fluorometholone: 9-Fluoro-11β,17-dihydroxy-6α-methylpregna-1,4-diene-3,20-dione.
Contains:
Active: fluorometholone 0.1%. **Preservative:** benzalkonium chloride 0.004%. **Inactives:** Edetate disodium; polysorbate 80; polyvinyl alcohol 1.4%; purified water; sodium chloride; sodium phosphate, dibasic; and sodium phosphate, monobasic; and sodium hydroxide to adjust the pH. FML® suspension is formulated with a pH from 6.2 to 7.5. It has an osmolality range of 290–350 mOsm/kg.
Clinical Pharmacology: Corticosteroids inhibit the inflammatory response to a variety of inciting agents and probably delay or slow healing. They inhibit the edema, fibrin deposition, capillary dilation, leukocyte migration, capillary proliferation, fibroblast proliferation, deposition of collagen, and scar formation associated with inflammation.
There is no generally accepted explanation for the mechanism of action of ocular corticosteroids. However, corticosteroids are thought to act by the induction of phospholipase A_2 inhibitory proteins, collectively called lipocortins. It is postulated that these proteins control the biosynthesis of potent mediators of inflammation such as prostaglandins and leukotrienes by inhibiting the release of their common precursor arachidonic acid. Arachidonic acid is released from membrane phospholipids by phospholipase A_2.
Corticosteroids are capable of producing a rise in intraocular pressure. In clinical studies of documented steroid-responders, fluorometholone demonstrated a significantly longer average time to produce a rise in intraocular pressure than dexamethasone phosphate; however, in a small percentage of individuals, a significant rise in intraocular pressure

occurred within one week. The ultimate magnitude of the rise was equivalent for both drugs.
Indications and Usage: FML® suspension is indicated for the treatment of corticosteroid-responsive inflammation of the palpebral and bulbar conjunctiva, cornea and anterior segment of the globe.
Contraindications: FML® suspension is contraindicated in most viral diseases of the cornea and conjunctiva, including epithelial herpes simplex keratitis (dendritic keratitis), vaccinia, and varicella, and also in mycobacterial infection of the eye and fungal diseases of ocular structures. FML® suspension is also contraindicated in individuals with known or suspected hypersensitivity to any of the ingredients of this preparation and to other corticosteroids.
Warnings: Prolonged use of corticosteroids may result in glaucoma with damage to the optic nerve, defects in visual acuity and fields of vision, and in posterior subcapsular cataract formation. Prolonged use may also suppress the host immune response and thus increase the hazard of secondary ocular infections.
Various ocular diseases and long-term use of topical corticosteroids have been known to cause corneal and scleral thinning. Use of topical corticosteroids in the presence of thin corneal or scleral tissue may lead to perforation.
Acute purulent infections of the eye may be masked or activity enhanced by presence of corticosteroid medication.
If this product is used for 10 days or longer, intraocular pressure should be routinely monitored even though it may be difficult in children and uncooperative patients. Steroids should be used with caution in the presence of glaucoma. Intraocular pressure should be checked frequently.
The use of steroids after cataract surgery may delay healing and increase the incidence of bleb formation.
Use of ocular steroids may prolong the course and may exacerbate the severity of many viral infections of the eye (including herpes simplex). Employment of a corticosteroid medication in the treatment of patients with a history of herpes simplex requires great caution; frequent slit lamp microscopy is recommended.
Corticosteroids are not effective in mustard gas keratitis and Sjögren's keratoconjunctivitis.
Precautions:
General: The initial prescription and renewal of the medication order beyond 20 milliliters of FML® suspension should be made by a physician only after examination of the patient with the aid of magnification, such as slit lamp biomicroscopy and, where appropriate, fluorescein staining. If signs and symptoms fail to improve after two days, the patient should be re-evaluated.
As fungal infections of the cornea are particularly prone to develop coincidentally with long-term local corticosteroid applications, fungal invasion should be suspected in any persistent corneal ulceration where a corticosteroid has been used or is in use. Fungal cultures should be taken when appropriate.
If this product is used for 10 days or longer, intraocular pressure should be monitored (see **Warnings**).
Information for Patients: If inflammation or pain persists longer than 48 hours or becomes aggravated, the patient should be advised to discontinue use of the medication and consult a physician.
This product is sterile when packaged. To prevent contamination, care should be taken to avoid touching the bottle tip to eyelids or to any other surface. The use of this bottle by

Continued on next page

FML Suspension—Cont.

more than one person may spread infection. Keep bottle tightly closed when not in use. Keep out of the reach of children.

The preservative in FML® suspension, benzalkonium chloride, may be absorbed by soft contact lenses. Patients wearing soft contact lenses should be instructed to wait at least 15 minutes after instilling FML® suspension to insert soft contact lenses.

Carcinogenesis, mutagenesis, impairment of fertility: No studies have been conducted in animals or in humans to evaluate the possibility of these effects with fluorometholone.

Pregnancy: Teratogenic effects. Pregnancy Category C: Fluorometholone has been shown to be embryocidal and teratogenic in rabbits when administered at low multiples of the human ocular dose. Fluorometholone was applied ocularly to rabbits daily on days 6–18 of gestation, and dose-related fetal loss and fetal abnormalities including cleft palate, deformed rib cage, anomalous limbs and neural abnormalities such as encephalocele, craniorachischisis, and spina bifida were observed. There are no adequate and well-controlled studies of fluorometholone in pregnant women, and it is not known whether fluorometholone can cause fetal harm when administered to a pregnant woman. Fluorometholone should be used during pregnancy only if the potential benefit justifies the potential risk to the fetus.

Nursing Mothers: It is not known whether topical ophthalmic administration of corticosteroids could result in sufficient systemic absorption to produce detectable quantities in human milk. Systemically administered corticosteroids appear in human milk and could suppress growth, interfere with endogenous corticosteroid production, or cause other untoward effects. Because of the potential for serious adverse reactions in nursing infants from fluorometholone, a decision should be made whether to discontinue nursing or to discontinue the drug, taking into account the importance of the drug to the mother.

Pediatric Use: Safety and effectiveness in infants below the age of 2 years have not been established.

Geriatric Use: No overall differences in safety or effectiveness have been observed between elderly and younger patients.

Adverse Reactions: Adverse reactions include, in decreasing order of frequency, elevation of intraocular pressure (IOP) with possible development of glaucoma and infrequent optic nerve damage, posterior subcapsular cataract formation, and delayed wound healing.

Although systemic effects are extremely uncommon, there have been rare occurrences of systemic hypercorticoidism after use of topical steroids.

Corticosteroid-containing preparations have also been reported to cause acute anterior uveitis and perforation of the globe. Keratitis, conjunctivitis, corneal ulcers, mydriasis, conjunctival hyperemia, loss of accommodation and ptosis have occasionally been reported following local use of corticosteroids.

The development of secondary ocular infection (bacterial, fungal and viral) has occurred. Fungal and viral infections of the cornea are particularly prone to develop coincidentally with long-term applications of steroids. The possibility of fungal invasion should be considered in any persistent corneal ulceration where steroid treatment has been used (see **Warnings**).

Transient burning and stinging upon instillation and other minor symptoms of ocular irritation have been reported with the use of FML® suspension. Other adverse events reported with the use of FML® suspension include: allergic reactions, visual disturbance (blurry vision) and taste perversion.

Dosage and Administration: Instill one drop into the conjunctival sac two to four times daily. During the initial 24 to 48 hours, the dosage may be increased to one application every four hours. Care should be taken not to discontinue therapy prematurely.

If signs and symptoms fail to improve after two days, the patient should be re-evaluated (see **Precautions**).

The dosing of FML® suspension may be reduced, but care should be taken not to discontinue therapy prematurely. In chronic conditions, withdrawal of treatment should be carried out by gradually decreasing the frequency of applications.

How Supplied: FML® (fluorometholone ophthalmic suspension, USP) 0.1% is supplied sterile in white LDPE plastic bottles with droppers with white high impact polystyrene (HIPS) caps as follows:
5 mL in 10 mL bottle – NDC 11980-211-05
10 mL in 15 mL bottle – NDC 11980-211-10
15 mL in 15 mL bottle – NDC 11980-211-15
Note: Store between 2° and 25°C (36°–77°F); protect from freezing. **Shake well before using.**
℞ only
©2003 Allergan, Inc.
Irvine, CA 92612
® Marks owned by Allergan, Inc.

FML® ℞
(fluorometholone ophthalmic ointment) 0.1% sterile

Description: FML® (fluorometholone ophthalmic ointment) 0.1% is a topical anti-inflammatory agent for ophthalmic use.
Chemical Name: Fluorometholone: 9-Fluoro-11β, 17-dihydroxy-6α-methylpregna-1,4-diene-3,20-dione.
Contains: Active: fluorometholone 0.1%. **Preservative:** phenylmercuric acetate (0.0008%). **Inactives:** mineral oil; petrolatum (and) lanolin alcohol; and white petrolatum.
Clinical Pharmacology: Corticosteroids inhibit the inflammatory response to a variety of inciting agents and probably delay or slow healing. They inhibit the edema, fibrin deposition, capillary dilation, leukocyte migration, capillary proliferation, fibroblast proliferation, deposition of collagen and scar formation associated with inflammation.

There is no generally accepted explanation for the mechanism of action of ocular corticosteroids. However, corticosteroids are thought to act by the induction of phospholipase A_2 inhibitory proteins, collectively called lipocortins. It is postulated that these proteins control the biosynthesis of potent mediators of inflammation such as prostaglandins and leukotrienes by inhibiting the release of their common precursor arachidonic acid. Arachidonic acid is released from membrane phospholipids by phospholipase A_2.

Corticosteroids are capable of producing a rise in intraocular pressure. In clinical studies of documented steroid-responders, fluorometholone demonstrated a significantly longer average time to produce a rise in intraocular pressure than dexamethasone phosphate; however, in a small percentage of individuals, a significant rise in intraocular pressure occurred within one week. The ultimate magnitude of the rise was equivalent for both drugs.

Indications and Usage: FML® ophthalmic ointment is indicated for the treatment of steroid-responsive inflammation of the palpebral and bulbar conjunctiva, cornea and anterior segment of the globe.
Contraindications: FML® ophthalmic ointment is contraindicated in most viral diseases of the cornea and conjunctiva, including epithelial herpes simplex keratitis (dendritic keratitis), vaccinia, and varicella and also in mycobacterial infection of the eye and fungal diseases of ocular structures. FML® ointment is also contraindicated in individuals with known or suspected hypersensitivity to any of the ingredients of this preparation and to other corticosteroids.

Warnings: Prolonged use of corticosteroids may result in glaucoma with damage to the optic nerve, defects in visual acuity and fields of vision, and in posterior subcapsular cataract formation. Prolonged use may also suppress the host immune response and thus increase the hazard of secondary ocular infections.

Various ocular diseases and long-term use of topical corticosteroids have been known to cause corneal and scleral thinning. Use of topical corticosteroids in the presence of thin corneal or scleral tissue may lead to perforation. Acute purulent infections of the eye may be masked or activity enhanced by the presence of corticosteroid medication.

If this product is used for 10 days or longer, intraocular pressure should be routinely monitored even though it may be difficult in children and uncooperative patients. Steroids should be used with caution in the presence of glaucoma. Intraocular pressure should be checked frequently.

The use of steroids after cataract surgery may delay healing and increase the incidence of bleb formation.

Use of ocular steroids may prolong the course and may exacerbate the severity of many viral infections of the eye (including herpes simplex). Employment of a corticosteroid medication in the treatment of patients with a history of herpes simplex requires great caution; frequent slit lamp microscopy is recommended. Corticosteroids are not effective in mustard gas keratitis and Sjögren's keratoconjunctivitis.

Precautions:
General: The initial prescription and renewal of the medication order beyond 8 grams of FML® ophthalmic ointment should be made by a physician only after examination of the patient with the aid of magnification, such as slit lamp biomicroscopy and, where appropriate, fluorescein staining. If signs and symptoms fail to improve after two days, the patient should be re-evaluated.

As fungal infections of the cornea are particularly prone to develop coincidentally with long-term local corticosteroid applications, fungal invasion should be suspected in any persistent corneal ulceration where a corticosteroid has been used or is in use. Fungal cultures should be taken when appropriate.

If this product is used for 10 days or longer, intraocular pressure should be monitored (see **Warnings**).

Ophthalmic ointments may retard corneal healing.

Information for Patients: If inflammation or pain persists longer than 48 hours or becomes aggravated, the patient should be advised to discontinue use of the medication and consult a physician.

This product is sterile when packaged. To prevent contamination, care should be taken to avoid touching the tube tip to eyelids or to any other surface. The use of this tube by more than one person may spread infection. Keep tube tightly closed when not in use. Keep out of the reach of children.

Carcinogenesis, mutagenesis, impairment of fertility: No studies have been conducted in animals or in humans to evaluate the possibility of these effects with fluorometholone.

Pregnancy: Teratogenic effects. Pregnancy Category C: Fluorometholone has been shown to be embryocidal and teratogenic in rabbits when administered at low multiples of the human ocular dose. Fluorometholone was applied ocularly to rabbits daily on days 6–18 of gestation, and dose-related fetal loss and fetal abnormalities including cleft palate, deformed rib cage, anamalous limbs and neural abnormalities such as encephalocele, craniorachischisis, and spina bifida were observed. There are no adequate and well-controlled studies of fluorometholone in pregnant women, and it is not known whether fluorometholone can cause fetal harm when administered to a pregnant woman. Fluorometholone should be used during pregnancy only if the potential benefit justifies the potential risk to the fetus.

Nursing Mothers: It is not known whether topical ophthalmic administration of corticosteroids could result in sufficient systemic absorption to produce detectable quantities in human milk. Systemically administered corticosteroids appear in human milk and could suppress growth, interfere with endogenous corticosteroid production, or cause other untoward effects. Because of the potential for serious adverse reactions in nursing infants from fluorometholone, a decision should be made whether to discontinue nursing or to discontinue the drug, taking into account the importance of the drug to the mother.

Pediatric Use: Safety and effectiveness in infants below the age of 2 years have not been established.

Geriatric Use: No overall differences in safety and effectiveness have been observed between elderly and younger patients.

Adverse Reactions: Adverse reactions include, in decreasing order of frequency, elevation of intraocular pressure (IOP) with possible development of glaucoma and infrequent optic nerve damage, posterior subcapsular cataract formation, and delayed wound healing.

Although systemic effects are extremely uncommon, there have been rare occurrences of systemic hypercorticoidism after use of topical steroids.

Corticosteroid-containing preparations have also been reported to cause acute anterior uveitis and perforation of the globe. Keratitis, conjunctivitis, corneal ulcers, mydriasis, conjunctival hyperemia, loss of accommodation and ptosis have occasionally been reported following local use of corticosteroids.

The development of secondary ocular infection (bacterial, fungal and viral) has occurred. Fungal and viral infections of the cornea are particularly prone to develop coincidentally with long-term applications of steroids. The possibility of fungal invasion should be considered in any persistent corneal ulceration where steroid treatment has been used (see **Warnings**).

Dosage and Administration: A small amount (approximately $1/2$ inch ribbon) of ointment should be applied to the conjunctival sac one to three times daily. During the initial 24 to 48 hours, the frequency of dosing may be increased to one application every four hours. Care should be taken not to discontinue therapy prematurely.

If signs and symptoms fail to improve after two days, the patient should be re-evaluated (see **Precautions**).

The dosing of FML® ophthalmic ointment may be reduced, but care should be taken not to discontinue therapy prematurely. In chronic conditions, withdrawal of treatment should be carried out by gradually decreasing the frequency of applications.

How Supplied: FML® (fluorometholone ophthalmic ointment) 0.1% is supplied in a collapsible aluminum tube with a black low density polyethylene screw cap in the following size:

3.5 g in 3.5 g tube—NDC 0023-0316-04

Note: Store at or below 25°C (77°F). Avoid exposure to temperatures above 40°C (104°F).

℞ only
©2001 Allergan, Inc.
Irvine, CA 92612
® Marks owned by Allergan, Inc.
Shown in Product Identification Guide, page 103

FML-S® ℞
(fluorometholone and sulfacetamide sodium ophthalmic suspension, USP) 0.1%/10% sterile

Description: FML-S® ophthalmic suspension is a topical anti-inflammatory/anti-infective product for ophthalmic use.

Chemical Names: Fluorometholone: 9-Fluoro-11β, 17-dihydroxy-6α-methylpregna-1,4-diene-3, 20-dione.

Sulfacetamide sodium: N-Sulfanilylacetamide monosodium salt monohydrate.

Contains: **Actives**: fluorometholone 0.1%; and sulfacetamide sodium 10%. **Preservative**: benzalkonium chloride 0.006%. **Inactives**: edetate disodium; polysorbate 80; polyvinyl alcohol (1.4%); povidone; purified water; sodium chloride; sodium phosphate dibasic; sodium phosphate, monobasic; sodium thiosulfate; and hydrochloric acid and/or sodium hydroxide to adjust the pH to 7.0 to 7.5.

Clinical Pharmacology: Corticosteroids suppress the inflammatory response to a variety of agents and they probably delay or slow healing. They inhibit the edema, fibrin deposition, capillary dilation, leukocyte migration, capillary proliferation, fibroblast proliferation, deposition of collagen, and scar formation associated with inflammation. Since corticosteroids may inhibit the body's defense mechanism against infection, a concomitant antimicrobial drug may be used when this inhibition is considered to be clinically significant in a particular case.

Corticosteroids are capable of producing a rise in intraocular pressure. In clinical studies of documented steroid-responders, fluorometholone demonstrated a significantly longer average time to produce a rise in intraocular pressure than dexamethasone phosphate; however, in a small percentage of individuals, a significant rise in intraocular pressure occurred within one week. The ultimate magnitude of the rise was equivalent for both drugs.

The anti-infective component in FML-S® ophthalmic suspension is included to provide action against specific organisms susceptible to it. Sulfacetamide sodium is active *in vitro* against susceptible strains of the following microorganisms: *Escherichia coli, Staphylococcus aureus, Streptococcus pneumoniae, Streptococcus* (*viridans* group), *Haemophilus influenzae, Klebsiella* species, and *Enterobacter* species. Some strains of these bacteria may be resistant to sulfacetamide or resistant strains may emerge *in vivo*.

When a decision to administer both a corticosteroid and an antimicrobial is made, the administration of such drugs in combination has the advantage of greater patient compliance and convenience, with the added assurance that the appropriate dosage of both drugs is administered. When both types of drugs are in the same formulation, compatibility of ingredients is assured and the correct volume of drug is delivered and retained.

The relative potency of corticosteroid formulations depends on the molecular structure, concentration, and release from the vehicle.

Indications and Usage: FML-S® ophthalmic suspension is indicated for steroid-responsive inflammatory ocular conditions for which a corticosteroid is indicated and where superficial bacterial ocular infection or a risk of bacterial ocular infection exists.

Ocular steroids are indicated in inflammatory conditions of the palpebral and bulbar conjunctiva, cornea, and anterior segment of the globe where the inherent risk of steroid use in certain infective conjunctivitides is accepted to obtain a diminution in edema and inflammation. They are also indicated in chronic anterior uveitis and corneal injury from chemical, radiation or thermal burns or penetration of foreign bodies.

The use of a combination drug with an anti-infective component is indicated where the risk of superficial ocular infection is high or where there is an expectation that potentially dangerous numbers of bacteria will be present in the eye.

The anti-infective drug in this product, sulfacetamide, is active against the following common bacterial eye pathogens: *Escherichia coli, Staphylococcus aureus, Streptococcus pneumoniae, Streptococcus* (*viridans* group), *Haemophilus influenzae, Klebsiella* species, and *Enterobacter* species.

The product does not provide adequate coverage against: *Neisseria* species and *Serratia marcescens*. A significant percentage of Staphylococcal isolates are completely resistant to sulfa drugs.

Contraindications: FML-S® ophthalmic suspension is contraindicated in most viral diseases of the cornea and conjunctiva, including epithelial herpes simplex keratitis (dendritic keratitis), vaccinia, and varicella, and also in mycobacterial infection of the eye and fungal diseases of ocular structures. FML-S® ophthalmic suspension is also contraindicated in individuals with known or suspected hypersensitivity to any of the ingredients of this preparation, to sulfonamides and to other corticosteroids.

Warnings:
Prolonged use of corticosteroids may result in glaucoma, with damage to the optic nerve, defects in visual acuity and fields of vision, and in posterior subcapsular cataract formation. Prolonged use may also suppress the host immune response in ocular tissues and thus increase the hazard of secondary ocular infections.

Various ocular diseases and long-term use of topical corticosteroids have been known to cause corneal and scleral thinning. Use of topical corticosteroids in the presence of thin corneal or scleral tissue may lead to perforation. Acute purulent infections of the eye may be masked or activity enhanced by the presence of corticosteroid medication.

If this product is used for 10 days or longer, intraocular pressure should be routinely monitored even though it may be difficult in children and uncooperative patients. Steroids should be used with caution in the presence of glaucoma. Intraocular pressure should be checked frequently.

The use of steroids after cataract surgery may delay healing and increase the incidence of bleb formation.

Use of ocular steroids may prolong the course and may exacerbate the severity of many viral infections of the eye. Employment of a corticosteroid medication in the treatment of patients with a history of herpes simplex requires great caution.

FML-S® ophthalmic suspension is not for injection. It should never be injected subconjunctivally, nor should it be directly introduced into the anterior chamber of the eye.

Corticosteroids are not effective in mustard gas keratitis and Sjögren's keratoconjunctivitis.

FATALITIES HAVE OCCURRED, ALTHOUGH RARELY, DUE TO SEVERE REACTIONS TO SULFONAMIDES INCLUDING STEVENS-JOHNSON SYNDROME, TOXIC EPIDERMAL NECROLYSIS, FULMINANT

Continued on next page

FML-S—Cont.

HEPATIC NECROSIS, AGRANULOCYTOSIS, APLASTIC ANEMIA, AND OTHER BLOOD DYSCRASIAS. Sensitizations may recur when a sulfonamide is readministered, irrespective of the route of administration. If signs of hypersensitivity or other serious reactions occur, discontinue use of this preparation (see **Adverse Reactions**).

Cross-sensitivity among corticosteroids has been demonstrated.

A significant percentage of staphylococcal isolates are completely resistant to sulfa drugs.

Precautions:
General: The initial prescription and renewal of the medication order beyond 20 milliliters should be made only by a physician after evaluation of the patient's intraocular pressure, examination of the patient with the aid of magnification, such as slit lamp biomicroscopy and, where appropriate, fluorescein staining. If signs and symptoms fail to improve after two days, the patient should be re-evaluated.

As fungal infections of the cornea are particularly prone to develop coincidentally with long-term local corticosteroid applications, fungal invasion should be suspected in any persistent corneal ulceration where a corticosteroid has been used or is in use. Fungal cultures should be taken when appropriate.

If this product is used for 10 days or longer, intraocular pressure should be monitored (see **WARNINGS**).

Information for Patients: If inflammation or pain persists longer than 48 hours or becomes aggravated, the patient should be advised to discontinue use of the medication and consult a physician.

This product is sterile when packaged. To prevent contamination, care should be taken to avoid touching the bottle tip to eyelids or to any other surface. The use of this bottle by more than one person may spread infection. Keep bottle tightly closed when not in use. Keep out of the reach of children.

Drug Interactions: Sulfacetamide preparations are incompatible with silver preparations.

Carcinogenesis, Mutagenesis, Impairment of Fertility: No studies have been conducted in animals or in humans to evaluate the possibility of these effects with fluorometholone or sulfacetamide.

Pregnancy: Teratogenic effects Pregnancy Category C: Animal studies have not been conducted with FML-S® Ophthalmic Suspension. Fluorometholone has been shown to be embryocidal and teratogenic in rabbits when administered at low multiples of the human dose. Fluorometholone was applied ocularly to rabbits daily on days 8–18 of gestation, and dose-related fetal loss and fetal abnormalities including cleft palate, deformed rib cage, anomalous limbs and neural abnormalities such as encephalocele, craniorachischisis, and spina bifida were observed. Kernicterus may be precipitated in infants by sulfonamides being given systemically during the third trimester of pregnancy. There are no adequate and well-controlled studies of FML-S® Ophthalmic Suspension in pregnant women, and it is not known whether FML-S® can cause fetal harm when administered to a pregnant woman. FML-S® ophthalmic suspension should be used during pregnancy only if the potential benefit justifies the potential risk to the fetus.

Nursing Mothers: It is not known whether topical administration of corticosteroids could result in sufficient systemic absorption to produce detectable quantities in breast milk. Systemically administered corticosteroids appear in breast milk and could suppress growth, interfere with endogenous corticosteroid production, or cause other untoward effects. Systemically administered sulfonamides are capable of producing kernicterus in infants of lactating women. Because of the potential for serious adverse reactions in nursing infants from FML-S® ophthalmic suspension, a decision should be made whether to discontinue nursing or to discontinue the medication.

Pediatric Use: Safety and effectiveness in pediatric patients have not been established.

Geriatric: No overall differences in safety or effectiveness have been observed between elderly and younger patients.

Adverse Reactions: Adverse reactions have occurred with corticosteroid/anti-infective combination drugs which can be attributed to the corticosteroid component, the anti-infective component, or the combination. Exact incidence figures are not available since no denominator of treated patients is available.

Reactions occurring most often from the presence of the anti-infective ingredient are allergic sensitizations. Fatalities have occurred, although rarely, due to severe reactions to sulfonamides including Stevens-Johnson syndrome, toxic epidermal necrolysis, fulminant hepatic necrosis, agranulocytosis, aplastic anemia, and other blood dyscrasias (see **Warnings**). Sulfacetamide sodium may cause local irritation.

The reactions due to the corticosteroid component in decreasing order of frequency are: elevation of intraocular pressure (IOP) with possible development of glaucoma, and infrequent optic nerve damage; posterior subcapsular cataract formation; and delayed wound healing.

Although systemic effects are extremely uncommon, there have been rare occurrences of systemic hypercorticoidism after use of topical steroids.

Corticosteroid-containing preparations have also been reported to cause acute anterior uveitis and perforation of the globe. Keratitis, conjunctivitis, corneal ulcers, mydriasis, conjunctival hyperemia, loss of accommodation and ptosis have occasionally been reported following local use of corticosteroids.

Secondary Infection: The development of secondary infection has occurred after use of combinations containing corticosteroids and antimicrobials. Fungal infections of the cornea are particularly prone to develop coincidentally with long-term application of corticosteroids. When signs of chronic ocular inflammation persist following prolonged corticosteroid dosing, the possibility of fungal infections of the cornea should be considered.

Secondary bacterial ocular infection following suppression of host responses also occurs.

Dosage and Administration: One drop of FML-S® ophthalmic suspension should be instilled into the conjunctival sac four times daily. Care should be taken not to discontinue therapy prematurely. If signs and symptoms fail to improve after two days, the patient should be re-evaluated (see **PRECAUTIONS**).

The dosing of FML-S® ophthalmic suspension may be reduced, but care should be taken not to discontinue therapy prematurely. In chronic conditions, withdrawal of treatment should be carried out by gradually decreasing the frequency of applications.

How Supplied: FML-S® (fluorometholone and sulfacetamide sodium ophthalmic suspension) is supplied sterile in opaque white LDPE plastic bottles with droppers with high impact polystyrene (HIPS) caps as follows:

5 mL in 10 mL bottle—NDC 11980-422-05
10 mL in 15 mL bottle—NDC 11980-422-10

Note: Store at 15°–30°C (59°–86°F). Protect from freezing and light. **SHAKE WELL BEFORE USING.** Do not use suspension if it is dark brown.

℞ only

©2002 Allergan, Inc.
Irvine, CA 92612
® Marks owned by Allergan, Inc.

GENOPTIC® ℞
(gentamicin sulfate ophthalmic solution, USP)
0.3%
Sterile

Description: GENOPTIC® (gentamicin sulfate ophthalmic solution; USP) is a sterile, topical anti-infective agent for ophthalmic use. The active ingredient, gentamicin sulfate, is a water-soluble antibiotic of the aminoglycoside group.

Gentamicin is obtained from cultures of *Micromonospora purpurea*. It is a mixture of the sulfate salts of gentamicin C_1, C_2, and C_{1A}. All three components appear to have similar antimicrobial activities. Gentamicin sulfate occurs as a white to buff powder and is soluble in water but insoluble in alcohol.

GENOPTIC® Solution:
Contains: Each mL contains—**Active:** gentamicin sulfate equivalent to 3 mg (0.3%) gentamicin base. **Preservative:** Benzalkonium chloride. **Inactives:** edetate disodium; polyvinyl alcohol 1.4%; purified water; sodium chloride; sodium phosphate, dibasic; and hydrochloric acid and/or sodium hydroxide to adjust the pH. The solution is an aqueous, buffered solution with a pH of 6.5–7.5.

Clinical Pharmacology: Microbiology: Gentamicin sulfate is active *in vitro* against many strains of the following microorganisms: *Staphylococcus aureus, Staphylococcus epidermidis, Streptococcus pyogenes, Streptococcus pneumoniae, Enterobacter aerogenes, Escherichia coli, Haemophilus influenzae, Klebsiella pneumoniae, Neisseria gonorrhoeae, Pseudomonas aeruginosa,* and *Serratia marcescens.*

Indications and Usage: GENOPTIC® (gentamicin sulfate ophthalmic solution; USP) is indicated in the topical treatment of ocular bacterial infections including conjunctivitis, keratitis, keratoconjunctivitis, corneal ulcers, blepharitis, blepharoconjunctivitis, acute meibomianitis, and dacryocystitis, caused by susceptible strains of the following microorganisms *Staphylococcus aureus, Staphylococcus epidermidis, Streptococcus pyogenes, Streptococcus pneumoniae, Enterobacter aerogenes, Escherichia coli, Haemophilus influenzae, Klebsiella pneumoniae, Neisseria gonorrhoeae, Pseudomonas aeruginosa,* and *Serratia marcescens.*

Contraindications: GENOPTIC® solution is contraindicated in patients with known hypersensitivity to any of the components.

Warnings
NOT FOR INJECTION INTO THE EYE.
Gentamicin solution is not for injection. It should never be injected subconjunctivally, nor should it be directly introduced into the anterior chamber of the eye.

Precautions:
General: Prolonged use of topical antibiotics may give rise to overgrowth of nonsusceptible microorganisms, including fungi. Bacterial resistance to gentamicin may also develop. If purulent discharge, inflammation or pain becomes aggravated, the patient should discontinue use of the medication and consult a physician.

If irritation or hypersensitivity to any component of the drug develops, the patient should discontinue use of this preparation, and appropriate therapy should be instituted.

Information for Patients: To avoid contamination, do not touch tip of container to the eye, eyelid or any surface.

Carcinogenesis, Mutagenesis, Impairment of Fertility: There are no published carcinogenicity or impairment of fertility studies on gentamicin. Aminoglycoside antibiotics have been found to be non-mutagenic.

Pregnancy: Pregnancy Category C. Gentamicin has been shown to depress body weights, kidney weights and median glomerular counts in newborn rats when administered systemically to pregnant rats in daily doses approximately 500 times the maximum recommended ophthalmic human dose. There are no adequate and well-controlled studies in pregnant women. Gentamicin should be used during pregnancy only if the potential benefit justifies the potential risk to the fetus.

Pediatric Use: Safety and effectiveness in neonates have not been established.

Adverse Reactions: Bacterial and fungal corneal ulcers have developed during treatment with gentamicin ophthalmic preparations.

The most frequently reported adverse reactions are ocular burning and irritation upon drug instillation, non-specific conjunctivitis, conjunctival epithelial defects and conjunctival hyperemia.

Other reactions which have occurred rarely are allergic reactions, thrombocytopenic purpura and hallucinations.

Dosage and Administration: Instill one or two drops into the affected eye(s) every four hours. In severe infections, dosage may be increased to as much as two drops every hour.

How Supplied: GENOPTIC® (gentamicin sulfate ophthalmic solution, USP) 0.3% is supplied sterile in white opaque LDPE plastic bottles and tips with white high impact polystyrene (HIPS) caps as follows:
1 mL in 5 mL bottle—NDC 11980-117-01

Note: Store at or below 25°C (77°F). Avoid exposure to excessive heat (104°F/40°C or above).

℞ only
©2003 Allergan, Inc.
Irvine, CA 92612 USA.
®Marks owned by Allergan, Inc.

HMS® ℞
(medrysone ophthalmic suspension) 1%
sterile

Description: HMS® (medrysone ophthalmic suspension) 1% is a topical anti-inflammatory agent for ophthalmic use.
Chemical Name: 11β-Hydroxy-6α-methyl-pregn-4-ene-3, 20-dione.
Contains: Active: medrysone 1%. **Preservative:** benzalkonium chloride 0.004%. **Inactives:** edetate disodium; hydroxypropyl methylcellulose; polyvinyl alcohol 1.4%; potassium chloride; purified water; sodium chloride; sodium phosphate, dibasic; sodium phosphate, monobasic; and sodium hydroxide to adjust the pH (6.2 – 7.5).
Clinical Pharmacology: HMS® (medrysone ophthalmic suspension) is a synthetic corticosteroid with topical anti-inflammatory activity. Corticosteroids inhibit the edema, fibrin deposition, capillary dilation, and phagocytic migration of the acute inflammatory response, as well as capillary proliferation, deposition of collagen, and scar formation. HMS® (medrysone ophthalmic suspension) has less anti-inflammatory potency than 0.1% dexamethasone.
Indications and Usage: HMS® (medrysone) is indicated for the treatment of allergic conjunctivitis, vernal conjunctivitis, episcleritis, and epinephrine sensitivity.
Contraindications: HMS® suspension is contraindicated in most viral diseases of the cornea and conjunctiva, including epithelial herpes simplex keratitis (dendritic keratitis), vaccinia, and varicella, and also in mycobacterial infection of the eye and fungal diseases of ocular structures. HMS® suspension is also contraindicated in individuals with known or suspected hypersensitivity to any of the ingredients of this preparation and to other corticosteroids.

Warnings:
HMS ophthalmic suspension is not recommended for use in iritis and uveitis as its therapeutic effectiveness has not been demonstrated in these conditions.
Prolonged use of corticosteroids may result in glaucoma with damage to the optic nerve, defects in visual acuity and fields of vision, and in posterior subcapsular cataract formation. Prolonged use may also suppress the host immune response and thus increase the hazard of secondary ocular infections.
Various ocular diseases and long-term use of topical corticosteroids have been known to cause corneal and scleral thinning. Use of topical corticosteroids in the presence of thin corneal or scleral tissue may lead to perforation.
Acute purulent infections of the eye may be masked or activity enhanced by the presence of corticosteroid medication.
If this product is used for 10 days or longer, intraocular pressure should be routinely monitored even though it may be difficult in children and uncooperative patients.
Steroids should be used with caution in the presence of glaucoma. Intraocular pressure should be checked frequently.
The use of steroids after cataract surgery may delay healing and increase the incidence of bleb formation.
Use of ocular steroids may prolong the course and may exacerbate the severity of many viral infections of the eye (including herpes simplex). Employment of a corticosteroid medication in the treatment of patients with a history of herpes simplex requires great caution; frequent slit lamp microscopy is recommended.
Corticosteroids are not effective in mustard gas keratitis and Sjögren's keratoconjunctivitis.

Precautions:
General: The initial prescription and renewal of the medication order beyond 20 milliliters of HMS® suspension should be made by a physician only after examination of the patient with the aid of magnification, such as slit lamp biomicroscopy and, where appropriate, fluorescein staining. If signs and symptoms fail to improve after 2 days, the patient should be re-evaluated.
As fungal infections of the cornea are particularly prone to develop coincidentally with long-term local corticosteroid applications, fungal invasion should be suspected in any persistent corneal ulceration where a corticosteroid has been used or is in use. Fungal cultures should be taken when appropriate.
If this product is used for 10 days or longer, intraocular pressure should be monitored (see **WARNINGS**).
Information for Patients: If inflammation or pain persists longer than 48 hours or becomes aggravated, the patient should be advised to discontinue use of the medication and consult a physician.
This product is sterile when packaged. To prevent contamination, care should be taken to avoid touching the bottle tip to eyelids or to any other surface. The use of this bottle by more than one person may spread infection. Keep bottle tightly closed when not in use. Keep out of the reach of children.
Carcinogenesis, Mutagenesis, Impairment of Fertility: No studies have been conducted in animals or in humans to evaluate the potential of these effects.
Pregnancy Teratogenic Effects Category C: Medrysone has been shown to be embryocidal in rabbits when given in doses 10 and 30 times the human dose. Two drops of medrysone were applied to both eyes of pregnant rabbits 4 times per day on day 6 through 18 of gestation. A significant increase in early resorptions was observed in the treated rabbits. There are no adequate and well-controlled studies of medrysone in pregnant women. Medrysone should be used during pregnancy only if the potential benefit justifies the potential risk to the fetus.
Nursing Mothers: It is not known whether topical ophthalmic administration of corticosteroids could result in sufficient systemic absorption to produce detectable quantities in human breast milk. Systemically administered corticosteroids appear in human milk and could suppress growth, interfere with endogenous corticosteroid production, or cause other untoward effects. Because of the potential for serious adverse reactions in nursing infants from medrysone, a decision should be made whether to discontinue nursing or to discontinue the drug, taking into account the importance of the drug to the mother.
Pediatric Use: Safety and effectiveness in pediatric patients below the age of 3 years have not been established.
Geriatric Use: No overall differences in safety or effectiveness have been observed between elderly and younger patients.
Adverse Reactions: Adverse reactions include, in decreasing order of frequency, elevation of intraocular pressure (IOP) with possible development of glaucoma and infrequent optic nerve damage, posterior subcapsular cataract formation, and delayed wound healing. Although systemic effects are extremely uncommon, there have been rare occurrences of systemic hypercorticoidism after use of topical steroids.
Corticosteroid-containing preparations have also been reported to cause acute anterior uveitis and perforation of the globe. Keratitis, conjunctivitis, corneal ulcers, mydriasis, conjunctival hyperemia, loss of accommodation and ptosis have occasionally been reported following local use of corticosteroids.
The development of secondary ocular infection (bacterial, fungal and viral) has occurred. Fungal and viral infections of the cornea are particularly prone to develop coincidentally with long-term application of steroids. The possibility of fungal invasion should be considered in any persistent corneal ulceration where steroid treatment has been used (see **WARNINGS**).
Transient burning and stinging upon instillation and other minor symptoms of ocular irritation have been reported with the use of HMS® suspension. Other adverse events reported with the use of HMS® suspension include: allergic reactions, foreign body sensation, and visual disturbance (blurry vision).
Overdosage: Overdosage will not ordinarily cause acute problems. If accidentally ingested, drink fluids to dilute.
Dosage and Administration: Shake well before using. Instill one drop in the conjunctival sac up to every four hours.
How Supplied: HMS® (medrysone ophthalmic suspension) 1% is supplied sterile in opaque white LDPE plastic bottles with droppers with white high impact polystyrene (HIPS) caps as follows:
5 mL in 10 mL bottle—NDC 11980-074-05
10 mL in 15 mL bottle—NDC 11980-074-10
Note: Store at temperature up to 25°C (77°F) Protect from freezing.
℞ only
©2002 Allergan, Inc.
Irvine, CA 92612 U.S.A.
® Marks owned by Allergan, Inc.

Continued on next page

LUMIGAN® ℞
(bimatoprost ophthalmic solution) 0.03%

Description: LUMIGAN® (bimatoprost ophthalmic solution) 0.03% is a synthetic prostamide analog with ocular hypotensive activity. Its chemical name is (Z)-7-[(1R,2R,3R,5S)-3,5-Dihydroxy-2-[1E,3S)-3-hydroxy-5-phenyl-1-pentenyl]cyclopentyl]-5-N-ethylheptenamide, and its molecular weight is 415.58. Its molecular formula is $C_{25}H_{37}NO_4$. Its chemical structure is:

Bimatoprost is a powder, which is very soluble in ethyl alcohol and methyl alcohol and slightly soluble in water. LUMIGAN® is a clear, isotonic, colorless, sterile ophthalmic solution with an osmolality of approximately 290 mOsmol/kg.
Each mL **contains: Active:** bimatoprost 0.3 mg; **Preservative:** Benzalkonium chloride 0.05 mg; **Inactives:** Sodium chloride; sodium phosphate, dibasic; citric acid; and purified water. Sodium hydroxide and/or hydrochloric acid may be added to adjust pH. The pH during its shelf life ranges from 6.8–7.8.

Clinical Pharmacology:
Mechanism of Action
Bimatoprost is a prostamide, a synthetic structural analog of prostaglandin with ocular hypotensive activity. It selectively mimics the effects of naturally occurring substances, prostamides. Bimatoprost is believed to lower intraocular pressure (IOP) in humans by increasing outflow of aqueous humor through both the trabecular meshwork and uveoscleral routes. Elevated IOP presents a major risk factor for glaucomatous field loss. The higher the level of IOP, the greater the likelihood of optic nerve damage and visual field loss.

Pharmacokinetics
Absorption: After one drop of bimatoprost ophthalmic solution 0.03% was administered once daily to both eyes of 15 healthy subjects for two weeks, blood concentrations peaked within 10 minutes after dosing and were below the lower limit of detection (0.025 ng/mL) in most subjects within 1.5 hours after dosing. Mean C_{max} and AUC_{0-24hr} values were similar on days 7 and 14 at approximately 0.08 ng/mL and 0.09 ng•hr/mL, respectively, indicating that steady state was reached during the first week of ocular dosing. There was no significant systemic drug accumulation over time.

Distribution
Bimatoprost is moderately distributed into body tissues with a steady-state volume of distribution of 0.67 L/kg. In human blood, bimatoprost resides mainly in the plasma. Approximately 12% of bimatoprost remains unbound in human plasma.

Metabolism
Bimatoprost is the major circulating species in the blood once it reaches the systemic circulation following ocular dosing. Bimatoprost then undergoes oxidation, N-deethylation and glucuronidation to form a diverse variety of metabolites.

Elimination
Following an intravenous dose of radiolabeled bimatoprost (3.12 μg/kg) to six healthy subjects, the maximum blood concentration of unchanged drug was 12.2 ng/mL and decreased rapidly with an elimination half-life of approximately 45 minutes. The total blood clearance of bimatoprost was 1.5 L/hr/kg. Up to 67% of the administered dose was excreted in the urine while 25% of the dose was recovered in the feces.

Clinical Studies:
In clinical studies of patients with open angle glaucoma or ocular hypertension with a mean baseline IOP of 26 mm Hg, the IOP-lowering effect of LUMIGAN® (bimatoprost ophthalmic solution) 0.03% once daily (in the evening) was 7–8 mm Hg.
In patients with a history of liver disease or abnormal ALT, AST and/or bilirubin at baseline, LUMIGAN® had no adverse effect on liver function over 24 months.

Indications and Usage: LUMIGAN® (bimatoprost ophthalmic solution) 0.03% is indicated for the reduction of elevated intraocular pressure in patients with open angle glaucoma or ocular hypertension who are intolerant of other intraocular pressure lowering medications or insufficiently responsive (failed to achieve target IOP determined after multiple measurements over time) to another intraocular pressure lowering medication.

Contraindications: LUMIGAN® (bimatoprost ophthalmic solution) 0.03% is contraindicated in patients with hypersensitivity to bimatoprost or any other ingredient in this product.

Warnings: LUMIGAN® (bimatoprost ophthalmic solution) 0.03% has been reported to cause changes to pigmented tissues. These reports include increased pigmentation and growth of eyelashes and increased pigmentation of the iris and periorbital tissue (eyelid). These changes may be permanent.
LUMIGAN® may gradually change eye color, increasing the amount of brown pigment in the iris by increasing the number of melanosomes (pigment granules) in melanocytes. The long-term effects on the melanocytes and the consequences of potential injury to the melanocytes and/or deposition of pigment granules to other areas of the eye are currently unknown. The change in iris color occurs slowly and may not be noticeable for several months to years. Patients should be informed of the possibility of iris color change.
Eyelid skin darkening has also been reported in association with the use of LUMIGAN®.
LUMIGAN® may gradually change eyelashes; these changes include increased length, thickness, pigmentation, and number of lashes.
Patients who are expected to receive treatment in only one eye should be informed about the potential for increased brown pigmentation of the iris, periorbital tissue, and eyelashes in the treated eye and thus, heterochromia between the eyes. They should also be advised of the potential for a disparity between the eyes in length, thickness, and/or number of eyelashes.

Precautions:
General:
There have been reports of bacterial keratitis associated with the use of multiple-dose containers of topical ophthalmic products. These containers had been inadvertently contaminated by patients who, in most cases, had a concurrent corneal disease or a disruption of the ocular epithelial surface (see Information for Patients).
Patients may slowly develop increased brown pigmentation of the iris. This change may not be noticeable for several months to years (see Warnings). Typically the brown pigmentation around the pupil is expected to spread concentrically towards the periphery in affected eyes, but the entire iris or parts of it may also become more brownish. Until more information about increased brown pigmentation is available, patients should be examined regularly and, depending on the clinical situation, treatment may be stopped if increased pigmentation ensues. The increase in brown iris pigment is not expected to progress further upon discontinuation of treatment, but the resultant color change may be permanent. Neither nevi nor freckles of the iris are expected to be affected by treatment.
LUMIGAN® (bimatoprost ophthalmic solution) 0.03% should be used with caution in patients with active intraocular inflammation (e.g., uveitis).
Macular edema, including cystoid macular edema, has been reported during treatment with bimatoprost ophthalmic solution. LUMIGAN® should be used with caution in aphakic patients, in pseudophakic patients with a torn posterior lens capsule, or in patients with known risk factors for macular edema.
LUMIGAN® has not been evaluated for the treatment of angle closure, inflammatory or neovascular glaucoma.
LUMIGAN® should not be administered while wearing contact lenses.

Information for Patients:
Patients should be informed that LUMIGAN® has been reported to cause increased growth and darkening of eyelashes and darkening of the skin around the eye in some patients. These changes may be permanent.
Some patients may slowly develop darkening of the iris, which may be permanent.
When only one eye is treated, patients should be informed of the potential for a cosmetic difference between the eyes in eyelash length, darkness or thickness, and/or color changes of the eyelid skin or iris.
Patients should be instructed to avoid allowing the tip of the dispensing container to contact the eye, surrounding structures, fingers, or any other surface in order to avoid contamination of the solution by common bacteria known to cause ocular infections. Serious damage to the eye and subsequent loss of vision may result from using contaminated solutions.
Patients should also be advised that if they develop an intercurrent ocular condition (e.g., trauma or infection) or have ocular surgery, they should immediately seek their physician's advice concerning the continued use of the multidose container.
Patients should be advised that if they develop any ocular reactions, particularly conjunctivitis and eyelid reactions, they should immediately seek their physician's advice.
Contact lenses should be removed prior to instillation of LUMIGAN® and may be reinserted 15 minutes following its administration. Patients should be advised that LUMIGAN® contains benzalkonium chloride, which may be absorbed by soft contact lenses. If more than one topical ophthalmic drug is being used, the drugs should be administered at least five (5) minutes between applications.

Carcinogenesis, Mutagenesis, Impairment of Fertility:
Carcinogenicity studies were not performed with bimatoprost.
Bimatoprost was not mutagenic or clastogenic in the Ames test, in the mouse lymphoma test, or in the *in vivo* mouse micronucleus tests.
Bimatoprost did not impair fertility in male or female rats up to doses of 0.6 mg/kg/day (approximately 103 times the recommended human exposure based on blood AUC levels).

Pregnancy: *Teratogenic Effects:* **Pregnancy Category C.**
In embryo/fetal developmental studies in pregnant mice and rats, abortion was observed at oral doses of bimatoprost which achieved at least 33 or 97 times, respectively, the intended human exposure based on blood AUC levels.
At doses 41 times the intended human exposure based on blood AUC levels, the gestation length was reduced in the dams, the incidence of dead fetuses, late resorptions, peri- and postnatal pup mortality was increased, and pup body weights were reduced.

There are no adequate and well-controlled studies of LUMIGAN® administration in pregnant women. Because animal reproductive studies are not always predictive of human response, LUMIGAN® should be administered during pregnancy only if the potential benefit justifies the potential risk to the fetus.

Nursing Mothers:
It is not known whether LUMIGAN® is excreted in human milk, although in animal studies, bimatoprost has been shown to be excreted in breast milk. Because many drugs are excreted in human milk, caution should be exercised when LUMIGAN® is administered to a nursing woman.

Pediatric Use:
Safety and effectiveness in pediatric patients have not been established.

Geriatric Use:
No overall clinical differences in safety or effectiveness have been observed between elderly and other adult patients.

Adverse Reactions: In clinical trials, the most frequent events associated with the use of LUMIGAN® (bimatoprost ophthalmic solution) 0.03% occurring in approximately 15% to 45% of patients, in descending order of incidence, included conjunctival hyperemia, growth of eyelashes, and ocular pruritus. Approximately 3% of patients discontinued therapy due to conjunctival hyperemia.
Ocular adverse events occurring in approximately 3 to 10% of patients, in descending order of incidence, included ocular dryness, visual disturbance, ocular burning, foreign body sensation, eye pain, pigmentation of the periocular skin, blepharitis, cataract, superficial punctate keratitis, eyelid erythema, ocular irritation, and eyelash darkening. The following ocular adverse events reported in approximately 1 to 3% of patients, in descending order of incidence, included: eye discharge, tearing, photophobia, allergic conjunctivitis, asthenopia, increases in iris pigmentation, and conjunctival edema. In less than 1% of patients, intraocular inflammation was reported as iritis.
Systemic adverse events reported in approximately 10% of patients were infections (primarily colds and upper respiratory tract infections). The following systemic adverse events reported in approximately 1 to 5% of patients, in descending order of incidence, included headaches, abnormal liver function tests, asthenia and hirsutism.

Overdosage: No information is available on overdosage in humans. If overdose with LUMIGAN® (bimatoprost ophthalmic solution) 0.03% occurs, treatment should be symptomatic.
In oral (by gavage) mouse and rat studies, doses up to 100 mg/kg/day did not produce any toxicity. This dose expressed as mg/m^2 is at least 70 times higher than the accidental dose of one bottle of LUMIGAN® for a 10 kg child.

Dosage and Administration: The recommended dosage is one drop in the affected eye(s) once daily in the evening. The dosage of LUMIGAN® (bimatoprost ophthalmic solution) 0.03% should not exceed once daily since it has been shown that more frequent administration may decrease the intraocular pressure lowering effect.
Reduction of the intraocular pressure starts approximately 4 hours after the first administration with maximum effect reached within approximately 8 to 12 hours.
LUMIGAN® may be used concomitantly with other topical ophthalmic drug products to lower intraocular pressure. If more than one topical ophthalmic drug is being used, the drugs should be administered at least five (5) minutes apart.

How Supplied: LUMIGAN® (bimatoprost ophthalmic solution) 0.03% is supplied sterile in opaque white low density polyethylene ophthalmic dispenser bottles and tips with turquoise polystyrene caps in the following sizes: 2.5 mL fill in 5 mL container — NDC 0023-9187-03; 5 mL fill in 8 mL container — NDC 0023-9187-05; or 7.5 mL fill in 8 mL container — NDC 0023-9187-07.
℞ only
Storage: LUMIGAN® should be stored in the original container at 2° to 25°C (36° to 77°F).
ALLERGAN
® Marks owned by Allergan, Inc.
US Pat. 5,688,819 and 6,403,649
July 2003
©Allergan, Inc., Irvine, CA 92612
Shown in Product Identification Guide, page 103

OCUFEN®   ℞
(flurbiprofen sodium ophthalmic solution, USP) 0.03%
sterile

Description: OCUFEN® (flurbiprofen sodium ophthalmic solution, USP) 0.03% is a sterile topical nonsteroidal anti-inflammatory product for ophthalmic use.
Chemical Name: Sodium (±)-2-(2-fluoro-4-biphenylyl)-propionate dihydrate.
Contains: Active: flurbiprofen sodium 0.03% (0.3 mg/mL).
Preservative: thimerosal 0.005%.
Inactives: citric acid; edetate disodium; polyvinyl alcohol 1.4%; potassium chloride; purified water; sodium chloride; and sodium citrate. May also contain hydrochloric acid and/or sodium hydroxide to adjust the pH. The pH of OCUFEN® ophthalmic solution is 6.0 to 7.0. It has an osmolality of 260-330 mOsm/kg.
Clinical Pharmacology: Flurbiprofen sodium is one of a series of phenylalkanoic acids that have shown analgesic, antipyretic, and anti-inflammatory activity in animal inflammatory diseases. Its mechanism of action is believed to be through inhibition of the cyclo-oxygenase enzyme that is essential in the biosynthesis of prostaglandins.
Prostaglandins have been shown in many animal models to be mediators of certain kinds of intraocular inflammation. In studies performed on animal eyes, prostaglandins have been shown to produce disruption of the blood-aqueous humor barrier, vasodilatation, increased vascular permeability, leukocytosis, and increased intraocular pressure.
Prostaglandins also appear to play a role in the miotic response produced during ocular surgery by constricting the iris sphincter independently of cholinergic mechanisms. In clinical studies, OCUFEN® ophthalmic solution has been shown to inhibit the miosis induced during the course of cataract surgery.
Results from clinical studies indicate that flurbiprofen sodium has no significant effect upon intraocular pressure.
Indications and Usage: OCUFEN® ophthalmic solution is indicated for the inhibition of intraoperative miosis.
Contraindications: OCUFEN® ophthalmic solution is contraindicated in individuals who are hypersensitive to any components of the medication.
Warnings: With nonsteroidal anti-inflammatory drugs, there exists the potential for increased bleeding due to interference with thrombocyte aggregation. There have been reports that OCUFEN® ophthalmic solution may cause increased bleeding of ocular tissues including hyphemas in conjunction with ocular surgery. There exists the potential for cross-sensitivity to acetylsalicylic acid and other nonsteroidal anti-inflammatory drugs. Therefore, caution should be used when treating individuals who have previously exhibited sensitivities to these drugs.

Precautions:
General: Wound healing may be delayed with the use of OCUFEN® ophthalmic solution. It is recommended that OCUFEN® ophthalmic solution be used with caution in surgical patients with known bleeding tendencies or who are receiving other medications which may prolong bleeding time.
Drug Interactions: Interaction of OCUFEN® ophthalmic solution with other topical ophthalmic medications has not been fully investigated. Although clinical studies with acetylcholine chloride and animal studies with acetylcholine chloride or carbachol revealed no interference, and there is no known pharmacological basis for an interaction, there have been reports that acetylcholine chloride and carbachol have been ineffective when used in patients treated with OCUFEN® ophthalmic solution.
Carcinogenesis, Mutagenesis, Impairment of Fertility: Long-term studies in mice and/or rats have shown no evidence of carcinogenicity with flurbiprofen.
Long-term mutagenicity studies in animals have not been performed.
Pregnancy: Pregnancy Category C. Flurbiprofen has been shown to be embryocidal, delay parturition, prolong gestation, reduce weight, and/or slightly retard growth of fetuses when given to rats in daily oral doses of 0.4 mg/kg (approximately 333 times the human daily topical dose) and above.
Nursing Mothers: It is not known whether this drug is excreted in human milk. Because many drugs are excreted in human milk and because of the potential for serious adverse reactions in nursing infants from flurbiprofen sodium, a decision should be made whether to discontinue nursing or to discontinue the drug, taking into account the importance of the drug to the mother.
Pediatric use: Safety and effectiveness in pediatric patients have not been established.
Geriatric Use: No overall differences in safety or effectiveness have been observed between elderly and younger patients.
Adverse Reactions: Transient burning and stinging upon instillation and other minor symptoms of ocular irritation have been reported with the use of OCUFEN® ophthalmic solution. Other adverse reactions reported with the use of OCUFEN® ophthalmic solution include: fibrosis, miosis, and mydriasis. Increased bleeding tendency of ocular tissues in conjunction with ocular surgery has also been reported.
Overdosage: Overdosage will not ordinarily cause acute problems. If accidentally ingested, drink fluids to dilute.
Dosage and Administration: A total of four (4) drops of OCUFEN® ophthalmic solution should be administered by instilling 1 drop approximately every $1/2$ hour beginning 2 hours before surgery.
How Supplied: OCUFEN® (flurbiprofen sodium ophthalmic solution, USP) is available for topical ophthalmic administration as a 0.03% sterile solution, and is supplied in a white opaque low density polyethylene bottle with a controlled dropper tip and a gray high impact polystyrene cap in the following size:
2.5 mL fill in 5 mL bottle—NDC 11980-801-03
Note: Store between 15°–25°C (59–77°F)
℞ only
©2004 Allergan, Inc.
Irvine, CA 92612
® Marks owned by Allergan, Inc.

Continued on next page

OPHTHETIC® ℞
(proparacaine HCl ophthalmic solution) 0.5% sterile

Description: OPHTHETIC® (proparacaine HCl ophthalmic solution) 0.5% is a topical local anesthetic for ophthalmic use.

Chemical Name:
Benzoic acid, 3-amino-4-propoxy-, 2-(diethylamino)ethyl ester, monohydrochloride.

Contains: Active: proparacaine HCl 0.5%
Preservative: benzalkonium chloride (0.01%)
Inactives: glycerin; purified water; sodium chloride; and hydrochloric acid and/or sodium hydroxide to adjust pH (5.0 to 6.0).

Clinical Pharmacology: OPHTHETIC® ophthalmic solution is a rapidly-acting topical anesthetic, with induced anesthesia lasting approximately 10–20 minutes.

Indications and Usage: OPHTHETIC® ophthalmic solution is indicated for procedures in which a topical ophthalmic anesthetic is indicated: corneal anesthesia of short duration, e.g., tonometry, gonioscopy, removal of corneal foreign bodies, and for short corneal and conjunctival procedures.

Contraindications: OPHTHETIC® ophthalmic solution should be considered contraindicated in patients with known hypersensitivity to any of the ingredients of this preparation.

Warnings: Prolonged use of a topical ocular anesthetic is not recommended. It may produce permanent corneal opacification with accompanying visual loss.

Precautions: Carcinogenesis, Mutagenesis, Impairment of Fertility: Long-term studies in animals have not been performed to evaluate carcinogenic potential, mutagenicity, or possible impairment of fertility in males or females.

Pregnancy: Pregnancy Category C: Animal reproduction studies have not been conducted with OPHTHETIC® (proparacaine hydrochloride ophthalmic solution) 0.5%. It is also not known whether proparacaine hydrochloride can cause fetal harm when administered to a pregnant woman or can affect reproduction capacity. Proparacaine hydrochloride should be administered to a pregnant woman only if clearly needed.

Nursing Mothers: It is not known whether this drug is excreted in human milk. Because many drugs are excreted in human milk, caution should be exercised when proparacaine hydrochloride is administered to a nursing mother.

Pediatric Use: Safety and effectiveness of proparacaine HCl ophthalmic solution in pediatric patients have been established. Use of proparacaine HCl is supported by evidence from adequate and well-controlled studies in adults and children over the age of twelve, and safety information in neonates and other pediatric patients.

Geriatric Use: No overall clinical differences in safety or effectiveness have been observed between the elderly and other adult patients.

Adverse Reactions: Occasional temporary stinging, burning, and conjunctival redness may occur with the use of proparacaine. A rare, severe, immediate-type, apparently hyperallergic corneal reaction, characterized by acute, intense and diffuse epithelial keratitis, a gray, ground glass appearance, sloughing of large areas of necrotic epithelium, corneal filaments and sometimes, iritis with descemetitis has been reported.

Allergic contact dermatitis from proparacaine with drying and fissuring of the fingertips has also been reported.

Dosage and Administration:
Usual Dosage: Removal of foreign bodies and sutures, and for tonometry: 1 to 2 drops (in single instillations) in each eye before operating.

Short corneal and conjunctival procedures: 1 drop in each eye every 5 to 10 minutes for 5–7 doses.

Note: OPHTHETIC® should be clear to straw-color. If the solution becomes darker, discard the solution.

How Supplied:
OPHTHETIC® (proparacaine HCl ophthalmic solution) 0.5% is supplied in opaque natural LDPE bottles with dropper tips and white high impact polystyrene (HIPS) cap as follows:

15 mL in 15 mL bottle—NDC 11980-048-15
Bottle must be stored in unit carton to protect contents from light. Store bottles under refrigeration at 2°C to 8°C (36°F to 46°F).

℞ only
©2002 Allergan, Inc.
Irvine CA 92612 U.S.A.
®Marks owned by Allergan, Inc.

POLY–PRED® ℞
(prednisolone acetate, neomycin sulfate, polymyxin B sulfate)
Liquifilm®
sterile ophthalmic suspension

Description: POLY-PRED® Liquifilm® sterile ophthalmic suspension is a topical anti-inflammatory/anti-infective combination product for ophthalmic use.

Chemical Name: Prednisolone acetate: 11β, 17, 21-Trihydroxypregna-1, 4-diene-3, 20-dione 21-acetate.

Neomycin sulfate is the sulfate salt of neomycin B and neomycin C which are produced by the growth of *Streptomyces fradiae* (Fam. *Streptomycetaceae*). It has a potency equivalent to not less than 600 micrograms per milligram of neomycin base, calculated on an anhydrous basis.

Polymyxin B sulfate is the sulfate salt of polymyxin B_1 and polymyxin B_2 which are produced by the growth of *Bacillus polymyxa* (Prazmowski) Migula (Fam. *Bacillaceae*). It has a potency of not less than 6,000 polymyxin B units per milligram, calculated on an anhydrous basis.

Contains: Actives: prednisolone acetate (microfine suspension) 0.5%, neomycin sulfate equivalent to 0.35% neomycin base, polymyxin B sulfate 10,000 units/mL. Preservative: thimerosal 0.001%. Inactives: Liquifilm® (polyvinyl alcohol) 1.4%; polysorbate 80; propylene glycol; sodium acetate; and purified water.

Clinical Pharmacology: Corticosteroids suppress the inflammatory response to a variety of agents and they probably delay or slow healing. Since corticosteroids may inhibit the body's defense mechanism against infection, a concomitant antimicrobial drug may be used when this inhibition is considered to be clinically significant in a particular case.

The anti-infective components in POLY-PRED® are included to provide action against specific organisms susceptible to them. Neomycin sulfate and polymyxin B sulfate are considered active against the following microorganisms: *Staphylococcus aureus*; *Escherichia coli*; *Haemophilus influenzae*; *Klebsiella / Enterobacter* species; *Neisseria* species; and *Pseudomonas aeruginosa*.

When a decision to administer both a corticosteroid and an antimicrobial is made, the administration of such drugs in combination has the advantage of greater patient compliance and convenience, with the added assurance that the appropriate dosage of both drugs is administered. When both types of drugs are in the same formulation, compatibility of ingredients is assured and the correct volume of drug is delivered and retained.

The relative potency of corticosteroids depends on the molecular structure, concentration and release from the vehicle.

Indications and Usage: A steroid/anti-infective combination is indicated for steroid-responsive inflammatory ocular conditions for which a corticosteroid is indicated and where bacterial infection or a risk of bacterial ocular infection exists.

Ocular steroids are indicated in inflammatory conditions of the palpebral and bulbar conjunctiva, cornea, and anterior segment of the globe where the inherent risk of steroid use in certain infective conjunctivitides is accepted to obtain a diminution in edema and inflammation. They are also indicated in chronic anterior uveitis and corneal injury from chemical, radiation or thermal burns or penetration of foreign bodies.

The use of a combination drug with an anti-infective component is indicated where the risk of infection is high or where there is an expectation that potentially dangerous numbers of bacteria will be present in the eye.

The particular anti-infective drugs in this product are active against the following common bacterial eye pathogens: *Staphylococcus aureus*; *Escherichia coli*; *Haemophilus influenzae*; *Klebsiella / Enterobacter* species; *Neisseria* species; and *Pseudomonas aeruginosa*.

The product does not provide adequate coverage against: *Serratia marcescens*; Streptococci, including *Streptococcus pneumoniae*.

Contraindications: Epithelial herpes simplex keratitis (dendritic keratitis), vaccinia, varicella, and many other viral diseases of the cornea and conjunctiva. Mycobacterial infection of the eye. Fungal diseases of the ocular structures. Hypersensitivity to a component of the medication. (Hypersensitivity to the antibiotic component occurs at a higher rate than for other components.)

The use of these combinations is always contraindicated after uncomplicated removal of a corneal foreign body.

Warnings: Prolonged use may result in glaucoma, with damage to the optic nerve, defects in visual acuity and fields of vision, and in posterior subcapsular cataract formation. Prolonged use may suppress the host response and thus increase the hazard of secondary ocular infections. In those diseases causing thinning of the cornea or sclera, perforations have been known to occur with the use of topical steroids. In acute purulent conditions of the eye, steroids may mask infection or enhance existing infection. If these products are used for 10 days or longer, intraocular pressure should be routinely monitored even though it may be difficult in children and uncooperative patients.

Employment of a steroid medication in the treatment of herpes simplex requires great caution.

There exists a potential for neomycin sulfate to cause cutaneous sensitization. The exact incidence of this reaction is unknown.

Precautions: The initial prescription and renewal of the medication order beyond 20 milliliters should be made by a physician only after examination of the patient with the aid of magnification, such as slit lamp biomicroscopy and, where appropriate, fluorescein staining.

The possibility of persistent fungal infections of the cornea should be considered after prolonged steroid dosing.

Adverse Reactions: Adverse reactions have occurred with steroid/anti-infective combination drugs which can be attributed to the steroid component, the anti-infective component, or the combination. Exact incidence figures are not available since no denominator of treated patients is available.

Reactions occurring most often from the presence of the anti-infective ingredients are allergic sensitizations. The reactions due to the steroid component in decreasing order of frequency are: elevation of intraocular pressure (IOP) with possible development of glaucoma, and infrequent optic nerve damage; posterior subcapsular cataract formation; and delayed wound healing.

Secondary Infection: The development of secondary infection has occurred after use of combinations containing steroids and antimicrobials. Fungal infections of the cornea are particularly prone to develop coincidentally with long-term applications of steroid. The possibility of fungal invasion must be considered in any persistent corneal ulceration where steroid treatment has been used.

Secondary bacterial ocular infection following suppression of host responses also occurs.

Dosage and Administration: TO TREAT THE EYE: 1 or 2 drops every 3 or 4 hours, or more frequently as required. Acute infections may require administration every 30 minutes, with frequency of administration reduced as the infection is brought under control. TO TREAT THE LIDS: Instill 1 or 2 drops in the eye every 3 to 4 hours, close the eye and rub the excess on the lids and lid margins.

Not more than 20 milliliters should be prescribed initially and the prescription should not be refilled without further evaluation as outlined in the **Precautions** section above.

How Supplied: POLY-PRED® Liquifilm® sterile ophthalmic suspension is supplied in plastic dropper bottles in the following sizes:
    5 mL—NDC 0023-0028-05
    10 mL—NDC 0023-0028-10

Note: Store at or below 25°C (77°F). Protect from freezing. **Shake well before using.**
℞ only

POLYTRIM® ℞
(trimethoprim sulfate and polymyxin B sulfate ophthalmic solution) Sterile

Description: POLYTRIM® (trimethoprim sulfate and polymyxin B sulfate ophthalmic solution) is a sterile antimicrobial solution for topical ophthalmic use. It has pH of 4.0 to 6.2 and osmolality of 270 to 310 mOsm/kg.

Chemical Names: Trimethoprim sulfate, 2,4-Diamino-5-(3,4,5-trimethoxybenzyl) pyrimidine sulfate, is a white, odorless, crystalline powder with a molecular weight of 678.72.

Polymyxin B sulfate is the sulfate salt of polymyxin B_1 and B_2 which are produced by the growth of *Bacillus polymyxa* (Prazmowski) Migula (Fam. Bacillaceae). It has a potency of not less than 6,000 polymyxin B units per mg, calculated on an anhydrous basis.

Contains: Actives: trimethoprim sulfate equivalent to 1 mg/mL; polymyxin B sulfate 10,000 units/mL. Preservative: benzalkonium chloride 0.04 mg/mL. Inactives: sodium chloride, sulfuric acid and purified water. May also contain sodium hydroxide for pH adjustment.

Clinical Pharmacology: Trimethoprim is a synthetic antibacterial drug active against a wide variety of aerobic gram-positive and gram-negative ophthalmic pathogens. Trimethoprim blocks the production of tetrahydrofolic acid from dihydrofolic acid by binding to and reversibly inhibiting the enzyme dihydrofolate reductase. This binding is stronger for the bacterial enzyme than for the corresponding mammalian enzyme and therefore selectively interferes with bacterial biosynthesis of nucleic acids and proteins.

Polymyxin B, a cyclic lipopeptide antibiotic, is bactericidal for a variety of gram-negative organisms, especially *Pseudomonas aeruginosa*. It increases the permeability of the bacterial cell membrane by interacting with the phospholipid components of the membrane.

Blood samples were obtained from 11 human volunteers at 20 minutes, 1 hour and 3 hours following instillation in the eye of 2 drops of ophthalmic solution containing 1 mg trimethoprim and 10,000 units polymyxin B per mL.

Peak serum concentrations were approximately 0.03 µg/mL trimethoprim and 1 unit/mL polymyxin B.

Microbiology: *In vitro* studies have demonstrated that the anti-infective components of POLYTRIM® are active against the following bacterial pathogens that are capable of causing external infections of the eye:

Trimethoprim: *Staphylococcus aureus* and *Staphylococcus epidermidis*, *Streptococcus pyogenes*, *Streptococcus faecalis*, *Streptococcus pneumoniae*, *Haemophilus influenzae*, *Haemophilus aegyptius*, *Escherichia coli*, *Klebsiella pneumoniae*, *Proteus mirabilis* (indole-negative), *Proteus vulgaris* (indole-positive), *Enterobacter aerogenes*, and *Serratia marcescens*.

Polymyxin B: *Pseudomonas aeruginosa*, *Escherichia coli*, *Klebsiella pneumoniae*, *Enterobacter aerogenes* and *Haemophilus influenzae*.

Indications and Usage: POLYTRIM® Ophthalmic Solution is indicated in the treatment of surface ocular bacterial infections, including acute bacterial conjunctivitis, and blepharoconjunctivitis, caused by susceptible strains of the following microorganisms: *Staphylococcus aureus*, *Staphylococcus epidermidis*, *Streptococcus pneumoniae*, *Streptococcus viridans*, *Haemophilus influenzae* and *Pseudomonas aeruginosa.**

*Efficacy for this organism in this organ system was studied in fewer than 10 infections.

Contraindications: POLYTRIM® Ophthalmic Solution is contraindicated in patients with known hypersensitivity to any of its components.

Warnings: NOT FOR INJECTION INTO THE EYE.

If a sensitivity reaction to POLYTRIM® occurs, discontinue use. POLYTRIM® Ophthalmic Solution is not indicated for the prophylaxis or treatment of ophthalmia neonatorum.

Precautions:

General: As with other antimicrobial preparations, prolonged use may result in overgrowth of nonsusceptible organisms, including fungi. If superinfection occurs, appropriate therapy should be initiated.

Information for Patients: Avoid contaminating the applicator tip with material from the eye, fingers, or other source. This precaution is necessary if the sterility of the drops is to be maintained.

If redness, irritation, swelling or pain persists or increases, discontinue use immediately and contact your physician. Patients should be advised not to wear contact lenses if they have signs and symptoms of ocular bacterial infections.

Carcinogenesis, Mutagenesis, Impairment of Fertility:

Carcinogenesis: Long-term studies in animals to evaluate carcinogenic potential have not been conducted with polymyxin B sulfate or trimethoprim.

Mutagenesis: Trimethoprim was demonstrated to be non-mutagenic in the Ames assay. In studies at two laboratories no chromosomal damage was detected in cultured Chinese hamster ovary cells at concentrations approximately 500 times human plasma levels after oral administration; at concentrations approximately 1000 times human plasma levels after oral administration in these same cells, a low level of chromosomal damage was induced at one of the laboratories. Studies to evaluate mutagenic potential have not been conducted with polymyxin B sulfate.

Impairment of Fertility: Polymyxin B sulfate has been reported to impair the motility of equine sperm, but its effects on male or female fertility are unknown.

No adverse effects on fertility or general reproductive performance were observed in rats given trimethoprim in oral dosages as high as 70 mg/kg/day for males and 14 mg/kg/day for females.

Pregnancy: *Teratogenic Effects: Pregnancy Category C.* Animal reproduction studies have not been conducted with polymyxin B sulfate. It is not known whether polymyxin B sulfate can cause fetal harm when administered to a pregnant woman or can affect reproduction capacity.

Trimethoprim has been shown to be teratogenic in the rat when given in oral doses 40 times the human dose. In some rabbit studies, the overall increase in fetal loss (dead and resorbed and malformed conceptuses) was associated with oral doses 6 times the human therapeutic dose.

While there are no large well-controlled studies on the use of trimethoprim in pregnant women, Brumfitt and Pursell, in a retrospective study, reported the outcome of 186 pregnancies during which the mother received either placebo or oral trimethoprim in combination with sulfamethoxazole. The incidence of congenital abnormalities was 4.5% (3 of 66) in those who received placebo and 3.3% (4 of 120) in those receiving trimethoprim and sulfamethoxazole. There were no abnormalities in the 10 children whose mothers received the drug during the first trimester. In a separate survey, Brumfitt and Pursell also found no congenital abnormalities in 35 children whose mothers had received oral trimethoprim and sulfamethoxazole at the time of conception or shortly thereafter.

Because trimethoprim may interfere with folic acid metabolism, trimethoprim should be used during pregnancy only if the potential benefit justifies the potential risk to the fetus.

Nonteratogenic Effects: The oral administration of trimethoprim to rats at a dose of 70 mg/kg/day commencing with the last third of gestation and continuing through parturition and lactation caused no deleterious effects on gestation or pup growth and survival.

Nursing Mothers: It is not known whether this drug is excreted in human milk. Because many drugs are excreted in human milk, caution should be exercised when POLYTRIM® Ophthalmic Solution is administered to a nursing woman.

Pediatric Use: Safety and effectiveness in children below the age of 2 months have not been established (see **Warnings**).

Geriatric Use: No overall differences in safety or effectiveness have been observed between elderly and other adult patients.

Adverse Reactions: The most frequent adverse reaction to POLYTRIM® Ophthalmic Solution is local irritation consisting of increased redness, burning, stinging, and/or itching. This may occur on instillation, within 48 hours, or at any time with extended use. There are also multiple reports of hypersensitivity reactions consisting of lid edema, itching, increased redness, tearing, and/or circumocular rash. Photosensitivity has been reported in patients taking oral trimethoprim.

Dosage and Administration: In mild to moderate infections, instill one drop in the affected eye(s) every three hours (maximum of 6 doses per day) for a period of 7 to 10 days.

How Supplied: Polytrim® (trimethoprim sulfate and polymyxin B sulfate ophthalmic solution) is supplied sterile in opaque white low density polyethylene ophthalmic dispenser bottles and tips with white high impact polystyrene (HIPS) caps as follows: 10 mL in 10 mL bottle—NDC 0023-7824-10.

Note: Store at 15°–25°C (59°–77°F) and protect from light.
℞ only

Continued on next page

Polytrim—Cont.

©2001 Allergan, Inc.
Irvine, CA 92612
® Marks owned by Allergan, Inc.

PRED FORTE® ℞
(prednisolone acetate ophthalmic suspension, USP) 1% sterile

Description: PRED FORTE® (prednisolone acetate ophthalmic suspension, USP) 1% is a topical anti-inflammatory agent for ophthalmic use.
Chemical Name: 11β, 17, 21-Trihydroxypregna-1,4-diene-3,20-dione 21-acetate.
Contains: Active: prednisolone acetate (microfine suspension) 1.0%. **Preservative:** benzalkonium chloride. **Inactives:** boric acid; edetate disodium; hydroxypropyl methylcellulose; polysorbate 80; purified water; sodium bisulfite; sodium chloride; and sodium citrate. The pH during its shelf life ranges from 5.0 to 6.0.
Clinical Pharmacology: Prednisolone acetate is a glucocorticoid that, on the basis of weight, has 3 to 5 times the anti-inflammatory potency of hydrocortisone. Glucocorticoids inhibit the edema, fibrin deposition, capillary dilation and phagocytic migration of the acute inflammatory response, as well as capillary proliferation, deposition of collagen, and scar formation.
Indications and Usage: PRED FORTE® is indicated for the treatment of steroid-responsive inflammation of the palpebral and bulbar conjunctiva, cornea and anterior segment of the globe.
Contraindications: PRED FORTE® suspension is contraindicated in most viral diseases of the cornea and conjunctiva including epithelial herpes simplex keratitis (dendritic keratitis), vaccinia, and varicella, and also in mycobacterial infection of the eye and fungal diseases of ocular structures. PRED FORTE® suspension is also contraindicated in individuals with known or suspected hypersensitivity to any of the ingredients of this preparation and to other corticosteroids.
Warnings: Prolonged use of corticosteroids may result in glaucoma with damage to the optic nerve, defects in visual acuity and fields of vision, and in posterior subcapsular cataract formation. Prolonged use may also suppress the host immune response and thus increase the hazard of secondary ocular infections.
Various ocular diseases and long-term use of topical corticosteroids have been known to cause corneal and scleral thinning. Use of topical corticosteroids in the presence of thin corneal or scleral tissue may lead to perforation.
Acute purulent infections of the eye may be masked or activity enhanced by the presence of corticosteroid medication.
If this product is used for 10 days or longer, intraocular pressure should be routinely monitored even though it may be difficult in children and uncooperative patients. Steroids should be used with caution in the presence of glaucoma. Intraocular pressure should be checked frequently.
The use of steroids after cataract surgery may delay healing and increase the incidence of bleb formation.
Use of ocular steroids may prolong the course and may exacerbate the severity of many viral infections of the eye (including herpes simplex). Employment of a corticosteroid medication in the treatment of patients with a history of herpes simplex requires great caution; frequent slit lamp microscopy is recommended.
Corticosteroids are not effective in mustard gas keratitis and Sjögren's keratoconjunctivitis.
Contains sodium bisulfite, a sulfite that may cause allergic-type reactions, including anaphylactic symptoms and life-threatening or less severe asthmatic episodes in certain susceptible people. The overall prevalence of sulfite sensitivity in the general population is unknown and probably low. Sulfite sensitivity is seen more frequently in asthmatic than in nonasthmatic people.
Precautions:
General: The initial prescription and renewal of the medication order beyond 20 milliliters of PRED FORTE® suspension should be made by a physician only after examination of the patient with the aid of magnification, such as slit-lamp biomicroscopy, and, where appropriate, fluorescein staining. If signs and symptoms fail to improve after 2 days, the patient should be re-evaluated.
As fungal infections of the cornea are particularly prone to develop coincidentally with long-term local corticosteroid applications, fungal invasion should be suspected in any persistent corneal ulceration where a corticosteroid has been used or is in use. Fungal cultures should be taken when appropriate.
If this product is used for 10 days or longer, intraocular pressure should be monitored (see **Warnings**).
Information for Patients: If inflammation or pain persists longer than 48 hours or becomes aggravated, the patient should be advised to discontinue use of the medication and consult a physician.
This product is sterile when packaged. To prevent contamination, care should be taken to avoid touching the bottle tip to eyelids or to any other surface. The use of this bottle by more than one person may spread infection. Keep bottle tightly closed when not in use. Keep out of the reach of children.
Carcinogenesis, Mutagenesis, Impairment of Fertility: No studies have been conducted in animals or in humans to evaluate the potential of these effects.
Pregnancy Category C: Prednisolone has been shown to be teratogenic in mice when given in doses 1–10 times the human dose. There are no adequate well-controlled studies in pregnant women. Prednisolone should be used during pregnancy only if the potential benefit justifies the potential risk to the fetus.
Dexamethasone, hydrocortisone and prednisolone were ocularly applied to both eyes of pregnant mice five times per day on days 10 through 13 of gestation. A significant increase in the incidence of cleft palate was observed in the fetuses of the treated mice.
Nursing Mothers: It is not known whether topical ophthalmic administration of corticosteroids could result in sufficient systemic absorption to produce detectable quantities in breast milk. Systemically administered corticosteroids appear in human milk and could suppress growth, interfere with endogenous corticosteroid production, or cause other untoward effects. Because of the potential for serious adverse reactions in nursing infants from prednisolone, a decision should be made whether to discontinue nursing or discontinue the drug, taking into account the importance of the drug to the mother.
Pediatric Use: Safety and effectiveness in pediatric patients have not been established.
Geriatric Use: No overall differences in safety or effectiveness have been observed between elderly and younger patients.
Adverse Reactions: Adverse reactions include, in decreasing order of frequency, elevation of intraocular pressure (IOP) with possible development of glaucoma and infrequent optic nerve damage, posterior subcapsular cataract formation, and delayed wound healing. Although systemic effects are extremely uncommon, there have been rare occurrences of systemic hypercorticoidism after use of topical steroids.
Corticosteroid-containing preparations have also been reported to cause acute anterior uveitis and perforation of the globe. Keratitis, conjunctivitis, corneal ulcers, mydriasis, conjunctival hyperemia, loss of accommodation and ptosis have occasionally been reported following local use of corticosteroids.
The development of secondary ocular infection (bacterial, fungal, and viral) have occurred. Fungal and viral infections of the cornea are particularly prone to develop coincidentally with long-term applications of steroid. The possibility of fungal invasion should be considered in any persistent corneal ulceration where steroid treatment has been used (see **Warnings**).
Transient burning and stinging upon instillation and other minor symptoms of ocular irritation have been reported with the use of PRED FORTE® suspension. Other adverse events reported with the use of PRED FORTE® suspension include: visual disturbance (blurry vision) and allergic reactions.
Overdosage: Overdosage will not ordinarily cause acute problems. If accidentally ingested, drink fluids to dilute.
Dosage and Administration: Shake well before using. Instill one to two drops into the conjunctival sac two to four times daily. During the initial 24 to 48 hours, the dosing frequency may be increased if necessary. Care should be taken not to discontinue therapy prematurely. If signs and symptoms fail to improve after 2 days, the patient should be re-evaluated (see **Precautions**).
How Supplied: PRED FORTE® (prednisolone acetate ophthalmic suspension, USP) 1% is supplied sterile in opaque white LDPE plastic bottles with droppers with white high impact polystyrene (HIPS) caps as follows:
1 mL in 5 mL bottle – NDC 11980-180-01
5 mL in 10 mL bottle – NDC 11980-180-05
10 mL in 15 mL bottle – NDC 11980-180-10
15 mL in 15 mL bottle – NDC 11980-180-15
Note: Store at temperatures up to 25°C (77°F). Protect from freezing. Store in an upright position.
℞ only
©2004 Allergan, Inc.
Irvine, CA 92612
® Marks owned by Allergan, Inc.
Shown in Product Identification Guide, page 103

PRED–G® ℞
(gentamicin and prednisolone acetate ophthalmic suspension, USP) 0.3%/1% sterile

Description: PRED-G® sterile ophthalmic suspension is a topical anti-inflammatory/anti-infective combination product for ophthalmic use.
Chemical Names: Prednisolone acetate: 11β, 17,21-Trihydroxypregna-1,4-diene-3,20-dione 21-acetate.
Gentamicin sulfate is the sulfate salt of gentamicin C_1, gentamicin C_2, and gentamicin C_{1A} which are produced by the growth of *Micromonospora purpurea*.
Contains: Actives: Gentamicin sulfate equivalent to 0.3% gentamicin base; prednisolone acetate (microfine suspension) 1.0%. **Preservative:** Benzalkonium chloride 0.005%. **Inactives:** Edetate disodium; hypromellose; polyvinyl alcohol 1.4%; polysorbate 80; purified water; sodium chloride; and sodium citrate, dihydrate. May contain sodium hydroxide and/or hydrochloric acid to adjust the pH (5.4 to 6.6).

PRED-G® suspension is formulated with a pH from 5.4 to 6.6 and its osmolality ranges from 260 to 340 mOsm/kg.

Clinical Pharmacology: Corticosteroids suppress the inflammatory response to a variety of agents and they probably delay or slow healing. Since corticosteroids may inhibit the body's defense mechanism against infection, a concomitant antimicrobial drug may be used when this inhibition is considered to be clinically significant in a particular case.

The anti-infective component in PRED-G® is included to provide action against specific organisms susceptible to it. Gentamicin sulfate is active *in vitro* against susceptible strains of the following microorganisms: *Staphylococcus aureus, Streptococcus pyogenes, Streptococcus pneumoniae, Enterobacter aerogenes, Escherichia coli, Haemophilus influenzae, Klebsiella pneumoniae, Neisseria gonorrhoeae, Pseudomonas aeruginosa, and Serratia marcescens.*

When a decision to administer both a corticosteroid and an antimicrobial is made, the administration of such drugs in combination has the advantage of greater patient compliance and convenience, with the added assurance that the appropriate dosage of both drugs is administered. When both types of drugs are in the same formulation, compatibility of ingredients is assured and the correct volume of drug is delivered and retained.

The relative potency of corticosteroids depends on the molecular structure, concentration, and release from the vehicle.

Indications and Usage: PRED-G® suspension is indicated for steroid-responsive inflammatory ocular conditions for which a corticosteroid is indicated and where superficial bacterial ocular infection or a risk of bacterial ocular infection exists.

Ocular steroids are indicated in inflammatory conditions of the palpebral and bulbar conjunctiva, cornea, and anterior segment of the globe where the inherent risk of steroid use in certain infective conjunctivitides is accepted to obtain a diminution in edema and inflammation. They are also indicated in chronic anterior uveitis and corneal injury from chemical, radiation, or thermal burns or penetration of foreign bodies.

The use of a combination drug with an anti-infective component is indicated where the risk of superficial ocular infection is high or where there is an expectation that potentially dangerous numbers of bacteria will be present in the eye.

The particular anti-infective drug in this product is active against the following common bacterial eye pathogens: *Staphylococcus aureus, Streptococcus pyogenes, Streptococcus pneumoniae, Enterobacter aerogenes, Escherichia coli, Haemophilus influenzae, Klebsiella pneumoniae, Neisseria gonorrhoeae, Pseudomonas aeruginosa, and Serratia marcescens.*

Contraindications: PRED-G® suspension is contraindicated in most viral diseases of the cornea and conjunctiva including epithelial herpes simplex keratitis (dendritic keratitis), vaccinia, and varicella, and also in mycobacterial infection of the eye and fungal diseases of the ocular structures. PRED-G® suspension is also contraindicated in individuals with known or suspected hypersensitivity to any of the ingredients of this preparation or to other corticosteroids.

Warnings: Prolonged use of corticosteroids may result in glaucoma with damage to the optic nerve, defects in visual acuity and fields of vision, and in posterior subcapsular cataract formation. Prolonged use of corticosteroids may suppress the host response and thus increase the hazard of secondary ocular infections.

Various ocular diseases and long-term use of topical corticosteroids have been known to cause corneal and scleral thinning. Use of topical corticosteroids in the presence of thin corneal or scleral tissue may lead to perforation. Acute purulent infections of the eye may be masked or enhanced by the presence of corticosteroid medication.

If this product is used for 10 days or longer, intraocular pressure should be routinely monitored even though it may be difficult in children and uncooperative patients. Steroids should be used with caution in the presence of glaucoma. Intraocular pressure should be checked frequently.

The use of steroids after cataract surgery may delay healing and increase the incidence of bleb formation.

Use of ocular steroids may prolong the course and may exacerbate the severity of many viral infections of the eye (including herpes simplex). Employment of a corticosteroid medication in the treatment of patients with a history of herpes simplex requires great caution; frequent slit lamp microscopy is recommended.

PRED-G® sterile ophthalmic suspension is not for injection. It should never be injected subconjunctivally, nor should it be directly introduced into the anterior chamber of the eye.

Precautions:

General: Ocular irritation and punctate keratitis have been associated with the use of PRED-G® suspension. The initial prescription and renewal of the medication order beyond 20 milliliters should be made by a physician only after examination of the patient's intraocular pressure, examination of the patient with the aid of magnification such as slit lamp biomicroscopy and, where appropriate, fluorescein staining.

As fungal infections of the cornea are particularly prone to develop coincidentally with long-term corticosteroid applications, fungal invasion should be suspected in any persistent corneal ulceration where a corticosteroid has been used or is in use. Fungal cultures should be taken when appropriate.

Information for Patients: If inflammation or pain persists longer than 48 hours or becomes aggravated, the patient should be advised to discontinue use of the medication and consult a physician.

This product is sterile when packaged. To prevent contamination, care should be taken to avoid touching the bottle tip to eyelids or to any other surface. The use of this bottle by more than one person may spread infection. Store at 15°–25°C (59°–77°F). Protect from freezing and from heat of 40°C (104°F) and above. Keep out of the reach of children. Shake well before using.

Carcinogenesis, mutagenesis, impairment of fertility: There are no published carcinogenicity or impairment of fertility studies on gentamicin. Aminoglycoside antibiotics have been found to be non-mutagenic.

There are no published mutagenicity or impairment of fertility studies on prednisolone. Prednisolone has been reported to be non-carcinogenic.

Pregnancy: Pregnancy Category C. Gentamicin has been shown to depress body weight, kidney weight, and median glomerular counts in newborn rats when administered systemically to pregnant rats in daily doses approximately 500 times the maximum recommended ophthalmic human dose. There are no adequate and well-controlled studies in pregnant women. Gentamicin should be used during pregnancy only if the potential benefit justifies the potential risk to the fetus.

Prednisolone has been shown to be teratogenic in mice when given in doses 1–10 times the human ocular dose. Dexamethasone, hydrocortisone and prednisolone were applied to both eyes of pregnant mice five times per day on days 10 through 13 of gestation. A significant increase in the incidence of cleft palate was observed in the fetuses of the treated mice. There are no adequate well-controlled studies in pregnant women. PRED-G® suspension should be used during pregnancy only if the potential benefit justifies the potential risk to the fetus.

Nursing Mothers: It is not known whether topical administration of corticosteroids could result in sufficient systemic absorption to produce detectable quantities in human milk. Systemically administered corticosteroids appear in human milk and could suppress growth, interfere with endogenous corticosteroid production, or cause other untoward effects. Because of the potential for serious adverse reactions in nursing infants from PRED-G® suspension, a decision should be made whether to discontinue nursing while the drug is being administered or to discontinue the medication.

Pediatric Use: Safety and effectiveness in pediatric patients have not been established.

Geriatric Use: No overall differences in safety or effectiveness have been observed between elderly and younger patients.

Adverse Reactions: Adverse reactions have occurred with steroid/anti-infective combination drugs which can be attributed to the steroid component, the anti-infective component, or the combination. Exact incidence figures are not available since no denominator of treated patients is available.

Reactions occurring most often from the presence of the anti-infective ingredient are allergic sensitizations. The reactions due to the steroid component in decreasing order of frequency are: elevation of intraocular pressure (IOP) with possible development of glaucoma, and infrequent optic nerve damage; posterior subcapsular cataract formation; and delayed wound healing.

Burning, stinging and other symptoms of irritation have been reported with PRED-G®. Superficial punctate keratitis has been reported occasionally with onset occurring typically after several days of use.

Secondary Infection: The development of secondary infection has occurred after use of combinations containing steroids and antimicrobials. Fungal and viral infections of the cornea are particularly prone to develop coincidentally with long-term applications of steroid. The possibility of fungal invasion should be considered in any persistent corneal ulceration where steroid treatment has been used. (See **Warnings**).

Secondary bacterial ocular infection following suppression of host responses also occurs.

Dosage and Administration: Instill one drop into the conjunctival sac two to four times daily. During the initial 24 to 48 hours, the dosing frequency may be increased, if necessary, up to 1 drop every hour. Care should be taken not to discontinue therapy prematurely. If signs and symptoms fail to improve after two days, the patient should be re-evaluated. (See **Precautions**)

Not more than 20 milliliters should be prescribed initially and the prescription should not be refilled without further evaluation as outlined in **Precautions** above.

How Supplied: PRED-G® (gentamicin and prednisolone acetate ophthalmic suspension, USP) 0.3%/1.0% is supplied sterile in opaque white LDPE plastic bottles with droppers with white high impact polystyrene (HIPS) caps as follows:

2 mL in 5 mL bottle – NDC 0023-0106-02
5 mL in 10 mL bottle – NDC 0023-0106-05
10 mL in 15 mL bottle – NDC 0023-0106-10

Note: Store at 15°–25°C (59°–77°F). Avoid excessive heat, 40° C (104° F) and above. Protect from freezing. **Shake well before using.**
℞ only

Continued on next page

Pred-G Suspension—Cont.

©Allergan, Inc.
Irvine, CA 92612
® Marks owned by Allergan, Inc.

PRED–G®
(gentamicin and prednisolone acetate ophthalmic ointment, USP) 0.3%/0.6% sterile

Description: PRED-G® sterile ophthalmic ointment is a topical anti-inflammatory/anti-infective combination product for ophthalmic use.
Chemical Names: Prednisolone acetate: 11β,17,21-Trihydroxypregna-1,4-diene-3, 20-dione 21-acetate.
Gentamicin sulfate is the sulfate salt of gentamicin C_1, gentamicin C_2, and gentamicin C_{1A} which are produced by the growth of *Micromonospora purpurea*.
Contains: Actives: gentamicin sulfate equivalent to 0.3% gentamicin base, prednisolone acetate 0.6%. **Preservative:** chlorobutanol (chloral derivative) 0.5%. **Inactives:** mineral oil; petrolatum (and) lanolin alcohol; purified water; and white petrolatum.
Clinical Pharmacology: Corticosteroids suppress the inflammatory response to a variety of agents and they probably delay or slow healing. Since corticosteroids may inhibit the body's defense mechanism against infection, a concomitant antimicrobial drug may be used when this inhibition is considered to be clinically significant in a particular case.
The anti-infective component in PRED-G® is included to provide action against specific organisms susceptible to it. Gentamicin sulfate is active *in vitro* against susceptible strains of the following microorganisms: *Staphylococcus aureus*, *Streptococcus pyogenes*, *Streptococcus pneumoniae*, *Enterobacter aerogenes*, *Escherichia coli*, *Haemophilus influenzae*, *Klebsiella pneumoniae*, *Neisseria gonorrhoeae*, *Pseudomonas aeruginosa*, and *Serratia marcescens*.
When a decision to administer both a corticosteroid and an antimicrobial is made, the administration of such drugs in combination has the advantage of greater patient compliance and convenience, with the added assurance that the appropriate dosage of both drugs is administered. When both types of drugs are in the same formulation, compatibility of ingredients is assured and the correct volume of drug is delivered and retained.
The relative potency of corticosteroids depends on the molecular structure, concentration, and release from the vehicle.
Indications and Usage: PRED-G® is indicated for steroid-responsive inflammatory ocular conditions for which a corticosteroid is indicated and where superficial bacterial ocular infection or a risk of bacterial ocular infection exists.
Ocular steroids are indicated in inflammatory conditions of the palpebral and bulbar conjunctiva, cornea, and anterior segment of the globe where the inherent risk of steroid use in certain infective conjunctivitides is accepted to obtain a diminution in edema and inflammation. They are also indicated in chronic anterior uveitis and corneal injury from chemical, radiation, or thermal burns or penetration of foreign bodies.
The use of a combination drug with an anti-infective component is indicated where the risk of superficial ocular infection is high or where there is an expectation that potentially dangerous numbers of bacteria will be present in the eye.
The particular anti-infective drug in this product is active against the following common bacterial eye pathogens: *Staphylococcus aureus*, *Streptococcus pyogenes*, *Streptococcus pneumoniae*, *Enterobacter aerogenes*, *Escherichia coli*, *Hemophilus influenzae*, *Klebsiella pneumoniae*, *Neisseria gonorrhoeae*, *Pseudomonas aeruginosa*, and *Serratia marcescens*.
Contraindications: PRED-G® ophthalmic ointment is contraindicated in most viral diseases of the cornea and conjunctiva including epithelial herpes simplex keratitis (dendritic keratitis), vaccinia and varicella, and also in mycobacterial infection of the eye and fungal diseases of ocular structures. Pred G® ointment is also contraindicated in individuals with known or suspected hypersensitivity to any of the ingredients of this preparation or to other corticosteroids.
Warnings: Prolonged use of corticosteroids may result in glaucoma, with damage to the optic nerve, defects in visual acuity and fields of vision, and in posterior subcapsular cataract formation. Prolonged use of corticosteroids may suppress the host immune response and thus increase the hazard of secondary ocular infections. Various ocular diseases and long term use of topical corticosteroids have been known to cause corneal and scleral thinning. Use of topical corticosteroids in the presence of thin corneal or scleral tissue may lead to perforation. Acute purulent infections of the eye may be masked or enhanced by the presence of corticosteroid medication.
If these products are used for 10 days or longer, intraocular pressure should be routinely monitored even though it may be difficult in children and uncooperative patients. Steroids should be used with caution in the presence of glaucoma. Intraocular pressure should be checked frequently.
The use of steroids after cataract surgery may delay healing and increase the incidence of bleb formation.
Use of ocular steroids may prolong the course and may exacerbate the severity of many viral infections of the eye (including herpes simplex). Employment of a corticosteroid medication in the treatment of patients with a history of herpes simplex requires great caution, frequent slit lamp microscopy is recommended.
Precautions:
General: Ocular irritation and punctate keratitis have been associated with the use of PRED-G® ophthalmic ointment. The initial prescription and renewal of the medication order beyond 8 grams should be made by a physician only after examination of the patient's intraocular pressure, examination of the patient with the aid of magnification, such as slit lamp biomicroscopy and, where appropriate, fluorescein staining. As fungal infections of the cornea are particularly prone to develop coincidentally with long term corticosteroid applications, fungal invasion should be suspected in any persistent corneal ulceration where a corticosteroid has been used or is in use. Fungal cultures should be taken when appropriate.
Information for Patients: If inflammation or pain persists longer than 48 hours or becomes aggravated the patient should be advised to discontinue use of the medication and consult a physician.
This product is sterile when packaged. To prevent contamination care should be taken to avoid touching the tip of the tube to eyelids or to any other surface. The use of this tube by more than one person may spread infection. Keep out of reach of children.
Carcinogenesis, mutagenesis, impairment of fertility: There are no published carcinogenicity or impairment of fertility studies on gentamicin. Aminoglycoside antibiotics have been found to be non-mutagenic.
There are no published mutagenicity or impairment of fertility studies on prednisolone. Prednisolone has been reported to be non-carcinogenic.
Pregnancy: Pregnancy Category C: Gentamicin has been shown to depress newborn body weights, kidney weights and median glomerular counts in newborn rats when administered systemically to pregnant rats in daily doses of approximately 500 times the maximum recommended ophthalmic dose in humans. There are no adequate and well-controlled studies in pregnant women. Gentamicin should be used during pregnancy only if the potential benefit justifies the potential risk to the fetus.
Prednisolone has been shown to be teratogenic in mice when given in doses 1–10 times the human dose. Dexamethasone, hydrocortisone and prednisolone were ocularly applied to both eyes of pregnant mice five times per day on days 10 through 13 of gestation. A significant increase in the incidence of cleft palate was observed in the fetuses of the treated mice. There are no adequate well-controlled studies in pregnant women. PRED-G® should be used during pregnancy only if the potential benefit justifies the potential risk to the fetus.
Nursing Mothers: It is not known whether topical administration of corticosteroids could result in sufficient systemic absorption to produce detectable quantities in breast milk. Systemically administered corticosteroids appear in breast milk and could suppress growth, interfere with endogenous corticosteroid production, or cause other untoward effects. Because of the potential for serious adverse reactions in nursing infants from PRED-G® a decision should be made whether to discontinue nursing or to discontinue the medication.
Pediatric Use: Safety and effectiveness in pediatric patients have not been established.
Geriatric Use: No overall differences in safety or effectiveness have been observed between elderly and young patients.
Adverse Reactions: Adverse reactions have occurred with steroid/anti-infective combination drugs which can be attributed to the steroid component, the anti-infective component, or the combination. Exact incidence figures are not available since no denominator of treated patients is available.
The most frequent reactions observed include ocular discomfort, irritation upon instillation of the medication and punctate keratitis. These reactions have resolved upon discontinuation of the medication.
Reactions occurring most often from the presence of the anti-infective ingredient are allergic sensitizations. The reactions due to the steroid component in decreasing order of frequency are: elevation of intraocular pressure (IOP) with possible development of glaucoma, and infrequent optic nerve damage; posterior subcapsular cataract formation; and delayed wound healing.
Secondary Infection: The development of secondary infection has occurred after use of combinations containing steroids and antimicrobials. Fungal and viral infections of the cornea are particularly prone to develop coincidentally with long-term applications of steroid. The possibility of fungal invasion must be considered in any persistent corneal ulceration where steroid treatment has been used. (See **Warnings**)
Secondary bacterial ocular infection following suppression of host responses also occurs.
Dosage and Administration: A small amount ($^1/_2$ inch ribbon) of ointment should be applied in the conjunctival sac one to three times daily. Care should be taken not to discontinue therapy prematurely.
Not more than 8 grams should be prescribed initially and the prescription should not be refilled without further evaluation as outlined in **Precautions** above. If signs and symptoms fail to improve after two days, the patient should be re-evaluated (see **Precautions**).
How Supplied: PRED-G® (gentamicin and prednisolone acetate ophthalmic ointment,

USP) 0.3%/0.6% is supplied sterile in collapsible aluminum tubes with epoxy-phenolic liners with tips with black LDPE caps of the following size:
3.5 g—NDC 0023-0066-04
Note: Store at 15°–25°C (59°–77°F).
℞ only
© 2004 Allergan, Inc.
Irvine, CA 92612
® Marks owned by Allergan, Inc.

PRED MILD® ℞
(prednisolone acetate ophthalmic suspension, USP) 0.12%
sterile

Description: PRED MILD® (prednisolone acetate ophthalmic suspension, USP) 0.12% is a topical anti-inflammatory agent for ophthalmic use.
Chemical Name: 11β,17,21-Trihydroxypregna-1,4-diene-3,20-dione 21-acetate.
Contains: Active: prednisolone acetate (microfine suspension) 0.12%. **Preservative:** benzalkonium chloride. **Inactives:** boric acid; edetate disodium; hydroxypropyl methylcellulose; polysorbate 80; purified water; sodium bisulfite; sodium chloride; and sodium citrate. The pH during its shelf life ranges from 5.0 to 6.0.
Clinical Pharmacology: Prednisolone acetate is a glucocorticoid that, on the basis of weight, has 3 to 5 times the anti-inflammatory potency of hydrocortisone. Glucocorticoids inhibit the edema, fibrin deposition, capillary dilation and phagocytic migration of the acute inflammatory response as well as capillary proliferation, deposition of collagen and scar formation.
Indications and Usage: PRED MILD® is indicated for the treatment of mild to moderate noninfectious allergic and inflammatory disorders of the lid, conjunctiva, cornea and sclera (including chemical and thermal burns).
Contraindications: PRED MILD® suspension is contraindicated in acute untreated purulent ocular infections, in most viral diseases of the cornea and conjunctiva including epithelial herpes simplex keratitis (dendritic keratitis), vaccinia, and varicella, and also in mycobacterial infection of the eye and fungal diseases of ocular structures. PRED MILD® suspension is also contraindicated in individuals with known or suspected hypersensitivity to any of the ingredients of this preparation and to other corticosteroids.
Warnings: Prolonged use of corticosteroids may result in glaucoma with damage to the optic nerve, defects in visual acuity and fields of vision, and in posterior subcapsular cataract formation. Prolonged use may also suppress the host immune response and thus increase the hazard of secondary ocular infections.
Various ocular diseases and long-term use of topical corticosteroids have been known to cause corneal and scleral thinning. Use of topical corticosteroids in the presence of thin corneal or scleral tissue may lead to perforation.
Acute purulent infections of the eye may be masked or activity enhanced by the presence of corticosteroid medication.
If this product is used for 10 days or longer, intraocular pressure should be routinely monitored even though it may be difficult in children and uncooperative patients. Steroids should be used with caution in the presence of glaucoma. Intraocular pressure should be checked frequently.
The use of steroids after cataract surgery may delay healing and increase the incidence of bleb formation.
Use of ocular steroids may prolong the course and may exacerbate the severity of many viral infections of the eye (including herpes simplex). Employment of a corticosteroid medication in the treatment of patients with a history of herpes simplex requires great caution; frequent slit lamp microscopy is recommended.
Corticosteroids are not effective in mustard gas keratitis and Sjögren's keratoconjunctivitis.
Contains sodium bisulfite, a sulfite that may cause allergic-type reactions, including anaphylactic symptoms and life-threatening or less severe asthmatic episodes in certain susceptible people. The overall prevalence of sulfite sensitivity in the general population is unknown and probably low. Sulfite sensitivity is seen more frequently in asthmatic than in nonasthmatic people.
Precautions:
General: The initial prescription and renewal of the medication order beyond 20 milliliters of PRED MILD® should be made by a physician only after examination of the patient with the aid of magnification, such as slit lamp biomicroscopy, and, where appropriate, fluorescein staining. If signs and symptoms fail to improve after 2 days, the patient should be re-evaluated.
As fungal infections of the cornea are particularly prone to develop coincidentally with long-term local corticosteroid applications, fungal invasion should be suspected in any persistent corneal ulceration where a corticosteroid has been used or is in use. Fungal cultures should be taken when appropriate.
If this product is used for 10 days or longer, intraocular pressure should be monitored (see **Warnings**).
Information for patients: If inflammation or pain persists longer than 48 hours or becomes aggravated, the patient should be advised to discontinue use of the medication and consult a physician.
This product is sterile when packaged. To prevent contamination, care should be taken to avoid touching the bottle tip to eyelids or to any other surface. The use of this bottle by more than one person may spread infection. Keep bottle tightly closed when not in use. Keep out of the reach of children.
Carcinogenesis, Mutagenesis, Impairment of Fertility: No studies have been conducted in animals or in humans to evaluate the potential of these effects.
Pregnancy Category C: Prednisolone has been shown to be teratogenic in mice when given in doses 1–10 times the human dose. There are no adequate well-controlled studies in pregnant women. Prednisolone should be used during pregnancy only if the potential benefit justifies the potential risk to the fetus.
Dexamethasone, hydrocortisone and prednisolone were ocularly applied to both eyes of pregnant mice five times per day on days 10 through 13 of gestation. A significant increase in the incidence of cleft palate was observed in the fetuses of the treated mice.
Nursing Mothers: It is not known whether topical ophthalmic administration of corticosteroids could result in sufficient systemic absorption to produce detectable quantities in breast milk. Systemically administered corticosteroids appear in human milk and could suppress growth, interfere with endogenous corticosteroid production, or cause other untoward effects. Because of the potential for serious adverse reactions in nursing infants from prednisolone, a decision should be made whether to discontinue nursing or to discontinue the drug, taking into account the importance of the drug to the mother.
Pediatric Use: Safety and effectiveness in pediatric patients have not been established.
Geriatric Use: No overall differences in safety or effectiveness have been observed between elderly and younger patients.
Adverse Reactions: Adverse reactions include, in decreasing order of frequency, elevation of intraocular pressure (IOP) with possible development of glaucoma and infrequent optic nerve damage, posterior subcapsular cataract formation, and delayed wound healing.
Although systemic effects are extremely uncommon, there have been rare occurrences of systemic hypercorticoidism after use of topical steroids.
Corticosteroid-containing preparations have also been reported to cause acute anterior uveitis and perforation of the globe. Keratitis, conjunctivitis, corneal ulcers, mydriasis, conjunctival hyperemia, loss of accommodation and ptosis have occasionally been reported following local use of corticosteroids.
The development of secondary ocular infection (bacterial, fungal, and viral) has occurred. Fungal and viral infections of the cornea are particularly prone to develop coincidentally with long-term applications of steroids. The possibility of fungal invasion should be considered in any persistent corneal ulceration where steroid treatment has been used (see **Warnings**).
Transient burning and stinging upon instillation and other minor symptoms of ocular irritation have been reported with the use of PRED MILD® suspension.
Overdosage: Overdosage will not ordinarily cause acute problems. If accidentally ingested, drink fluids to dilute.
Dosage and Administration: Shake well before using. Instill one to two drops into the conjunctival sac two to four times daily. During the initial 24 to 48 hours, the dosing frequency may be increased if necessary. Care should be taken not to discontinue therapy prematurely. If signs and symptoms fail to improve after 2 days, the patient should be re-evaluated (see **Precautions**).
How Supplied: PRED MILD® (prednisolone acetate ophthalmic suspension, USP) 0.12% is supplied sterile in opaque white LDPE plastic bottles with droppers with white high impact polystyrene (HIPS) caps as follows:
5 mL in 10 mL bottle – NDC 11980-174-05
10 mL in 15 mL bottle – NDC 11980-174-10
Note: Store between 15°C–30°C (59°F–86°F). Protect from freezing. Store in an upright position.
Rx only
©Allergan, Inc.
Irvine, CA 92612
® Marks owned by Allergan, Inc.

PROPINE® ℞
(dipivefrin hydrochloride)
ophthalmic solution, USP, 0.1% sterile

Description: PROPINE® contains dipivefrin hydrochloride in a sterile, isotonic solution. Dipivefrin HCl is a white, crystalline powder, freely soluble in water with an osmolality of approx. 250–330 mOsmol/kg.
Empirical Formula: $C_{19}H_{29}O_5N \cdot HCl$
Chemical Name: (±)-3,4-Dihydroxy-α-[(methylamino)methyl]benzyl alcohol 3,4-dipivalate hydrochloride.
Contains:
Active: dipivefrin HCl 0.1%
Preservative: benzalkonium chloride
Inactives: edetate disodium; sodium chloride; hydrochloric acid to adjust pH; and purified water. The pH during its shelf life ranges from 2.5–3.5.
Clinical Pharmacology: PROPINE® (dipivefrin HCl ophthalmic solution, USP) is a member of a class of drugs known as prodrugs. Prodrugs are usually not active in themselves and require biotransformation to the parent com-

Continued on next page

Propine—Cont.

pound before therapeutic activity is seen. These modifications are undertaken to enhance absorption, decrease side effects and enhance stability and comfort, thus making the parent compound a more useful drug. Enhanced absorption makes the prodrug a more efficient delivery system for the parent drug because less drug will be needed to produce the desired therapeutic response.

PROPINE® ophthalmic solution is a prodrug of epinephrine formed by the diesterification of epinephrine and pivalic acid. The addition of pivaloyl groups to the epinephrine molecule enhances its lipophilic character and, as a consequence, its penetration into the anterior chamber.

PROPINE® is converted to epinephrine inside the human eye by enzyme hydrolysis. The liberated epinephrine, an adrenergic agonist, appears to exert its action by decreasing aqueous production and by enhancing outflow facility. The PROPINE® prodrug delivery system is a more efficient way of delivering the therapeutic effects of epinephrine, with fewer side effects than are associated with conventional epinephrine therapy.

The onset of action with one drop of PROPINE® occurs about 30 minutes after treatment, with maximum effect seen at about one hour.

Using a prodrug means that less drug is needed for therapeutic effect since absorption is enhanced with the prodrug. PROPINE® ophthalmic solution at 0.1% dipivefrin was judged less irritating than a 1% solution of epinephrine hydrochloride or bitartrate. In addition, only 8 of 455 patients (1.8%) treated with PROPINE® reported discomfort due to photophobia, glare or light sensitivity.

Indications: PROPINE® (dipivefrin HCl ophthalmic solution, USP) is indicated as initial therapy for the control of intraocular pressure in chronic open-angle glaucoma. Patients responding inadequately to other antiglaucoma therapy may respond to addition of PROPINE®.

In controlled and open-label studies of glaucoma, PROPINE® ophthalmic solution demonstrated a statistically significant intraocular pressure-lowering effect. Patients using PROPINE® twice daily in studies with mean durations of 76–146 days experienced mean pressure reductions ranging from 20–24%.

Therapeutic response to PROPINE® ophthalmic solution twice daily is somewhat less than 2% epinephrine twice daily. Controlled studies showed statistically significant differences in lowering of intraocular pressure between PROPINE® and 2% epinephrine. In controlled studies in patients with a history of epinephrine intolerance, only 3% of patients treated with PROPINE® ophthalmic solution exhibited intolerance, while 55% of those treated with epinephrine again developed intolerance. Therapeutic response to PROPINE® twice daily therapy is comparable to 2% pilocarpine 4 times daily. In controlled clinical studies comparing PROPINE® ophthalmic solution and 2% pilocarpine, there were no statistically significant differences in the maintenance of IOP levels for the two medications. PROPINE® does not produce miosis or accommodative spasm which cholinergic agents are known to produce. Night blindness often associated with miotic agents is not present with PROPINE® therapy. Patients with cataracts avoid the inability to see around lenticular opacities caused by constricted pupil.

Contraindications: PROPINE® should not be used in patients with narrow angles since any dilation of the pupil may predispose the patient to an attack of angle-closure glaucoma. This product is contraindicated in patients who are hypersensitive to any of its components.

Precautions: Aphakic Patients. Macular edema has been shown to occur in up to 30% of aphakic patients treated with epinephrine. Discontinuation of epinephrine generally results in reversal of the maculopathy.

Pregnancy: Pregnancy Category B. Reproduction studies have been performed in rats and rabbits at daily oral doses up to 10 mg/kg body weight (5 mg/kg in teratogenicity studies), and have revealed no evidence of impaired fertility or harm to the fetus due to dipivefrin HCl. There are, however, no adequate and well-controlled studies in pregnant women. Because animal reproduction studies are not always predictive of human response, this drug should be used during pregnancy only if clearly needed.

Nursing Mothers. It is not known whether this drug is excreted in human milk. Because many drugs are excreted in human milk, caution should be exercised when PROPINE® ophthalmic solution is administered to a nursing woman.

Pediatric Use: Safety and effectiveness in pediatric patients have not been established.

Geriatric Use. No overall clinical differences in safety or effectiveness have been observed between elderly and other adult patients.

Animal Studies. Rabbit studies indicated a dose-related incidence of meibomian gland retention cysts following topical administration of both dipivefrin hydrochloride and epinephrine.

Adverse Reactions:

Cardiovascular Effects. Tachycardia, arrhythmias and hypertension have been reported with ocular administration of epinephrine.

Local Effects. The most frequent side effects reported with PROPINE® alone were injection in 6.5% of patients and burning and stinging in 6%. Follicular conjunctivitis, eye pain, mydriasis, blurry vision, eye pruritus, headache, and allergic reaction to PROPINE® ophthalmic solution have been reported. Epinephrine therapy can lead to adrenochrome deposits in the conjunctiva and cornea.

Dosage and Administration:

Initial Glaucoma Therapy. The usual dosage of PROPINE® is one drop in the eye(s) every 12 hours.

Replacement with PROPINE®. When patients are being transferred to PROPINE® from antiglaucoma agents other than epinephrine, on the first day continue the previous medication and add one drop of PROPINE® ophthalmic solution in each eye every 12 hours. On the following day, discontinue the previously used antiglaucoma agent and continue with PROPINE®.

In transferring patients from conventional epinephrine therapy to PROPINE® ophthalmic solution, simply discontinue the epinephrine medication and institute the PROPINE® regimen.

Addition of PROPINE®. When patients on other antiglaucoma agents require additional therapy, add one drop of PROPINE® every 12 hours.

Concomitant Therapy. For difficult to control patients, the addition of PROPINE® ophthalmic solution to other agents such as pilocarpine, carbachol, echothiophate iodide or acetazolamide has been shown to be effective.

Note: Not for injection.

How Supplied: PROPINE® (dipivefrin HCl ophthalmic solution, USP) 0.1%, is supplied sterile in opaque white low density polyethylene ophthalmic dispenser bottles and tips with purple polystyrene caps as follows:

5mL in 10mL bottle—NDC 0023-9208-05
10mL in 10mL bottle—NDC 0023-9208-10
15mL in 15mL bottle—NDC 0023-9208-15

Note: Store in a tight, light-resistant container at 15° to 25°C (59° to 77°F).
℞ only
©Allergan, Inc.
Irvine, CA 92612
® Marks owned by Allergan, Inc.

REFRESH® CELLUVISC® OTC
(carboxymethylcellulose sodium) 1%
Lubricant Eye Drops
Preservative-Free

Soothing Relief For Dry, Irritated Eyes.
Due to its thicker formula, REFRESH® CELLUVISC® Lubricant Eye Drops is an ideal eye drop for persistent dry eye conditions. REFRESH® CELLUVISC® restores the moisture your eyes crave with a gentle protecting and lubricating formula that has some of the same healthy qualities as natural tears. So, you can enjoy long-lasting relief from the irritating, scratchy feeling of dry, irritated eyes.

To avoid the use of potentially irritating preservatives found in some bottled eye drops, REFRESH® CELLUVISC® Lubricant Eye Drops comes in preservative-free, air-tight, single-use containers. So you can apply REFRESH® CELLUVISC® as often as necessary to provide 24-hour comfort.

Drug Facts
Active Ingredient: **Purpose:**
Carboxymethylcellulose .... Eye Lubricant sodium (CMC) 1.0%

Uses
- For the temporary relief of burning, irritation and discomfort due to dryness of the eye or to exposure to wind or sun.
- May be used as a protectant against further irritation.

Warnings:
- For external use only.
- To avoid contamination, do not touch tip of container to any surface. Do not reuse. Once opened, discard.
- Do not touch unit-dose tip to eye.
- Do not use if solution changes color or becomes cloudy.

Stop use and ask a doctor if you experience eye pain, changes in vision, continued redness or irritation of the eye, or if the condition worsens or persists for more than 72 hrs.

Keep out of the reach of children. If swallowed, get medical help or contact a Poison Control Center right away.

Other Information:
- Use only if single-use container is intact.
- REFRESH® CELLUVISC® may cause temporary blurring due to its viscosity.
- RETAIN CARTON FOR FUTURE REFERENCE.

Inactive ingredients:
Calcium chloride, potassium chloride, purified water, sodium chloride, and sodium lactate.

How Supplied: REFRESH® CELLUVISC® (carboxymethylcellulose sodium) 1.0% Lubricant Eye Drops are supplied in sterile, preservative-free, disposable, single-use containers of 0.4 mL (0.01 fl. oz.) each, in the following size:
30 Sterile Single-Use Containers—NDC 0023-4554-30
®Marks owned by Allergan, Inc.
©Allergan, Inc.
Irvine, CA 92612

Shown in Product Identification Guide, page 103

REFRESH ENDURA® OTC
Lubricant Eye Drops

Breakthrough technology for complete relief plus protection. With its unique formulation, REFRESH ENDURA® does more than wet the

eye. It is the first eye drop which benefits all three layers of the tear film.
REFRESH ENDURA® Lubricant Eye Drops create a soothing shield with a long lasting layer of moisture for sustained relief of persistent dry eye symptoms.
The unique formulation of REFRESH ENDURA® appears as a light milky eye drop. It looks and feels different because it is different.
Technologically advanced REFRESH ENDURA® Lubricant Eye Drops are safe to use as often as necessary and provides 24-hour comfort for dry, irritated eyes.

Drug Facts
Active Ingredients: **Purpose:**
Glycerin 1% .... Eye lubricant
Polysorbate 80 1% .... Eye lubricant

Uses:
- For the temporary relief of burning, irritation, and discomfort due to the dryness of the eye or exposure to wind or sun.
- May be used as a protectant against further irritation.

Warnings:
- **For external use only.**
- **To avoid contamination, do not touch tip of container to any surface. Do not reuse. Once opened, discard.**
- **Do not touch unit-dose tip to eye.**
- **Do not use if solution changes color.**

Stop use and ask a doctor if you experience eye pain, changes in vision, continued redness or irritation of the eye, or if the condition worsens or persists for more than 72 hours.
Keep out of the reach of children. If swallowed, get medical help or contact a Poison Control Center right away.
Directions To open, **TWIST AND PULL TAB TO REMOVE.** Instill 1 to 2 drops in the affected eye(s) as needed and discard container.

Other Information
- **Use only if single-use container is intact.**
- **RETAIN CARTON FOR FUTURE REFERENCE.**

Inactive Ingredients:
Carbomer; castor oil; mannitol; purified water; and sodium hydroxide.
How Supplied: In sterile, preservative-free, disposable, single-use containers of 0.01 fluid ounces each in the following size:
20 sterile single-use containers—NDC 0023-9235-20
®Marks owned by Allergan, Inc.
©Allergan, Inc.
Irvine, CA 92612

Shown in Product Identification Guide, page 103

REFRESH LIQUIGEL®   OTC
(carboxymethylcellulose sodium) 1%
Lubricant Eye Drops

REFRESH LIQUIGEL® Lubricant Eye Drops is a unique, extra-strength eye drop, specially formulated to provide added moisture for immediate relief of moderate-to-severe dry eye symptoms. REFRESH LIQUIGEL® works like your own natural tears; it is safe to use as often as needed.

Drug Facts
Active Ingredients: **Purpose:**
carboxymethylcellulose
  sodium 1.0% .... Eye Lubricant

Uses:
- For the temporary relief of burning, irritation, and discomfort due to the dryness of the eye or exposure to the wind or sun.
- May be used as a protectant against further irritation.

Warnings:
- **For external use only**
- **To avoid contamination, do not touch the tip of the container to any surface. Replace cap after using.**

- **If solution changes color or becomes cloudy, do not use.**

Stop use and ask a doctor if you experience eye pain, changes in vision, continued redness or irritation of the eye, or if the condition worsens or persists for more than 72 hours.
Keep out of the reach of children. If swallowed, get medical help or contact a Poison Control Center right away.
Directions: Instill 1 or 2 drops in the affected eye(s) as needed.

Other Information:
- **Use only if imprinted tape seals on top and bottom flaps are intact and clearly legible.**
- **RETAIN CARTON FOR FUTURE REFERENCE.**

Inactive Ingredients:
Boric acid, calcium chloride, magnesium chloride, potassium chloride, purified water, PURITE® (stabilized oxychloro complex), sodium borate, and sodium chloride.
How Supplied: REFRESH LIQUIGEL® (carboxymethylcellulose sodium) 1.0% Lubricant Eye Drops are supplied in the following sizes:
15 mL bottle — NDC 0023-9205-15
30 mL bottle — NDC 0023-9205-30
®Marks owned by Allergan, Inc.
© Allergan, Inc.
Irvine, CA 92612

Shown in Product Identification Guide, page 103

REFRESH PLUS®
(carboxymethylcellulose sodium) 0.5%
Lubricant Eye Drops
Preservative-Free

Immediate, Long-Lasting Relief Plus Protection.
Many things can make your eyes feel dry, scratchy, burning or uncomfortable. Air conditioners or heaters. Computer use. Reading. Some medications. Wind. LASIK procedures.* Or a reduction in the amount of tears your body produces—tears which help to lubricate and nourish your eyes. REFRESH PLUS® Lubricant Eye Drops restores the moisture your eyes crave with a special formula that has some of the same healthy qualities as natural tears.
Since REFRESH PLUS® is preservative-free, it also avoids the potential irritation to your eyes caused by some preservatives found in bottled eye drops. REFRESH PLUS® is formulated for the mild-to-moderate dry eye, and can be used as often as needed to provide 24-hour comfort.

Drug Facts
Active Ingredient: **Purpose:**
Carboxymethylcellulose   Eye lubricant
  sodium (CMC) 0.5%

Uses:
- For the temporary relief of burning, irritation, and discomfort due to dryness of the eye or exposure to wind or sun
- May be used as a protectant against further irritation.

Warnings:
- **For external use only.**
- **To avoid contamination, do not touch tip of container to any surface. Do not reuse. Once opened, discard.**
- **Do not touch unit-dose tip to eye.**
- **Do not use if solution changes color or becomes cloudy**

Stop use and ask a doctor if you experience eye pain, changes in vision, continued redness or irritation of the eye, or if the condition worsens or persists for more than 72 hours.

Keep out of the reach of children. If swallowed, get medical help or contact a Poison Control Center right away.

---

*If used for post-operative (e.g. LASIK) dryness and discomfort, follow your eye doctor's instructions.

Other Information:
- **Use only if single-use container is intact.**
- **RETAIN CARTON FOR FUTURE REFERENCE.**

Inactive Ingredients: Calcium chloride, magnesium chloride, potassium chloride, purified water, sodium chloride, and sodium lactate. May also contain hydrochloric acid and/or sodium hydroxide to adjust pH.
How Supplied: In sterile, preservative-free, disposable, single-use containers of 0.01 fluid ounces each in the following sizes:
30 single-use containers—NDC 0023-0403-30.
50 single-use containers—NDC 0023-0403-50.
70 single-use containers—NDC 0023-0403-70.
®Marks owned by Allergan, Inc.
©Allergan, Inc.
Irvine, CA 92612

Shown in Product Identification Guide, page 103

REFRESH P.M.®   OTC
Lubricant Eye Ointment
Preservative-Free Formula

Nighttime relief and protection for dry eyes. Strong relief for dry, irritated eyes.
REFRESH P.M.® has been specially formulated to soothe, moisturize and protect dry, irritated eyes. REFRESH P.M.® is ideal for use at bedtime.
Just as important, REFRESH P.M.® is preservative-free to avoid the risk of preservative-induced irritation.

Active Ingredients: Mineral Oil 42.5% and White Petrolatum 57.3%
Purpose: Eye Lubricant
Uses: For the temporary relief of burning, irritation, and discomfort due to the dryness of the eye or exposure to wind or sun. May be used as a protectant against further irritation.
Warnings: For external use only. To avoid contamination, do not touch tip of container to any surface. Replace cap after using.
Stop use and ask a doctor if you experience eye pain, changes in vision, continued redness or irritation of the eye, or if the condition worsens or persists for more than 72 hrs.
Keep out of the reach of children. If swallowed, get medical help or contact a Poison Control Center right away.
Directions: Pull down the lower lid of the affected eye and apply a small amount (one fourth inch) of ointment to the inside of the eyelid. Replace cap after using.
Other Information: Store away from heat. Protect from freezing. Use only if imprinted tape seals on top and bottom flaps are intact and clearly legible.
RETAIN CARTON FOR FUTURE REFERENCE
Inactive Ingredients: Lanolin alcohols
How Supplied: As a sterile eye lubricant in 3.5 g tube—UPC 0023-0667-04; NDC 0023-0240-04
®Marks owned by Allergan, Inc.
©Allergan, Inc.
Irvine, CA 92612

Shown in Product Identification Guide, page 103

Continued on next page

REFRESH TEARS® OTC
(carboxymethylcellulose sodium) 0.5%
Lubricant Eye Drops

For mild-to-moderate dry eye, REFRESH TEARS® Lubricant Eye Drops restores the moisture your eyes crave with a special formula that has many of the same healthy qualities as your own natural tears.

Drug Facts

Active Ingredient	Purpose
Carboxymethylcellulose sodium 0.5%	Eye lubricant

Uses:
- For the temporary relief of burning, irritation, and discomfort due to the dryness of the eye or exposure to wind or sun.
- May be used as a protectant against further irritation.

Warnings:
- **For external use only.**
- **To avoid contamination, do not touch tip of container to any surface. Replace cap after using.**
- **Do not use if solution changes color or becomes cloudy.**

Stop use and ask a doctor if you experience eye pain, changes in vision, continued redness or irritation of the eye, or if the condition worsens or persists for more than 72 hours.

Keep out of the reach of children. If swallowed, get medical help or contact a Poison Control Center right away.

Directions: Instill 1 or 2 drops in the affected eye(s) as needed

Other Information:
- Use only if imprinted tape seals on top and bottom flaps are intact and clearly legible.
- RETAIN CARTON FOR FUTURE REFERENCE.

Inactive Ingredients: Boric acid; calcium chloride; magnesium chloride; potassium chloride; purified water; PURITE® (stabilized oxychloro complex); sodium borate and sodium chloride. May also contain hydrochloric acid and/or sodium hydroxide to adjust pH

How Supplied: REFRESH TEARS® (carboxymethylcellulose sodium) 0.5% Lubricant Eye Drops are supplied in the following sizes:
15-mL bottle – NDC 0023-0798-15.
30-mL bottle – NDC 0023-0798-30.
Two – 30-mL bottles – NDC 0023-0798-60
®Marks owned by Allergan, Inc.
©Allergan, Inc.
Irvine, CA 92612

Shown in Product Identification Guide, page 103

RESTASIS® ℞
[rĕ'stă-sĭs]
(cyclosporine ophthalmic emulsion) 0.05%
Sterile, Preservative-Free

Description: RESTASIS® (cyclosporine ophthalmic emulsion) 0.05% contains a topical immunomodulator with anti-inflammatory effects. Cyclosporine's chemical name is Cyclo[[(E)-(2S,3R,4R)-3-hydroxy-4-methyl-2-(methylamino)-6-octenoyl]-L-2-aminobutyryl-N-methylglycyl-N-methyl-L-leucyl-L-valyl-N-methyl-L-leucyl-L-alanyl-D-alanyl- N-methyl-L-leucyl-N-methyl-L-leucyl-N-methyl-L-valyl] and it has the following structure:

[See chemical structure at top of next column]
Cyclosporine is a fine white powder. RESTASIS® appears as a white opaque to slightly translucent homogeneous emulsion. It has an osmolality of 230 to 320 mOsmol/kg and a pH of 6.5-8.0.

Each mL of RESTASIS® ophthalmic emulsion contains: **Active:** cyclosporine 0.05%. **Inactives:** glycerin; castor oil; polysorbate 80; carbomer 1342; purified water and sodium hydroxide to adjust the pH.

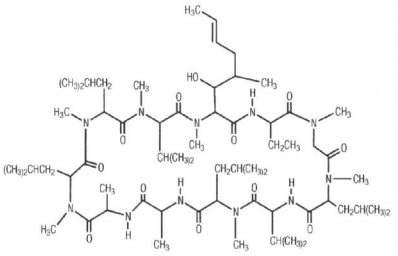

Clinical Pharmacology:
Mechanism of action:
Cyclosporine is an immunosuppressive agent when administered systemically.
In patients whose tear production is presumed to be suppressed due to ocular inflammation associated with keratoconjunctivitis sicca, cyclosporine emulsion is thought to act as a partial immunomodulator. The exact mechanism of action is not known.

Pharmacokinetics:
Blood cyclosporin A concentrations were measured using a specific high pressure liquid chromatography-mass spectrometry assay.
Blood concentrations of cyclosporine, in all the samples collected, after topical administration of RESTASIS® 0.05%, BID, in humans for up to 12 months, were below the quantitation limit of 0.1 ng/mL. There was no detectable drug accumulation in blood during 12 months of treatment with RESTASIS® ophthalmic emulsion.

Clinical Evaluations:
Four multicenter, randomized, adequate and well-controlled clinical studies were performed in approximately 1200 patients with moderate to severe keratoconjunctivitis sicca. RESTASIS® demonstrated statistically significant increases in Schirmer wetting of 10 mm versus vehicle at six months in patients whose tear production was presumed to be suppressed due to ocular inflammation. This effect was seen in approximately 15% of RESTASIS® ophthalmic emulsion treated patients versus approximately 5% of vehicle treated patients. Increased tear production was not seen in patients currently taking topical anti-inflammatory drugs or using punctal plugs. No increase in bacterial or fungal ocular infections was reported following administration of RESTASIS®.

Indications and Usage: RESTASIS® ophthalmic emulsion is indicated to increase tear production in patients whose tear production is presumed to be suppressed due to ocular inflammation associated with keratoconjunctivitis sicca. Increased tear production was not seen in patients currently taking topical anti-inflammatory drugs or using punctal plugs.

Contraindications: RESTASIS® is contraindicated in patients with active ocular infections and in patients with known or suspected hypersensitivity to any of the ingredients in the formulation.

Warning: RESTASIS® ophthalmic emulsion has not been studied in patients with a history of herpes keratitis.

Precautions:
General: For ophthalmic use only.
Information for Patients:
The emulsion from one individual single-use vial is to be used immediately after opening for administration to one or both eyes, and the remaining contents should be discarded immediately after administration.
Do not allow the tip of the vial to touch the eye or any surface, as this may contaminate the emulsion.
RESTASIS® should not be administered while wearing contact lenses. Patients with decreased tear production typically should not wear contact lenses. If contact lenses are worn, they should be removed prior to the administration of the emulsion. Lenses may be reinserted 15 minutes following administration of RESTASIS® ophthalmic emulsion.

Carcinogenesis, Mutagenesis, and Impairment of Fertility:
Systemic carcinogenicity studies were carried out in male and female mice and rats. In the 78-week oral (diet) mouse study, at doses of 1, 4, and 16 mg/kg/day, evidence of a statistically significant trend was found for lymphocytic lymphomas in females, and the incidence of hepatocellular carcinomas in mid-dose males significantly exceeded the control value.
In the 24-month oral (diet) rat study, conducted at 0.5, 2, and 8 mg/kg/day, pancreatic islet cell adenomas significantly exceeded the control rate in the low dose level. The hepatocellular carcinomas and pancreatic islet cell adenomas were not dose related. The low doses in mice and rats are approximately 1000 and 500 times greater, respectively, than the daily human dose of one drop (28 μL) of 0.05% RESTASIS® BID into each eye of a 60 kg person (0.001 mg/kg/day), assuming that the entire dose is absorbed.
Cyclosporine has not been found mutagenic/genotoxic in the Ames Test, the V79-HGPRT Test, the micronucleus test in mice and Chinese hamsters, the chromosome-aberration tests in Chinese hamster bone-marrow, the mouse dominant lethal assay, and the DNA-repair test in sperm from treated mice. A study analyzing sister chromatid exchange (SCE) induction by cyclosporine using human lymphocytes in vitro gave indication of a positive effect (i.e., induction of SCE). No impairment in fertility was demonstrated in studies in male and female rats receiving oral doses of cyclosporine up to 15 mg/kg/day (approximately 15,000 times the human daily dose of 0.001 mg/kg/day) for 9 weeks (male) and 2 weeks (female) prior to mating.

Pregnancy-Teratogenic effects:
Pregnancy category C.
Teratogenic effects: No evidence of teratogenicity was observed in rats or rabbits receiving oral doses of cyclosporine up to 300 mg/kg/day during organogenesis. These doses in rats and rabbits are approximately 300,000 times greater than the daily human dose of one drop (28 μL) 0.05% RESTASIS® BID into each eye of a 60 kg person (0.001mg/kg/day), assuming that the entire dose is absorbed.

Non-Teratogenic effects: Adverse effects were seen in reproduction studies in rats and rabbits only at dose levels toxic to dams. At toxic doses (rats at 30 mg/kg/day and rabbits at 100 mg/kg/day), cyclosporine oral solution, USP, was embryo- and fetotoxic as indicated by increased pre- and postnatal mortality and reduced fetal weight together with related skeletal retardations. These doses are 30,000 and 100,000 times greater, respectively, than the daily human dose of one-drop (28 μL) of 0.05% RESTASIS® BID into each eye of a 60 kg person (0.001 mg/kg/day), assuming that the entire dose is absorbed. No evidence of embryofetal toxicity was observed in rats or rabbits receiving cyclosporine at oral doses up to 17 mg/kg/day or 30 mg/kg/day, respectively, during organogenesis. These doses in rats and rabbits are approximately 17,000 and 30,000 times greater, respectively, than the daily human dose.
Offspring of rats receiving a 45 mg/kg/day oral dose of cyclosporine from Day 15 of pregnancy until Day 21 post partum, a maternally toxic level, exhibited an increase in postnatal mortality; this dose is 45,000 times greater than the daily human topical dose, 0.001 mg/kg/day, assuming that the entire dose is absorbed. No adverse events were observed at oral doses up to 15 mg/kg/day (15,000 times greater than the daily human dose).

There are no adequate and well-controlled studies of RESTASIS® in pregnant women. RESTASIS® should be administered to a pregnant woman only if clearly needed.
Nursing Mothers:
Cyclosporine is known to be excreted in human milk following systemic administration but excretion in human milk after topical treatment has not been investigated. Although blood concentrations are undetectable after topical administration of RESTASIS® ophthalmic emulsion, caution should be exercised when RESTASIS® is administered to a nursing woman.
Pediatric Use:
The safety and efficacy of RESTASIS® ophthalmic emulsion have not been established in pediatric patients below the age of 16.
Geriatric Use:
No overall difference in safety or effectiveness has been observed between elderly and younger patients.
Adverse Reactions: The most common adverse event following the use of RESTASIS® was ocular burning (17%). Other events reported in 1% to 5% of patients included conjunctival hyperemia, discharge, epiphora, eye pain, foreign body sensation, pruritus, stinging, and visual disturbance (most often blurring).
Dosage and Administration: Invert the unit dose vial a few times to obtain a uniform, white, opaque emulsion before using. Instill one drop of RESTASIS® ophthalmic emulsion twice a day in each eye approximately 12 hours apart. RESTASIS® can be used concomitantly with artificial tears, allowing a 15 minute interval between products. Discard vial immediately after use.
How Supplied: RESTASIS® ophthalmic emulsion is packaged in single use vials. Each vial contains 0.4 mL fill in a 0.9 mL LDPE vial; 32 vials are packaged in a polypropylene tray with an aluminum peelable lid.
RESTASIS® 32 Vials 0.4 mL each - NDC 0023-9163-32
Storage: Store RESTASIS® ophthalmic emulsion at 15° to 25° C (59°-77° F).
KEEP OUT OF THE REACH OF CHILDREN.
Rx Only
© 2004 Allergan, Inc., Irvine, CA 92612, U.S.A.
® Marks owned by Allergan, Inc.
U.S. Pat. 4,649,047; 4,839,342; 5,474,979.
INSPIRE PHARMACEUTICALS, INC.
Inspire and the Inspire logo are registered trademarks of Inspire Pharmaceuticals, Inc.
Shown in Product Identification Guide, page 103

ZYMAR™ ℞
[zi-mar]
(gatifloxacin ophthalmic solution) 0.3%
Sterile
Description: ZYMAR™ (gatifloxacin ophthalmic solution) 0.3% is a sterile ophthalmic solution. It is an 8-methoxy fluoroquinolone anti-infective for topical ophthalmic use.
Structure and Empirical Formula:

$C_{19}H_{22}FN_3O_4 \cdot 1.5\ H_2O$ Mol Wt 402.42

Chemical Name: (±)-1-cyclopropyl-6-fluoro-1,4-dihydro-8-methoxy-7-(3-methyl-1-piperazinyl)-4-oxo-3-quinolinecarboxylic acid sesquihydrate

Contains: Active: gatifloxacin 0.3% (3 mg/mL).
Preservative: benzalkonium chloride 0.005%.
Inactives: edetate disodium; purified water and sodium chloride. May contain hydrochloric acid and/or sodium hydroxide to adjust pH to approximately 6.
ZYMAR™ is a sterile, clear, pale yellow colored isotonic unbuffered solution. It has an osmolality of 260-330 mOsm/kg.
Clinical Pharmacology:
Pharmacokinetics: Gatifloxacin ophthalmic solution 0.3% or 0.5% was administered to one eye of 6 healthy male subjects each in an escalated dosing regimen starting with a single 2 drop dose, then 2 drops 4 times daily for 7 days and finally 2 drops 8 times daily for 3 days. At all time points, serum gatifloxacin levels were below the lower limit of quantification (5 ng/mL) in all subjects.
Microbiology: Gatifloxacin is an 8-methoxy fluoroquinolone with a 3-methylpiperazinyl substituent at C7. The antibacterial action of gatifloxacin results from inhibition of DNA gyrase and topoisomerase IV. DNA gyrase is an essential enzyme that is involved in the replication, transcription and repair of bacterial DNA. Topoisomerase IV is an enzyme known to play a key role in the partitioning of the chromosomal DNA during bacterial cell division.
The mechanism of action of fluoroquinolones including gatifloxacin is different from that of aminoglycoside, macrolide, and tetracycline antibiotics. Therefore, gatifloxacin may be active against pathogens that are resistant to these antibiotics and these antibiotics may be active against pathogens that are resistant to gatifloxacin. There is no cross-resistance between gatifloxacin and the aforementioned classes of antibiotics. Cross resistance has been observed between systemic gatifloxacin and some other fluoroquinolones.
Resistance to gatifloxacin *in vitro* develops via multiple step mutations. Resistance to gatifloxacin *in vitro* occurs at a general frequency of between 1×10^{-7} to 10^{-10}.
Gatifloxacin has been shown to be active against most strains of the following organisms both *in vitro* and clinically, in conjunctival infections as described in the INDICATIONS AND USAGE section.
Aerobes, Gram-Positive:
*Corynebacterium propinquum**
Staphylococcus aureus
Staphylococcus epidermidis
*Streptococcus mitis**
Streptococcus pneumoniae
Aerobes, Gram-Negative:
Haemophilus influenzae

---
* Efficacy for this organism was studied in fewer than 10 infections.
The following *in vitro* data are available, **but their clinical significance in ophthalmic infections is unknown.** The safety and effectiveness of ZYMAR™ in treating ophthalmic infections due to the following organisms have not been established in adequate and well-controlled clinical trials.
The following organisms are considered susceptible when evaluated using systemic breakpoints. However, a correlation between the *in vitro* systemic breakpoint and ophthalmological efficacy has not been established. The following list of organisms is provided as guidance only in assessing the potential treatment of conjunctival infections.
Gatifloxacin exhibits *in vitro* minimal inhibitory concentrations (MICs) of 2µg/mL or less (systemic susceptible breakpoint) against most (≥ 90%) strains of the following ocular pathogens.
Aerobes, Gram-Positive:
Listeria monocytogenes
Staphylococcus saprophyticus

Streptococcus agalactiae
Streptococcus pyogenes
Streptococcus viridans Group
Streptococcus Groups C, F, G
Aerobes, Gram-Negative:
Acinetobacter lwoffii
Enterobacter aerogenes
Enterobacter cloacae
Escherichia coli
Citrobacter freundii
Citrobacter koseri
Haemophilus parainfluenzae
Klebsiella oxytoca
Klebsiella pneumoniae
Moraxella catarrhalis
Morganella morganii
Neisseria gonorrhoeae
Neisseria meningitidis
Proteus mirabilis
Proteus vulgaris
Serratia marcescens
Vibrio cholerae
Yersinia enterocolitica
Other Microorganisms:
Chlamydia pneumoniae
Legionella pneumophila
Mycobacterium marinum
Mycobacterium fortuitum
Mycoplasma pneumoniae
Anaerobic Microorganisms:
Bacteroides fragilis
Clostridium perfringens
Clinical Studies:
In a randomized, double-masked, multicenter clinical trial, where patients were dosed for 5 days, ZYMAR™ solution was superior to its vehicle on day 5-7 in patients with conjunctivitis and positive conjunctival cultures. Clinical outcomes for the trial demonstrated clinical cure of 77% (40/52) for the gatifloxacin treated group versus 58% (28/48) for the placebo treated group. Microbiological outcomes for the same clinical trial demonstrated a statistically superior eradication rate for causative pathogens of 92% (48/52) for gatifloxacin vs. 72% (34/48) for placebo. Please note that microbiologic eradication does not always correlate with clinical outcome in anti-infective trials.
Indications and Usage: ZYMAR™ solution is indicated for the treatment of bacterial conjunctivitis caused by susceptible strains of the following organisms:
Aerobic Gram-Positive Bacteria:
*Corynebacterium propinquum**
Staphylococcus aureus
Staphylococcus epidermidis
*Streptococcus mitis**
Streptococcus pneumoniae
Aerobic Gram-Negative Bacteria:
Haemophilus influenzae

---
* Efficacy for this organism was studied in fewer than 10 infections.
Contraindications: ZYMAR™ solution is contraindicated in patients with a history of hypersensitivity to gatifloxacin, to other quinolones, or to any of the components in this medication.
Warnings: NOT FOR INJECTION.
ZYMAR™ solution should not be injected subconjunctivally, nor should it be introduced directly into the anterior chamber of the eye.
In patients receiving systemic quinolones, including gatifloxacin, serious and occasionally fatal hypersensitivity (anaphylactic) reactions, some following the first dose, have been reported. Some reactions were accompanied by cardiovascular collapse, loss of consciousness, angioedema (including laryngeal, pharyngeal or facial edema), airway obstruction, dyspnea,

Continued on next page

Zymar—Cont.

urticaria, and itching. If an allergic reaction to gatifloxacin occurs, discontinue the drug. Serious acute hypersensitivity reactions may require immediate emergency treatment. Oxygen and airway management should be administered as clinically indicated.

Precautions:

General: As with other anti-infectives, prolonged use may result in overgrowth of non-susceptible organisms, including fungi. If superinfection occurs discontinue use and institute alternative therapy. Whenever clinical judgment dictates, the patient should be examined with the aid of magnification, such as slit lamp biomicroscopy and, where appropriate, fluorescein staining.

Patients should be advised not to wear contact lenses if they have signs and symptoms of bacterial conjunctivitis.

Information for Patients: Avoid contaminating the applicator tip with material from the eye, fingers or other source.

Systemic quinolones, including gatifloxacin, have been associated with hypersensitivity reactions, even following a single dose. Discontinue use immediately and contact your physician at the first sign of a rash or allergic reaction.

Drug Interactions: Specific drug interaction studies have not been conducted with ZYMAR™ ophthalmic solution. However, the systemic administration of some quinolones has been shown to elevate plasma concentrations of theophylline, interfere with the metabolism of caffeine, and enhance the effects of the oral anticoagulant warfarin and its derivatives, and has been associated with transient elevations in serum creatinine in patients receiving systemic cyclosporine concomitantly.

Carcinogenesis, Mutagenesis, Impairment of Fertility

There was no increase in neoplasms among B6C3F1 mice given gatifloxacin in the diet for 18 months at doses averaging 81 mg/kg/day in males and 90 mg/kg/day in females. These doses are approximately 2000-fold higher than the maximum recommended ophthalmic dose of 0.04 mg/kg/day in a 50 kg human.

There was no increase in neoplasms among Fischer 344 rats given gatifloxacin in the diet for 2 years at doses averaging 47 mg/kg/day in males and 139 mg/kg/day in females (1000 and 3000-fold higher, respectively, than the maximum recommended ophthalmic dose). A statistically significant increase in the incidence of large granular lymphocyte (LGL) leukemia was seen in males treated with a high dose of approximately 2000-fold higher than the maximum recommended ophthalmic dose. Fischer 344 rats have a high spontaneous background rate of LGL leukemia and the incidence in high-dose males only slightly exceeded the historical control range established for this strain.

In genetic toxicity tests, gatifloxacin was positive in 1 of 5 strains used in bacterial reverse mutation assays; Salmonella strain TA102. Gatifloxacin was positive in *in vitro* mammalian cell mutation and chromosome aberration assays. Gatifloxacin was positive in *in vitro* unscheduled DNA synthesis in rat hepatocytes but not human leukocytes. Gatifloxacin was negative in *in vivo* micronucleus tests in mice, cytogenetics test in rats, and DNA repair test in rats. The findings may be due to the inhibitory effects of high concentrations on eukaryotic type II DNA topoisomerase.

There were no adverse effects on fertility or reproduction in rats given gatifloxacin orally at doses up to 200 mg/kg/day (approximately 4500-fold higher than the maximum recommended ophthalmic dose for ZYMAR™).

Pregnancy: Teratogenic Effects. Pregnancy Category C:

There were no teratogenic effects observed in rats or rabbits following oral gatifloxacin doses up to 50 mg/kg/day (approximately 1000-fold higher than the maximum recommended ophthalmic dose). However, skeletal/craniofacial malformations or delayed ossification, atrial enlargement, and reduced fetal weight were observed in fetuses from rats given ≥150 mg/kg/day (approximately 3000-fold higher than the maximum recommended ophthalmic dose). In a perinatal/postnatal study, increased late post-implantation loss and neonatal/perinatal mortalities were observed at 200 mg/kg/day (approximately 4500 times the maximum recommended ophthalmic dose).

Because there are no adequate and well-controlled studies in pregnant women, ZYMAR™ solution should be used during pregnancy only if the potential benefit justifies the potential risk to the fetus.

Nursing Mothers: Gatifloxacin is excreted in the breast milk of rats. It is not known whether this drug is excreted in human milk. Because many drugs are excreted in human milk, caution should be exercised when gatifloxacin is administered to a nursing woman.

Pediatric Use: Safety and effectiveness in infants below the age of one year have not been established.

Geriatric use: No overall differences in safety or effectiveness have been observed between elderly and younger patients.

Adverse Reactions:

Ophthalmic Use: The most frequently reported adverse events in the overall study population were conjunctival irritation, increased lacrimation, keratitis, and papillary conjunctivitis. These events occurred in approximately 5-10% of patients. Other reported reactions occurring in 1-4% of patients were chemosis, conjunctival hemorrhage, dry eye, eye discharge, eye irritation, eye pain, eyelid edema, headache, red eye, reduced visual acuity and taste disturbance.

Dosage and Administration: The recommended dosage regimen for the treatment of bacterial conjunctivitis is:

Days 1 and 2: Instill one drop every two hours in the affected eye(s) while awake, up to 8 times daily.

Days 3 through 7: Instill one drop up to four times daily while awake.

How Supplied: ZYMAR™ (gatifloxacin ophthalmic solution) 0.3% is supplied sterile in a white, low density polyethylene (LDPE) bottle with a controlled dropper tip and a tan, high impact polystyrene (HIPS) cap in the following size:

5 mL in an 8 mL bottle- NDC 0023-9218-05

Note: Store at 15°–25°C (59°–77°F). Protect from freezing.

Animal Pharmacology: Quinolone antibacterials have been shown to cause bone or cartilage changes in immature animals. There was no evidence of bone cartilage changes following ocular administration of gatifloxacin in rabbits or dogs.

Rx only
October 2003
©2003 Allergan, Inc., Irvine, CA 92612, U.S.A.
® and ™ Marks owned by Allergan, Inc.
Licensed from: Kyorin Pharmaceuticals Co., Ltd.
U.S. PAT. 4,980,470; 5,880,283
9415X 71706US11M

Shown in Product Identification Guide, page 103

Bausch & Lomb, Incorporated
180 EAST VIA VERDE
SAN DIMAS, CA 91773

Direct Inquiries to:
Customer Services (800) 338-2020

INTRAOCULAR PRODUCTS
Please see Section 8, "Intraocular Product Information," for information on Bausch & Lomb Inc., Surgical Division's intraocular products.

Bausch & Lomb Incorporated
8500 HIDDEN RIVER PARKWAY
TAMPA, FL 33637

NDC 24208	PRODUCT	
-353-	**ALREX®** loteprednol etabonate ophthalmic suspension, 0.2% 5 mL: -05 10 mL: -10	℞
-825-55	**ATROPINE SULFATE OPHTHALMIC OINTMENT USP, 1%** 3.5 gram tubes	℞
-750-	**ATROPINE SULFATE OPHTHALMIC SOLUTION USP, 1%** 5mL: -60 15mL: -06	℞
555-55	**BACITRACIN ZINC & POLYMYXIN B SULFATE OPHTHALMIC OINTMENT USP** 3.5 g tube	℞
367-	**CARTEOLOL HYDROCHLORIDE OPHTHALMIC SOLUTION, USP, 1%** 5 mL: -05 10 mL: -10 15 mL: -15	℞
300-10	**CROLOM®** cromolyn sodium ophthalmic solution USP, 4% 10 mL	℞
-735-	**CYCLOPENTOLATE HYDROCHLORIDE OPHTHALMIC SOLUTION USP, 1%** 2mL: -01 15mL: -06	℞
-720-02	**DEXAMETHASONE SODIUM PHOSPHATE** Ophthalmic Solution, USP, 0.1% 5 mL	℞
540	**DIPIVEFRIN HYDROCHLORIDE** Ophthalmic Solution USP, 0.1% 5 mL: -05 10 mL: -10 15 mL: -15	℞
910-	**ERYTHROMYCIN OPHTHALMIC** Ointment USP, 0.5% 50 × 1 g tube -19 3.5 g tube -55	℞

BAUSCH & LOMB / 245

Code	Product
732-05	**FLUORESCEIN SODIUM & BENOXINATE HCl OPHTHALMIC SOLUTION** ℞ USP, 0.25%/0.4% 5 ml
390-83	**FLUOR-I-STRIP®** ℞ 9mg Fluorescein Sodium Ophthalmic Strips Box of 300
391-83	**FLUOR-I-STRIP® A.T.** ℞ 1 mg Fluorescein Sodium Ophthalmic Strips Box of 300
288-	**FLUOROMETHOLONE OPHTHALMIC** ℞ Suspension USP, 0.1% 5 mL -05 10 mL -10 15 mL -15
314-25	**FLURBIPROFEN** ℞ Sodium Ophthalmic Solution USP, 0.03% 2.5 ml
-580-	**GENTAMICIN SULFATE** ℞ Ophthalmic Solution USP, 0.3% 5mL: -60 15mL: -64
-545-	**LEVOBUNOLOL HYDROCHLORIDE OPHTHALMIC SOLUTION USP, 0.25%** ℞ 5mL: -05 10mL: -10
-505-	**LEVOBUNOLOL HYDROCHLORIDE OPHTHALMIC SOLUTION USP, 0.5%** ℞ 5mL: -05 10mL: -10 15 mL: -15
-299-	**LOTEMAX®** ℞ loteprednol etabonate opthalmic suspension, 0.5% 5 mL -05 10 mL -10 15 mL -15
-402-	**METIPRANOLOL OPHTHALMIC SOLUTION 0.3%** ℞ 5 mL -05 10 mL -10
-280-15	**MUROCEL®** OTC Methylcellulose Lubricant Ophthalmic Solution USP, 1% 15 mL
-278-05	**MUROCOLL® 2** ℞ Phenylephrine Hydrochloride 10% and Scopolamine Hydrobromide 0.3% Ophthalmic Solution 5 mL
-385	**MURO 128® 5% OINTMENT** OTC Sodium Chloride Hypertonicity Ophthalmic Ointment, 5% 3.5g: -55 TWIN PACK 2×3.5g: -56
-276-15	**MURO 128® 2%** OTC Sodium Chloride Hypertonicity Ophthalmic Solution, 2% 15 mL
-277-	**MURO 128® 5% SOLUTION** OTC Sodium Chloride Hypertonicity Ophthalmic Solution, 5% 15 mL: -15 30 mL: -30
-725-06	**NAPHAZOLINE HYDROCHLORIDE OPHTHALMIC SOLUTION** ℞ USP, 0.1% 15mL
-785-55	**NEOMYCIN & POLYMYXIN B SULFATES, BACITRACIN ZINC AND HYDROCORTISONE OPHTHALMIC** ℞ Ointment USP 3.5 g tube
-780-55	**NEOMYCIN AND POLYMYXIN B SULFATES AND BACITRACIN ZINC OPHTHALMIC** ℞ Ointment USP 3.5 gram tubes
-795-35	**NEOMYCIN AND POLYMYXIN B SULFATES AND DEXAMETHASONE OPHTHALMIC OINTMENT USP** ℞ 3.5 gram tubes
830-60	**NEOMYCIN AND POLYMYXIN B SULFATES AND DEXAMETHASONE** ℞ Ophthalmic Suspension USP 5 mL
790-62	**NEOMYCIN AND POLYMYXIN B SULFATES AND GRAMICIDIN** ℞ Ophthalmic Solution USP 10 mL
377-11	**MOISTURE EYES LIQUID GEL** OTC Lubricating Eye Drops 15 mL
384-48	**MOISTURE EYES LIQUID GEL PF** OTC Lubricating Eye Drops 28 × 0.5 mL Unit Dose
387-60	**OCUVITE®** OTC Vitamin and Mineral Supplement Bottle of 60 tablets
387-62	**OCUVITE®** OTC Antioxidant Vitamin and Mineral Supplement Bottle of 120 tablets
388-19	**OCUVITE® extra®** OTC Antioxidant Vitamin and Mineral Supplement Bottle of 50 tablets
403-19	**OCUVITE® Lutein** OTC Vitamin and Mineral Supplement Bottle of 36 capsules
432-62	**OCUVITE PRESERVISION** 120s
432-72	**OCUVITE PRESERVISION** 240s
434-05	**OFLOXACIN OPHTHALMIC SOLUTION** 5 mL
434-10	**OFLOXACIN OPHTHALMIC SOLUTION** 10 mL
-275-	**OPTIPRANOLOL®** ℞ (metipranolol ophthalmic solution) 0.3% 5 mL: -07 10 mL: -09
-740-	**PHENYLEPHRINE HYDROCHLORIDE OPHTHALMIC SOLUTION USP, 2.5%** ℞ 2mL: -59 5mL: -02 15mL: -06
-806-15	**PILOCARPINE HYDROCHLORIDE OPHTHALMIC SOLUTION USP, 0.5%** ℞ 15mL
-676-	**PILOCARPINE HYDROCHLORIDE OPHTHALMIC SOLUTION USP, 1%** ℞ 15mL: -15 TWIN PACK 2×15 mL: -30
-681-	**PILOCARPINE HYDROCHLORIDE OPHTHALMIC SOLUTION USP, 2%** ℞ 15mL: -15 TWIN PACK 2×15 mL: -30
-811-15	**PILOCARPINE HYDROCHLORIDE OPHTHALMIC SOLUTION USP, 3%** ℞ 15mL
-686-	**PILOCARPINE HYDROCHLORIDE OPHTHALMIC SOLUTION USP, 4%** ℞ 15mL: -15 TWIN PACK 2×15 mL: -30
-821-15	**PILOCARPINE HYDROCHLORIDE OPHTHALMIC SOLUTION USP, 6%** ℞ 15mL
315-10	**POLYMYXIN B SULFATE AND TRIMETHOPRIM SULFATE OPHTHALMIC SOLUTION USP** ℞ 10mL
715-	**PREDNISOLONE SODIUM PHOSPHATE OPHTHALMIC SOLUTION USP, 1%** ℞ 5 mL: -02 10 mL: -10 15 mL: -06
730-06	**PROPARACAINE HYDROCHLORIDE OPHTHALMIC SOLUTION USP, 0.5%** ℞ 15 mL
394-07	**REV-EYES®** ℞ Dapiprazole HCl Ophthalmic Solution 0.5% 25 mg Vial
317-	**SULFACETAMIDE SODIUM AND PREDNISOLONE SODIUM PHOSPHATE** ℞ Ophthalmic Solution 10%/0.23% (prednisolone phosphate) 5 mL: -05 10 mL: -10

Continued on next page

Product List-B & L—Cont.

-670-04	SULFACETAMIDE SODIUM OPHTHALMIC SOLUTION USP, 10% 15mL	℞
-920-64	TETRACAINE HYDRO-CHLORIDE OPHTHALMIC SOLUTION USP, 0.5% 15mL	℞
-330-	TIMOLOL MALEATE OPHTHALMIC SOLUTION USP, 0.25% 5 mL: -05 10 mL: -10 15 mL: -15	℞
-324-	TIMOLOL MALEATE OPHTHALMIC SOLUTION USP, 0.5% 5 mL: -05 10 mL: -10 15 mL: -15	℞
-290-05	TOBRAMYCIN OPHTHALMIC SOLUTION USP, 0.3% 5mL	℞
-590-64	TROPICAMIDE OPHTHALMIC SOLUTION, USP 0.5% 15 mL	℞
-585-	TROPICAMIDE OPHTHALMIC SOLUTION, USP 1% 2 × 12 mL: -59 15 mL: -64	℞

ALREX®
[ăl rĕx]
loteprednol etabonate
ophthalmic suspension 0.2%
STERILE OPHTHALMIC SUSPENSION
℞ only

Description: ALREX® (loteprednol etabonate ophthalmic suspension) contains a sterile, topical anti-inflammatory corticosteroid for ophthalmic use. Loteprednol etabonate is a white to off-white powder.
Loteprednol etabonate is represented by the following structural formula:

$C_{24}H_{31}ClO_7$ Mol. Wt. 466.96

Chemical name:
chloromethyl 17α[(ethoxycarbonyl)oxy]-11β-hydroxy-3-oxoandrosta-1,4-diene-17β-carboxylate.
Each mL contains:
ACTIVE: Loteprednol Etabonate 2 mg (0.2%); INACTIVES: Edetate Disodium, Glycerin, Povidone, Purified Water and Tyloxapol. Hydrochloric Acid and/or Sodium Hydroxide may be added to adjust the pH to 5.3–5.6. The suspension is essentially isotonic with a tonicity of 250 to 310 mOsmol/kg.
PRESERVATIVE ADDED: Benzalkonium Chloride 0.01%.
Clinical Pharmacology: Corticosteroids inhibit the inflammatory response to a variety of inciting agents and probably delay or slow healing. They inhibit the edema, fibrin deposition, capillary dilation, leukocyte migration, capillary proliferation, fibroblast proliferation, deposition of collagen, and scar formation associated with inflammation. There is no generally accepted explanation for the mechanism of action of ocular corticosteroids. However, corticosteroids are thought to act by the induction of phospholipase A_2 inhibitory proteins, collectively called lipocortins. It is postulated that these proteins control the biosynthesis of potent mediators of inflammation such as prostaglandins and leukotrienes by inhibiting the release of their common precursor arachidonic acid. Arachidonic acid is released from membrane phospholipids by phospholipase A_2. Corticosteroids are capable of producing a rise in intraocular pressure.
Loteprednol etabonate is structurally similar to other corticosteroids. However, the number 20 position ketone group is absent. It is highly lipid soluble which enhances its penetration into cells. Loteprednol etabonate is synthesized through structural modifications of prednisolone-related compounds so that it will undergo a predictable transformation to an inactive metabolite. Based upon *in vivo* and *in vitro* preclinical metabolism studies, loteprednol etabonate undergoes extensive metabolism to inactive carboxylic acid metabolites.
Results from a bioavailability study in normal volunteers established that plasma levels of loteprednol etabonate and Δ^1 cortienic acid etabonate (PJ 91), its primary, inactive metabolite, were below the limit of quantitation (1 ng/mL) at all sampling times. The results were obtained following the ocular administration of one drop in each eye of 0.5% loteprednol etabonate 8 times daily for 2 days or 4 times daily for 42 days. This study suggests that limited (<1 ng/mL) systemic absorption occurs with ALREX.
Clinical Studies:
In two double-masked, placebo-controlled six-week environmental studies of 268 patients with seasonal allergic conjunctivitis, ALREX, when dosed four times per day was superior to placebo in the treatment of the signs and symptoms of seasonal allergic conjunctivitis. ALREX provided reduction in bulbar conjunctival injection and itching, beginning approximately 2 hours after instillation of the first dose and throughout the first 14 days of treatment.
Indications and Usage: ALREX Ophthalmic Suspension is indicated for the temporary relief of the signs and symptoms of seasonal allergic conjunctivitis.
Contraindications: ALREX, as with other ophthalmic corticosteroids, is contraindicated in most viral diseases of the cornea and conjunctiva including epithelial herpes simplex keratitis (dendritic keratitis), vaccinia, and varicella, and also in mycobacterial infection of the eye and fungal diseases of ocular structures. ALREX is also contraindicated in individuals with known or suspected hypersensitivity to any of the ingredients of this preparation and to other corticosteroids.
Warnings: Prolonged use of corticosteroids may result in glaucoma with damage to the optic nerve, defects in visual acuity and fields of vision, and in posterior subcapsular cataract formation. Steroids should be used with caution in the presence of glaucoma.
Prolonged use of corticosteroids may suppress the host response and thus increase the hazard of secondary ocular infections. In those diseases causing thinning of the cornea or sclera, perforations have been known to occur with the use of topical steroids. In acute purulent conditions of the eye, steroids may mask infection or enhance existing infection.
Use of ocular steroids may prolong the course and may exacerbate the severity of many viral infections of the eye (including herpes simplex). Employment of a corticosteroid medication in the treatment of patients with a history of herpes simplex requires great caution.

Precautions:
General: For ophthalmic use only. The initial prescription and renewal of the medication order beyond 14 days should be made by a physician only after examination of the patient with the aid of magnification, such as slit lamp biomicroscopy and, where appropriate, fluorescein staining.
If signs and symptoms fail to improve after two days, the patient should be re-evaluated.
If this product is used for 10 days or longer, intraocular pressure should be monitored.
Fungal infections of the cornea are particularly prone to develop coincidentally with long-term local steroid application. Fungus invasion must be considered in any persistent corneal ulceration where a steroid has been used or is in use. Fungal cultures should be taken when appropriate.
Information for Patients: This product is sterile when packaged. Patients should be advised not to allow the dropper tip to touch any surface, as this may contaminate the suspension. If redness or itching becomes aggravated, the patient should be advised to consult a physician.
Patients should be advised not to wear a contact lens if their eye is red. ALREX should not be used to treat contact lens related irritation. The preservative in ALREX, benzalkonium chloride, may be absorbed by soft contact lenses. Patients who wear soft contact lenses **and whose eyes are not red**, should be instructed to wait at least ten minutes after instilling ALREX before they insert their contact lenses.
Carcinogenesis, mutagenesis, impairment of fertility: Long-term animal studies have not been conducted to evaluate the carcinogenic potential of loteprednol etabonate. Loteprednol etabonate was not genotoxic *in vitro* in the Ames test, the mouse lymphoma tk assay, or in a chromosome aberration test in human lymphocytes, or *in vivo* in the single dose mouse micronucleus assay. Treatment of male and female rats with up to 50 mg/kg/day and 25 mg/kg/day of loteprednol etabonate, respectively, (1500 and 750 times the maximum clinical dose, respectively) prior to and during mating did not impair fertility in either gender.
Pregnancy: Teratogenic effects: Pregnancy Category C. Loteprednol etabonate has been shown to be embryotoxic (delayed ossification) and teratogenic (increased incidence of meningocele, abnormal left common carotid artery, and limb flexures) when administered orally to rabbits during organogenesis at a dose of 3 mg/kg/day (85 times the maximum daily clinical dose), a dose which caused no maternal toxicity. The no-observed-effect-level (NOEL) for these effects was 0.5 mg/kg/day (15 times the maximum daily clinical dose). Oral treatment of rats during organogenesis resulted in teratogenicity (absent innominate artery at ≥5mg/kg/day doses, and cleft palate and umbilical hernia at ≥50 mg/kg/day) and embryotoxicity (increased post-implantation losses at 100 mg/kg/day and decreased fetal body weight and skeletal ossification with ≥50 mg/kg/day). Treatment of rats with 0.5 mg/kg/day (15 times the maximum clinical dose) during organogenesis did not result in any reproductive toxicity. Loteprednol etabonate was maternally toxic (significantly reduced body weight gain during treatment) when administered to pregnant rats during organogenesis at doses of ≥5 mg/kg/day.
Oral exposure of female rats to 50 mg/kg/day of loteprednol etabonate from the start of the fetal period through the end of lactation, a maternally toxic treatment regimen (significantly decreased body weight gain), gave rise to decreased growth and survival, and retarded development in the offspring during lactation; the NOEL for these effects was 5 mg/kg/day. Loteprednol etabonate had no effect on the du-

ration of gestation or parturition when administered orally to pregnant rats at doses up to 50 mg/kg/day during the fetal period.

Nursing Mothers: It is not known whether topical ophthalmic administration of corticosteroids could result in sufficient systemic absorption to produce detectable quantities in human milk. Systemic steroids appear in human milk and could suppress growth, interfere with endogenous corticosteroid production, or cause other untoward effects. Caution should be exercised when ALREX is administered to a nursing woman.

Pediatric Use: Safety and effectiveness in pediatric patients have not been established.

Adverse Reactions: Reactions associated with ophthalmic steroids include elevated intraocular pressure, which may be associated with optic nerve damage, visual acuity and field defects, posterior subcapsular cataract formation, secondary ocular infection from pathogens including herpes simplex, and perforation of the globe where there is thinning of the cornea or sclera.

Ocular adverse reactions occurring in 5–15% of patients treated with loteprednol etabonate ophthalmic suspension (0.2%–0.5%) in clinical studies included abnormal vision/blurring, burning on instillation, chemosis, discharge, dry eyes, epiphora, foreign body sensation, itching, injection, and photophobia. Other ocular adverse reactions occurring in less than 5% of patients include conjunctivitis, corneal abnormalities, eyelid erythema, keratoconjunctivitis, ocular irritation/pain/discomfort, papillae, and uveitis. Some of these events were similar to the underlying ocular disease being studied.

Non-ocular adverse reactions occurred in less than 15% of patients. These include headache, rhinitis and pharyngitis.

In a summation of controlled, randomized studies of individuals treated for 28 days or longer with loteprednol etabonate, the incidence of significant elevation of intraocular pressure ($\geq$10 mm Hg) was 2% (15/901) among patients receiving loteprednol etabonate, 7% (11/164) among patients receiving 1% prednisolone acetate and 0.5% (3/583) among patients receiving placebo. Among the smaller group of patients who were studied with ALREX, the incidence of clinically significant increases in IOP ($\geq$10 mm Hg) was 1% (1/133) with ALREX and 1% (1/135) with placebo.

Dosage and Administration: SHAKE VIGOROUSLY BEFORE USING.
One drop instilled into the affected eye(s) four times daily.

How Supplied: ALREX® (loteprednol etabonate ophthalmic suspension, 0.2%) is supplied in a plastic bottle with a controlled drop tip in the following sizes:
2.5 mL bottle (NDC 24208-353-25)-AB35304
 5 mL bottle (NDC 24208-353-05)-AB35307
10 mL bottle (NDC 24208-353-10)-AB35309

DO NOT USE IF NECKBAND IMPRINTED WITH "Protective Seal" AND YELLOW IS NOT INTACT.

Storage: Store upright between 15°–25°C (59°–77°F). DO NOT FREEZE.

KEEP OUT OF REACH OF CHILDREN
Bausch & Lomb Incorporated,
Tampa, Florida 33637
U.S. Patent No. 4,996,335
U.S. Patent No. 5,540,930
©Bausch & Lomb Incorporated
® Alrex is a trademark of Bausch & Lomb Incorporated
Rev. 12/03-83
Shown in Product Identification Guide, page 104

BRIMONIDINE TARTRATE ℞
Ophthalmic Solution 0.2%
STERILE OPHTHALMIC SOLUTION
℞ only

Description: Brimonidine Tartrate Ophthalmic Solution 0.2% is a relatively selective alpha-2 adrenergic agonist for ophthalmic use. In solution, brimonidine tartrate ophthalmic solution 0.2% has a clear, greenish-yellow color. It has an osmolality of 280-330 mOsml/kg and a pH of 5.6–6.6 The structural formula is

$C_{11}H_{10}BrN_5 \cdot C_4H_6O_6$

Mol. Wt. 442.24 (as the tartrate salt)

Chemical Name: 5-bromo-6-(2-imidazolidinylideneamino) quinoxaline L-tartrate.
CAS Number 59803-98-4
Each mL Contains:
ACTIVE: Brimonidine tartrate: 0.2% (2 mg/mL).
INACTIVES: Citric Acid, Polyvinyl Alcohol, Sodium Chloride, Sodium Citrate, Purified Water. Hydrochloric Acid and/or Sodium Hydroxide may be added to adjust pH.
PRESERVATIVE ADDED: Benzalkonium Chloride (0.05 mg).

Clinical Pharmacology
Mechanism of Action: Brimonidine tartrate ophthalmic solution 0.2% is an alpha adrenergic receptor agonist. It has a peak ocular hypotensive effect occurring at two hours post-dosing. Fluorophotometric studies in animals and humans suggest that brimonidine tartrate has a dual mechanism of action by reducing aqueous humor production and increasing uveoscleral outflow.

Pharmacokinetics: After ocular administration of a 0.2% solution, plasma concentrations peaked within 1 to 4 hours and declined with a systemic half-life of approximately 3 hours. In humans, systemic metabolism of brimonidine is extensive. It is metabolized primarily by the liver. Urinary excretion is the major route of elimination of the drug and its metabolites. Approximately 87% of an orally-administered radioactive dose was eliminated within 120 hours, with 74% found in the urine.

Clinical Evaluations: Elevated IOP presents a major risk factor in glaucomatous field loss. The higher the level of IOP, the greater the likelihood of optic nerve damage and visual field loss. Brimonidine tartrate has the action of lowering intraocular pressure with minimal effect on cardiovascular and pulmonary parameters.

In comparative clinical studies with timolol 0.5%, lasting up to one year, the IOP lowering effect of brimonidine tartrate ophthalmic solution 0.2% was approximately 4-6 mmHg compared with approximately 6 mmHg for timolol. In these studies, both patient groups were dosed BID; however, due to the duration of action of brimonidine tartrate ophthalmic solution 0.2%, it is recommended that brimonidine tartrate ophthalmic solution 0.2% be dosed TID. Eight percent of subjects were discontinued from studies due to inadequately controlled intraocular pressure, which in 30% of these patients occurred within the first month of therapy. Approximately 20% were discontinued due to adverse experiences.

Indications and Usage: Brimonidine tartrate ophthalmic solution 0.2% is indicated for lowering intraocular pressure in patients with open-angle glaucoma or ocular hypertension.

The IOP lowering efficacy of brimonidine tartrate ophthalmic solution 0.2% diminishes over time in some patients. This loss of effect appears with a variable time of onset in each patient and should be closely monitored.

Contraindications: Brimonidine tartrate ophthalmic solution 0.2% is contraindicated in patients with hypersensitivity to brimonidine tartrate or any component of this medication. It is also contraindicated in patients receiving monoamine oxidase (MAO) inhibitor therapy.

Precautions:
General: Although brimonidine tartrate ophthalmic solution 0.2% had minimal effect on blood pressure of patients in clinical studies, caution should be exercised in treating patients with severe cardiovascular disease.
Brimonidine tartrate ophthalmic solution 0.2% has not been studied in patients with hepatic or renal impairment; caution should be used in treating such patients.
Brimonidine tartrate ophthalmic solution 0.2% should be used with caution in patients with depression, cerebral or coronary insufficiency, Raynaud's phenomenon, orthostatic hypotension or thromboangitis obliterans.
During the studies there was a loss of effect in some patients. The IOP-lowering efficacy observed with brimonidine tartrate opthalmic solution 0.2% during the first month of therapy may not always reflect the long-term level of IOP reduction. Patients prescribed IOP-lowering medication should be routinely monitored for IOP.

Information for Patients: The preservative in brimonidine tartrate ophthalmic solution 0.2%, benzalkonium chloride, may be absorbed by soft contact lenses. Patients wearing soft contact lenses should be instructed to wait at least 15 minutes after instilling brimonidine tartrate ophthalmic solution 0.2% to insert soft contact lenses.

As with other drugs in this class, brimonidine tartrate ophthalmic solution 0.2% may cause fatigue and/or drowsiness in some patients. Patients who engage in hazardous activities should be cautioned of the potential for a decrease in mental alertness.

Drug Interactions: Although specific drug interaction studies have not been conducted with brimonidine tartrate ophthalmic solution 0.2%, the possibility of an additive or potentiating effect with CNS depressants (alcohol, barbiturates, opiates, sedatives, or anesthetics) should be considered. Alpha-agonists, as a class, may reduce pulse and blood pressure. Caution in using concomitant drugs such as beta-blockers (ophthalmic and systemic), antihypertensives and/or cardiac glycosides is advised.

Tricyclic antidepressants have been reported to blunt the hypotensive effect of systemic clonidine. It is not known whether the concurrent use of these agents with brimonidine tartrate ophthalmic solution 0.2% in humans can lead to resulting interference with the IOP lowering effect. No data on the level of circulating catecholamines after brimonidine tartrate ophthalmic solution 0.2% are available. Caution, however, is advised in patients taking tricyclic antidepressants which can affect the metabolism and uptake of circulating amines.

Carcinogenesis, mutagenesis, impairment of fertility: No compound-related carcinogenic effects were observed in either mice or rats following a 21-month and 24-month study, respectively. In these studies, dietary administration of brimonidine tartrate at doses up to 2.5 mg/kg/day in mice and 1.0 mg/kg/day in rats achieved ~77 and 118 times, respectively, the plasma drug concentration estimated in humans treated with one drop brimonidine tartrate ophthalmic solution 0.2% in both eyes 3 times per day.

Continued on next page

Brimonidine Tartrate—Cont.

Brimonidine tartrate was not mutagenic or cytogenic in a series of in vitro and in vivo studies including the Ames test, chromosomal aberation assay in Chinese Hamster Ovary (CHO) cells, a host-mediated assay and cytogenic studies in mice, and dominant lethal assay.

Reproductive studies performed in rats with oral doses of 0.66 mg base/kg revealed no evidence of harm to the fetus due to brimonidine tartrate ophthalmic solution 0.2%.

Pregnancy: Teratogenic Effects: Pregnancy Category B.

Reproductive studies performed in rats with oral doses of 0.66 mg base/kg revealed no evidence of harm to the fetus due to brimonidine tartrate ophthalmic solution 0.2%. Dosing at this level produced 100 times the plasma drug concentration level seen in humans following multiple ophthalmic doses.

There are no adequate and well-controlled studies in pregnant women. In animal studies, brominidine crossed the placenta and entered into the fetal circulation to a limited extent. Brimonidine tartrate ophthalmic solution 0.2% should be used during pregnancy only if the potential benefit to the mother justifies the potential risk to the fetus.

Nursing Mothers: It is not known whether this drug is excreted in human milk; in animal studies brimonidine tartrate was excreted in breast milk. A decision should be made whether to discontinue nursing or to discontinue the drug, taking into account the importance of the drug to the mother.

Pediatric Use: In a well-controlled clinical study conducted in pediatric glaucoma patients (ages 2 to 7 years) the most commonly observed adverse events with brimonidine tartrate ophthalmic solution 0.2% dosed three times daily were somnolence (50% – 83% in patients ages 2 to 6 years) and decreased alertness. In pediatric patients 7 years of age or older (>20kg), somnolence appears to occur less frequently (25%). The most commonly observed adverse event was somnolence. Approximately 16% of patients on brimonidine tartrate ophthalmic solution discontinued from the study due to somnolence.

The safety and effectiveness of brimonidine tartrate ophthalmic solution 0.2% have not been studied in pediatric patients below the age of 2 years. Brimonidine tartrate ophthalmic solution 0.2% is not recommended for use in pediatric patients under the age of 2 years. (Also refer to Adverse Reactions section).

Geriatric Use: No overall differences in safety or effectiveness have been observed between elderly and other adult patients.

Adverse Reactions: Adverse events occurring in approximately 10-30% of the subjects, in descending order of incidence, included oral dryness, ocular hyperemia, burning and stinging, headache, blurring, foreign body sensation, fatigue/drowsiness, conjunctival follicles, ocular allergic reactions, and ocular pruritus. Events occurring in approximately 3-9% of the subjects, in descending order included corneal staining/erosion, photophobia, eyelid erythema, ocular ache/pain, ocular dryness, tearing, upper respiratory symptoms, eyelid edema, conjunctival edema, dizziness, blepharitis, ocular irritation, gastrointestinal symptoms, asthenia, conjunctival blanching, abnormal vision and muscular pain.

The following adverse reactions were reported in less than 3% of the patients: lid crusting, conjunctival hemorrhage, abnormal taste, insomnia, conjunctival discharge, depression, hypertension, anxiety, palpitations/arrhythmias, nasal dryness and syncope.

The following events have been identified during post-marketing use of brimonidine tartrate ophthalmic solution 0.2% in clinical practice. Because they are reported voluntarily from a population of unknown size, estimates and frequency cannot be made. The events, which have been chosen for inclusion due to either their seriousness, frequency of reporting, possible causal connection to brimonidine tartrate ophthalmic solution 0.2%, or a combination of these factors, include: bradycardia; hypotension; iritis; miosis; skin reactions (including erythema, eyelid pruritus, rash, and vasodilation); and tachycardia. Apnea, bradycardia, hypotension, hypothermia, hypotonia, and somnolence have been reported in infants receiving brimonidine tartrate ophthalmic solution 0.2%.

Overdosage: No information is available on overdosage in humans. Treatment of an oral overdose includes supportive and symptomatic therapy; a patent airway should be maintained.

Dosage and Administration: The recommended dose is one drop of brimonidine tartrate ophthalmic solution 0.2% in the affected eye(s) three times daily, approximately 8 hours apart.

Brimonidine tartrate ophthalmic solution 0.2% may be used concomitantly with other topical ophthalmic drug products to lower intraocular pressure. If more than one topical ophthalmic product is being used, the products should be administered at least 5 minutes apart.

How Supplied: Brimonidine Tartrate Ophthalmic Solution 0.2% is supplied sterile in a plastic bottle with a controlled drop tip in the following sizes:
5 mL bottles – Prod. No. 41107
10 mL bottles – Prod. No. 41109
15 mL bottles – Prod. No. 41111
Storage: Store between 15° – 25°C (59° – 77°F).
KEEP OUT OF THE REACH OF CHILDREN.
DO NOT USE IF IMPRINTED "Protective Seal" WITH YELLOW ☛ IS NOT INTACT.
Bausch & Lomb
Pharmaceuticals, Inc.
Tampa, FL 33637
©Bausch & Lomb Incorporated
XO50280 (Folded) XM10082 (Flat)
REV. 2/04-02
Prod. No. 411

Shown in Product Identification Guide, page 104

CARTEOLOL HYDROCHLORIDE ℞
Ophthalmic Solution USP, 1%
STERILE OPHTHALMIC SOLUTION

Rx only
FOR USE IN THE EYES ONLY

Description: Carteolol Hydrochloride Ophthalmic Solution, 1%, is a nonselective beta-adrenoceptor blocking agent for ophthalmic use. Carteolol hydrochloride is represented by the following structural formula:

$C_{16}H_{24}N_2O_3 \cdot HCl$ Mol. Wt. 328.84

Chemical Name: (+)-5-[3-[(1, 1-dimethylethyl) amino]-2-hydroxypropoxy]-3, 4-dihydro-2(1H)-quinolinone monohydrochloride.

Each mL of sterile solution contains:
ACTIVE: Carteolol Hydrochloride 10mg (1%).
INACTIVES: Sodium Chloride, Monobasic and Dibasic Sodium Phosphate, Purified Water.
PRESERVATIVE ADDED: Benzalkonium Chloride 0.005%. The product has a pH range of 6.2–7.2.

Clinical Pharmacology: Carteolol is a nonselective beta-adrenergic blocking agent with associated intrinsic sympathomimetic activity and without significant membrane-stabilizing activity.

Carteolol hydrochloride reduces normal and elevated intraocular pressure (IOP) whether or not accompanied by glaucoma. The exact mechanism of the ocular hypotensive effect of beta-blockers has not been definitely demonstrated.

In general, beta-adrenergic blockers reduce cardiac output in patients in good and poor cardiovascular health. In patients with severe impairment of myocardial function, beta-blockers may inhibit the sympathetic stimulation necessary to maintain adequate cardiac function. Beta-adrenergic blockers may also increase airway resistance in the bronchi and bronchioles due to unopposed parasympathetic activity.

Given topically twice daily in controlled domestic clinical trials ranging from 1.5 to 3 months, carteolol hydrochloride ophthalmic solution, 1% produced a median percent reduction of IOP 22% to 25%. No significant effects were noted on corneal sensitivity, tear secretion, or pupil size.

Indications And Usage: Carteolol hydrochloride ophthalmic solution, 1%, has been shown to be effective in lowering intraocular pressure and may be used in patients with chronic open-angle glaucoma and intraocular hypertension. It may be used alone or in combination with other intraocular pressure lowering medications.

Contraindications: Carteolol is contraindicated in those individuals with bronchial asthma or with a history of bronchial asthma, or severe chronic obstructive pulmonary disease (see Warnings); sinus bradycardia; second- and third-degree atrioventricular block; overt cardiac failure (see Warnings); cardiogenic shock; or hypersensitivity to any component of this product.

Warnings: Carteolol has not been detected in plasma following ocular instillation. However, as with other topically applied ophthalmic preparations, carteolol may be absorbed systemically. The same adverse reactions found with systemic administration of beta-adrenergic blocking agents may occur with topical administration. For example, severe respiratory reactions and cardiac reactions, including death due to bronchospasm in patients with asthma and rarely death in association with cardiac failure, have been reported with topical application of beta-adrenergic blocking agents (see Contraindications).

Cardiac Failure: Sympathetic stimulation may be essential for support of the circulation in individuals with diminished myocardial contractility, and its inhibition by beta-adrenergic receptor blockade may precipitate more severe failure.

In Patients Without a History of Cardiac Failure: Continued depression of the myocardium with beta-blocking agents over a period of time can, in some cases, lead to cardiac failure. At the first sign or symptom of cardiac failure, carteolol hydrochloride should be discontinued.

Non-allergic Bronchospasm: In patients with non-allergic bronchospasm or with a history of non-allergic bronchospasm (e.g., chronic bronchitis, emphysema), carteolol should be administered with caution since it may block bronchodilation produced by endogenous and exogenous catecholamine stimulation of beta$_2$ receptors.

Major Surgery: The necessity or desirability of withdrawal of beta-adrenergic blocking agents prior to major surgery is controversial.

Beta-adrenergic receptor blockade impairs the ability of the heart to respond to beta-adrenergically mediated reflex stimuli. This may augment the risk of general anesthesia in surgical procedures. Some patients receiving beta-adrenergic receptor blocking agents have been subject to protracted severe hypotension during anesthesia. For these reasons, in patients undergoing elective surgery, gradual withdrawal of beta-adrenergic receptor blocking agents may be appropriate.

If necessary during surgery, the effects of beta-adrenergic blocking agents may be reversed by sufficient doses of such agonists as isoproterenol, dopamine, dobutamine or levarterenol (see Overdosage).

Diabetes Mellitus: Beta-adrenergic blocking agents should be administered with caution in patients subject to spontaneous hypoglycemia or to diabetic patients (especially those with labile diabetes) who are receiving insulin or oral hypoglycemic agents. Beta-adrenergic receptor blocking agents may mask the signs and symptoms of acute hypoglycemia.

Thyrotoxicosis: Beta-adrenergic blocking agents may mask certain clinical signs (e.g., tachycardia) of hyperthyroidism. Patients suspected of developing thyrotoxicosis should be managed carefully to avoid abrupt withdrawal of beta-adrenergic blocking agents which might precipitate a thyroid storm.

Precautions: General: Carteolol hydrochloride ophthalmic solution should be used with caution in patients with known hypersensitivity to other beta-adrenoceptor blocking agents. Use with caution in patients with known diminished pulmonary function.

In patients with angle-closure glaucoma, the immediate objective of treatment is to reopen the angle. This requires constricting the pupil with a miotic. Carteolol has little or no effect on the pupil. When carteolol is used to reduce elevated intraocular pressure in angle-closure glaucoma, it should be used with a miotic and not alone.

Information to the Patient: For topical use only. To prevent contaminating the dropper tip and solution, care should be taken not to touch the eyelids or surrounding areas with the dropper tip of the bottle. Keep bottle tightly closed when not in use. Protect from light.

Risk from Anaphylactic Reaction: While taking beta-blockers, patients with a history of atopy or a history of severe anaphylactic reaction to a variety of allergens may be more reactive to repeated accidental, diagnostic or therapeutic challenge with such allergens. Such patients may be unresponsive to the usual doses of epinephrine used to treat anaphylactic reactions.

Muscle Weakness: Beta-adrenergic blockade has been reported to potentiate muscle weakness consistent with certain myasthenic symptoms (e.g., diplopia, ptosis and generalized weakness).

Drug Interactions: Carteolol should be used with caution in patients who are receiving a beta-adrenergic blocking agent orally, because of the potential for additive effects on systemic beta-blockade.

Close observation of the patient is recommended when a beta-blocker is administered to patients receiving catecholamine-depleting drugs such as reserpine, because of possible additive effects and the production of hypotension and/or marked bradycardia, which may produce vertigo, syncope, or postural hypotension.

Carcinogenesis, Mutagenesis, Impairment of Fertility: Carteolol hydrochloride did not produce carcinogenic effects at doses up to 40 mg/kg/day in two-year oral rat and mouse studies. Tests of mutagenicity, including the Ames Test, recombinant (rec)-assay, *in vivo* cytogenetics and dominant lethal assay demonstrated no evidence for mutagenic potential. Fertility of male and female rats and male and female mice was unaffected by administration of carteolol hydrochloride dosages up to 150 mg/kg/day.

Pregnancy: Teratogenic Effects: Pregnancy Category C: Carteolol hydrochloride increased resorptions and decreased fetal weights in rabbits and rats at maternally toxic doses approximately 1052 and 5264 times the maximum recommended human oral dose (10 mg/70 kg/day), respectively. A dose-related increase in wavy ribs was noted in the developing rat fetus when pregnant females received daily doses of approximately 212 times the maximum recommended human oral dose. No such effects were noted in pregnant mice subjected to up to 1052 times the maximum recommended human oral dose. There are no adequate and well-controlled studies in pregnant women. Carteolol hydrochloride ophthalmic solution should be used during pregnancy only if the potential benefit justifies the potential risk to the fetus.

Nursing Mothers: It is not known whether this drug is excreted in human milk, although in animal studies carteolol has been shown to be excreted in breast milk. Caution should be exercised when carteolol hydrochloride ophthalmic solution is administered to nursing mothers.

Pediatric Use: Safety and effectiveness in pediatric patients have not been established.

Adverse Reactions: The following adverse reactions have been reported in clinical trials with carteolol hydrochloride ophthalmic solution:

Ocular: Transient eye irritation, burning, tearing, conjunctival hyperemia and edema occurred in about 1 of 4 patients. Ocular symptoms including blurred and cloudy vision, photophobia, decreased night vision, and ptosis and ocular signs including blepharoconjunctivitis, abnormal corneal staining, and corneal sensitivity occurred occasionally.

Systemic: As is characteristic of nonselective adrenergic blocking agents, carteolol may cause bradycardia and decreased blood pressure (see Warnings). The following systemic events have occasionally been reported with the use of carteolol hydrochloride: cardiac arrhythmia, heart palpitation, dyspnea, asthenia, headache, dizziness, insomnia, sinusitis, and taste perversion.

The following additional adverse reactions have been reported with ophthalmic use of beta$_1$ and beta$_2$ (nonselective) adrenergic receptor blocking agents:

Body As a Whole: Headache
Cardiovascular: Arrhythmia, syncope, heart block, cerebral vascular accident, cerebral ischemia, congestive heart failure, palpitation (see Warnings).
Digestive: Nausea
Psychiatric: Depression
Skin: Hypersensitivity, including localized and generalized rash
Respiratory: Bronchospasm (predominantly in patients with pre-existing bronchospastic disease), respiratory failure (see Warnings)
Endocrine: Masked symptoms of hypoglycemia in insulin-dependent diabetics (see Warnings)
Special Senses: Signs and symptoms of keratitis, blepharoptosis, visual disturbances including refractive changes (due to withdrawal of miotic therapy in some cases), diplopia, ptosis.

Other reactions associated with the oral use of nonselective adrenergic receptor blocking agents should be considered potential effects with ophthalmic use of these agents.

Overdosage: No specific information on emergency treatment of overdosage in humans is available. Should accidental ocular overdosage occur, flush eye(s) with water or normal saline. The most common effects expected with overdosage of a beta-adrenergic blocking agent are bradycardia, bronchospasm, congestive heart failure and hypotension.

In case of ingestion, treatment with carteolol hydrochloride ophthalmic solution should be discontinued and gastric lavage considered. The patient should be closely observed and vital signs carefully monitored. The prolonged effects of carteolol must be considered when determining the duration of corrective therapy. On the basis of the pharmacologic profile, the following additional measures should be considered as appropriate:

Symptomatic Sinus Bradycardia or Heart Block: Administer atropine. If there is no response to vagal blockade, administer isoproterenol cautiously.

Bronchospasm: Administer a beta$_2$-stimulating agent such as isoproterenol and/or a theophylline derivative.

Congestive Heart Failure: Administer diuretics and digitalis glycosides as necessary.

Hypotension: Administer vasopressors such as intravenous dopamine, epinephrine or norepinephrine bitartrate.

Dosage and Administration: The usual dose is one drop of carteolol hydrochloride ophthalmic solution, 1%, in the affected eye(s) twice a day.

If the patient's IOP is not at a satisfactory level on this regimen, concomitant therapy with pilocarpine and other miotics, and/or epinephrine or dipivefrin, and/or systemically administered carbonic anhydrase inhibitors, such as acetazolamide, can be instituted.

How Supplied: Carteolol Hydrochloride Ophthalmic Solution, 1% is supplied as a sterile ophthalmic solution in a plastic bottle with a controlled drop tip in the following sizes:
  5 mL bottles - Prod. No. 36707
  10 mL bottles - Prod. No. 36709
  15 mL bottles - Prod. No. 36711

Storage: Store between 15°–30°C (59°–86°F). Protect from light.

DO NOT USE IF IMPRINTED NECKBAND IS NOT INTACT

KEEP OUT OF REACH OF CHILDREN
Bausch & Lomb
Incorporated
Tampa, Florida 33637   REV. 2/04-92

CROLOM® ℞
cromolyn sodium
ophthalmic solution USP, 4%
STERILE OPHTHALMIC SOLUTION
℞ Only

Description: Crolom® (cromolyn sodium ophthalmic solution USP, 4%) is a clear, colorless, sterile solution for topical ophthalmic use. Cromolyn sodium is represented by the following structural formula:

$C_{23}H_{14}Na_2O_{11}$ Mol. Wt. 512.34

Chemical Name: Disodium 5,5'- [(2-hydroxytrimethylene)dioxy]bis[4-oxo-4*H*-1-benzopyran-2-carboxylate]

Pharmacologic Category: Mast cell stabilizer.
EACH mL CONTAINS: ACTIVE: Cromolyn Sodium 40 mg (4%); INACTIVES: Edetate Disodium 0.1% and Purified Water. Hydrochloric Acid and/or Sodium Hydroxide may be added to adjust pH (4.0–7.0). PRESERVATIVE ADDED: Benzalkonium Chloride 0.01%.

Continued on next page

Crolom—Cont.

Clinical Pharmacology: *In vitro* and *in vivo* animal studies have shown that cromolyn sodium inhibits the degranulation of sensitized mast cells which occurs after exposure to specific antigens. Cromolyn sodium acts by inhibiting the release of histamine and SRS-A (slow-reacting substance of anaphylaxis) from the mast cell.

Another activity demonstrated *in vitro* is the capacity of cromolyn sodium to inhibit the degranulation of nonsensitized rat mast cells by phospholipase A and the subsequent release of chemical mediators. Another study showed that cromolyn sodium did not inhibit the enzymatic activity of released phospholipase A on its specific substrate.

Cromolyn sodium has no intrinsic vasoconstrictor, antihistamine or anti-inflammatory activity.

Cromolyn sodium is poorly absorbed. When multiple doses of cromolyn sodium ophthalmic solution are instilled into normal rabbit eyes, less than 0.07% of the administered dose of cromolyn sodium is absorbed into the systemic circulation (presumably by way of the eye, nasal passages, buccal activity and gastrointestinal tract). Trace amounts (less than 0.01%) of the cromolyn sodium dose penetrate into the aqueous humor and clearance from this chamber is virtually complete within 24 hours after treatment is stopped.

In normal volunteers, analysis of drug excretion indicates that approximately 0.03% of cromolyn sodium is absorbed following administration to the eye.

Indications and Usage: Cromolyn sodium ophthalmic solution is indicated in the treatment of vernal keratoconjunctivitis, vernal conjunctivitis, and vernal keratitis.

Contraindications: Cromolyn sodium ophthalmic solution is contraindicated in those patients who have shown hypersensitivity to cromolyn sodium or to any of the other ingredients.

Precautions: General: Patients may experience a transient stinging or burning sensation following application of cromolyn sodium ophthalmic solution.

The recommended frequency of administration should not be exceeded (see **Dosage and Administration**).

Information for Patients: Patients should be advised to follow the patient instructions listed on the Information for Patients sheet.

Users of contact lenses should refrain from wearing lenses while exhibiting the signs and symptoms of vernal keratoconjunctivitis, vernal conjunctivitis, or vernal keratitis. Do not wear contact lenses during treatment with cromolyn sodium ophthalmic solution.

Carcinogenesis, Mutagenesis, and Impairment of Fertility: Long-term studies of cromolyn sodium in mice (12 months intraperitoneal administration at doses up to 150 mg/kg three days per week), hamsters (intraperitoneal administration at doses up to 52.6 mg/kg three days per week for 15 weeks followed by 17.5 mg/kg three days per week for 37 weeks), and rats (18 months subcutaneous administration at doses up to 75 mg/kg six days per week) showed no neoplastic effects. The average daily maximum dose levels administered in these studies were 192.9 mg/m^2 for mice, 47.2 mg/m^2 for hamsters and 385.8 mg/m^2 for rats. These doses correspond to approximately 6.8, 1.7, and 14 times the maximum daily human dose of 28 mg/m^2.

Cromolyn sodium showed no mutagenic potential in the Ames *Salmonella*/microsome plate assays, mitotic gene conversion in *Saccharomyces cerevisiae* and in an *in vitro* cytogenetic study in human peripheral lymphocytes.

No evidence of impaired fertility was shown in laboratory reproduction studies conducted subcutaneously in rats at the highest doses tested, 175 mg/kg/day (1050 mg/m^2) in males and 100 mg/kg/day (600 mg/m^2) in females. These doses are approximately 37 and 21 times the maximum daily human dose, respectively, based on mg/m^2.

Pregnancy: Teratogenic effects: Pregnancy Category B: Reproduction studies with cromolyn sodium administered subcutaneously to pregnant mice and rats at maximum daily doses of 540 mg/kg (1620 mg/m^2) and 164 mg/kg (984 mg/m^2), respectively, and intravenously to rabbits at a maximum daily dose of 485 mg/kg (5820 mg/m^2) produced no evidence of fetal malformation. These doses represent approximately 57, 35, and 205 times the maximum daily human dose, respectively, on a mg/m^2 basis. Adverse fetal effects (increased resorption and decreased fetal weight) were noted only at the very high parenteral doses that produced maternal toxicity. There are, however, no adequate and well-controlled studies in pregnant women. Because animal reproduction studies are not always predictive of human response, this drug should be used during pregnancy only if clearly needed.

Nursing Mothers It is not known whether this drug is excreted in human milk. Because many drugs are excreted in human milk, caution should be exercised when cromolyn sodium ophthalmic solution is administered to a nursing woman.

Pediatric Use: Safety and effectiveness in pediatric patients below the age of 4 years have not been established.

Geriatric Use: No overall differences in safety or effectiveness have been observed between elderly and younger patients.

Adverse Reactions: The most frequently reported adverse reaction attributed to the use of cromolyn sodium ophthalmic solution, on the basis of reoccurrence following readministration, is transient ocular stinging or burning upon instillation.

The following adverse reactions have been reported as infrequent events. It is unclear whether they are attributed to the drug:

Conjunctival injection; watery eyes; itchy eyes; dryness around the eye; puffy eyes; eye irritation; and styes.

Immediate hypersensitivity reactions have been reported rarely and include dyspnea, edema, and rash.

Dosage and Administration: The dose is 1–2 drops in each eye 4–6 times day at regular intervals.

One drop contains approximately 1.6 mg cromolyn sodium.

Patients should be advised that the effect of cromolyn sodium ophthalmic solution therapy is dependent upon its administration at regular intervals, as directed.

Symptomatic response to therapy (decreased itching, tearing, redness, and discharge) is usually evident within a few days, but longer treatment for up to six weeks is sometimes required. Once symptomatic improvement has been established, therapy should be continued for as long as needed to sustain improvement. If required, corticosteroids may be used concomitantly with cromolyn sodium ophthalmic solution.

FOR OPHTHALMIC USE ONLY

How Supplied: Crolom® (cromolyn sodium ophthalmic solution USP, 4%) is supplied in a plastic bottle individually cartoned with a controlled drop tip in the following sizes:
10 mL bottle (NDC 24208-300-10) - AB30709

> **DO NOT USE IF IMPRINTED NECKBAND IS NOT INTACT.**

Storage: Store between 15°–30°C (59°–86°F). Protect from light – store in original carton.

Keep tightly closed. Replace cap immediately after use.

KEEP OUT OF REACH OF CHILDREN

Bausch & Lomb
Incorporated
Tampa, Florida 33637
©Bausch & Lomb Incorporated
Rev. 1/04–83

Information for the Patient
Crolom®
(cromolyn sodium ophthalmic solution USP, 4%)
Sterile

It is important to use Crolom® **regularly**, as directed by your physician.

1. Thoroughly wash your hands.
2. Remove safety seal (Figure 1).

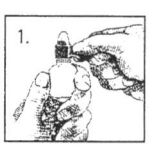

3. Remove cap (Figure 2).

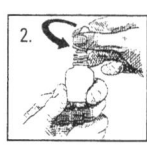

4. Sit or stand comfortably, with your head tilted back (Figure 3).

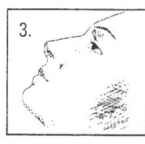

5. Open eyes, look up, and draw the lower lid of your eye down gently with your index finger (Figure 4).

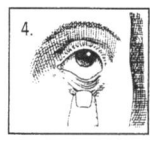

6. Hold the Crolom® bottle upside down. Place dropper tip as close as possible to the lower eyelid and gently squeeze out the prescribed number of drops (Figure 5).

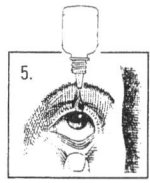

7. Do not touch the eye or eyelid with the dropper tip.
8. Blink a few times to make sure the eye is covered with the solution.
9. Close your eye and remove any excess solution with a clean tissue.
10. Repeat process in the other eye.

SPECIAL TIPS
1. Avoid placing Crolom® solution directly on the cornea (the area just over the pupil), because it is especially sensitive. You will find the administration of eye drops more comfortable if you place the drops just inside the lower eyelid as shown in Figure 5.

2. To avoid contamination of the solution, do not touch dropper tip to the eye, fingers or any other surface. Replace cap after use. It is recommended that any remaining contents be discarded after the treatment period prescribed by your physician.
3. Store between 15°–30°C (59°–86°F). Protect from light – store in original carton. Keep tightly closed. Replace cap immediately after use.
4. Keep out of the reach of children.
5. Do not use with any other ocular medication unless directed by your physician. Do not wear contact lenses during treatment with Crolom®.

Bausch & Lomb
Pharmaceuticals, Inc.
Tampa, Florida 33637
©Bausch & Lomb Pharmaceuticals, Inc.
Rev. 3/02-8I
Shown in Product Identification Guide, page 104

FLUOR–I–STRIP® ℞
[floo-or 'a "strip]
(Fluorescein Sodium Ophthalmic Strips)

Composition (per strip):
Diagnostic dye: Fluorescein Sodium 9 mg
Preservative: Chlorobutanol (chloral derivative) 0.5%
Surface active agent: Polysorbate 80
Buffering agents: Potassium Chloride, Boric Acid, Sodium Carbonate
Description: FLUOR-I-STRIP is a specially prepared sterile ophthalmic strip for diagnostic use.
Indications: For staining the anterior segment of the eye when:
a) delineating a corneal injury, herpetic lesion or foreign body,
b) determining the site of an intraocular injury,
c) fitting contact lenses,
d) making the fluorescein test to ascertain postoperative closure of the sclerocorneal (also referred to as corneoscleral) wound in delayed anterior chamber reformation,
e) making the lacrimal drainage test.
Directions for Use: To open envelope, grasp pull-tabs firmly and separate slowly. Separate the two strips by tearing off white tab end. Moisten end of strip with a drop of sterile water. Place moistened strip at the fornix in the lower cul-de-sac close to the punctum. For best results, patient should close lid tightly over strip until desired amount of staining is obtained. Another method is to retract upper lid and touch tip of strip to the bulbar conjunctiva on the temporal side until an adequate amount of stain is available for a clearly defined endpoint reading.
Warning: Never use fluorescein while the patient is wearing *soft contact lenses* because the lenses may become stained. Whenever fluorescein is used, flush the eyes with sterile, normal saline solution, and wait at least one hour before replacing the lenses.
Storage: Store at room temperature (approximately 25°C).
How Supplied: Boxes of 300 strips in individual envelopes (NDC 24208-390-83).
Manufactured by
Wyeth Ayerst Laboratories
Rouses Point, NY 12979
Marketed by
Bausch & Lomb Incorporated
Tampa, FL 33637
Shown in Product Identification Guide, page 104

FLUOR–I–STRIP® -A.T. ℞
[floo-or 'a "strip]
(Fluorescein Sodium Ophthalmic Strips)
For Applanation Tonometry

Composition (Per Strip):
Diagnostic dye: Fluorescein Sodium 1 mg
Preservative: Chlorobutanol (chloral derivative) 0.5%
Surface active agent: Polysorbate 80
Buffering agents: Potassium Chloride, Boric Acid, Sodium Carbonate
Description: FLUOR-I-STRIP-A.T. consists of sterile ophthalmic strips, specially prepared for diagnostic use in applanation tonometry.
Indications: For staining the anterior segment of the eye when:
a) delineating a corneal injury, herpetic lesion or foreign body,
b) determining the site of an intraocular injury,
c) fitting contact lenses,
d) making the fluorescein test to ascertain postoperative closure of the sclerocorneal (also referred to as corneoscleral) wound in delayed anterior chamber reformation,
e) making the lacrimal drainage test.
Directions for Use: To open envelope, grasp pull-tabs firmly and separate slowly. Separate the two strips by tearing off white tab end. Anesthetize the eyes. Retract upper lid and touch tip of strip to the bulbar conjunctiva on the temporal side until an adequate amount of stain is available for a clearly defined endpoint reading.
Warning: Never use fluorescein while the patient is wearing *soft contact lenses* because the lenses may become stained. Whenever fluorescein is used, flush the eyes with sterile, normal saline solution, and wait at least one hour before replacing the lenses.
Storage: Store at room temperature (approximately 25°C).
How Supplied: Boxes of 300 strips, 2 in each envelope NDC 24208-391-83
Manufactured by
Wyeth-Ayerst Laboratories
Rouses Point, NY 12979
Marketed by
Bausch & Lomb Incorporated
Tampa, FL 33637
Shown in Product Identification Guide, page 104

LOTEMAX® ℞
[Lō tĕ max]
loteprednol etabonate ophthalmic suspension 0.5%
STERILE OPHTHALMIC SUSPENSION
℞ only

Description: LOTEMAX® (loteprednol etabonate ophthalmic suspension) contains a sterile, topical anti-inflammatory corticosteroid for ophthalmic use. Loteprednol etabonate is a white to off-white powder.
Loteprednol etabonate is represented by the following structural formula:

$C_{24}H_{31}ClO_7$ Mol. Wt. 466.96

Chemical name:
chloromethyl 17α-[(ethoxycarbonyl)oxy]-11β-hydroxy-3-oxoandrosta-1,4-diene-17β-carboxylate

Each mL contains:
ACTIVE: Loteprednol Etabonate 5 mg (0.5%).
INACTIVES: Edetate Disodium, Glycerin, Povidone, Purified Water and Tyloxapol. Hydrochloric Acid and/or Sodium Hydroxide may be added to adjust the pH to 5.3–5.6. The suspension is essentially isotonic with a tonicity of 250 to 310 mOsmol/kg.
PRESERVATIVE ADDED: Benzalkonium Chloride 0.01%.
Clinical Pharmacology: Corticosteroids inhibit the inflammatory response to a variety of inciting agents and probably delay or slow healing. They inhibit the edema, fibrin deposition, capillary dilation, leukocyte migration, capillary proliferation, fibroblast proliferation, deposition of collagen, and scar formation associated with inflammation. There is no generally accepted explanation for the mechanism of action of ocular corticosteroids. However, corticosteroids are thought to act by the induction of phospholipase A_2 inhibitory proteins, collectively called lipocortins. It is postulated that these proteins control the biosynthesis of potent mediators of inflammation such as prostaglandins and leukotrienes by inhibiting the release of their common precursor, arachidonic acid. Arachidonic acid is released from membrane phospholipids by phospholipase A_2. Corticosteroids are capable of producing a rise in intraocular pressure.
Loteprednol etabonate is structurally similar to other corticosteroids. However, the number 20 position ketone group is absent. It is highly lipid soluble which enhances its penetration into cells. Loteprednol etabonate is synthesized through structural modifications of prednisolone-related compounds so that it will undergo a predictable transformation to an inactive metabolite. Based upon *in vivo* and *in vitro* preclinical metabolism studies, loteprednol etabonate undergoes extensive metabolism to inactive carboxylic acid metabolites.
Results from a bioavailability study in normal volunteers established that plasma levels of loteprednol etabonate and Δ^1 cortienic acid etabonate (PJ 91), its primary, inactive metabolite, were below the limit of quantitation (1 ng/mL) at all sampling times. The results were obtained following the ocular administration of one drop in each eye of 0.5% loteprednol etabonate 8 times daily for 2 days or 4 times daily for 42 days. This study suggests that limited (<1 ng/mL) systemic absorption occurs with LOTEMAX.
Clinical Studies:
Post-Operative Inflammation: Placebo-controlled clinical studies demonstrated that LOTEMAX is effective for the treatment of anterior chamber inflammation as measured by cell and flare.
Giant Papillary Conjunctivitis: Placebo-controlled clinical studies demonstrated that LOTEMAX was effective in reducing the signs and symptoms of giant papillary conjunctivitis after 1 week of treatment and continuing for up to 6 weeks while on treatment.
Seasonal Allergic Conjunctivitis: A placebo-controlled clinical study demonstrated that LOTEMAX was effective in reducing the signs and symptoms of allergic conjunctivitis during peak periods of pollen exposure.
Uveitis: Controlled clinical studies of patients with uveitis demonstrated that LOTEMAX was less effective than prednisolone acetate 1%. Overall, 72% of patients treated with LOTEMAX experienced resolution of anterior chamber cell by day 28, compared to 87% of patients treated with 1% prednisolone acetate. The incidence of patients with clinically significant increases in IOP (≥10 mmHg) was 1% with LOTEMAX and 6% with prednisolone acetate 1%.

Continued on next page

Lotemax—Cont.

Indications and Usage: LOTEMAX is indicated for the treatment of steroid responsive inflammatory conditions of the palpebral and bulbar conjunctiva, cornea and anterior segment of the globe such as allergic conjunctivitis, acne rosacea, superficial punctate keratitis, herpes zoster keratitis, iritis, cyclitis, selected infective conjunctivitides, when the inherent hazard of steroid use is accepted to obtain an advisable diminution in edema and inflammation.

LOTEMAX is less effective than prednisolone acetate 1% in two 28-day controlled clinical studies in acute anterior uveitis, where 72% of patients treated with LOTEMAX experienced resolution of anterior chamber cells, compared to 87% of patients treated with prednisolone acetate 1%. The incidence of patients with clinically significant increases in IOP (≥ 10 mmHg) was 1% with LOTEMAX and 6% with prednisolone acetate 1%. LOTEMAX should not be used in patients who require a more potent corticosteroid for this indication. LOTEMAX is also indicated for the treatment of post-operative inflammation following ocular surgery.

Contraindications: LOTEMAX, as with other ophthalmic corticosteroids, is contraindicated in most viral diseases of the cornea and conjunctiva including epithelial herpes simplex keratitis (dendritic keratitis), vaccinia, and varicella, and also in mycobacterial infection of the eye and fungal diseases of ocular structures. LOTEMAX is also contraindicated in individuals with known or suspected hypersensitivity to any of the ingredients of this preparation and to other corticosteroids.

Warnings: Prolonged use of corticosteroids may result in glaucoma with damage to the optic nerve, defects in visual acuity and fields of vision, and in posterior subcapsular cataract formation. Steroids should be used with caution in the presence of glaucoma.

Prolonged use of corticosteroids may suppress the host response and thus increase the hazard of secondary ocular infections. In those diseases causing thinning of the cornea or sclera, perforations have been known to occur with the use of topical steroids. In acute purulent conditions of the eye, steroids may mask infection or enhance existing infection.

Use of ocular steroids may prolong the course and may exacerbate the severity of many viral infections of the eye (including herpes simplex). Employment of a corticosteroid medication in the treatment of patients with a history of herpes simplex requires great caution.

The use of steroids after cataract surgery may delay healing and increase the incidence of bleb formation.

Precautions:
General: For ophthalmic use only. The initial prescription and renewal of the medication order beyond 14 days should be made by a physician only after examination of the patient with the aid of magnification, such as slit lamp biomicroscopy and, where appropriate, fluorescein staining.

If signs and symptoms fail to improve after two days, the patient should be re-evaluated.

If this product is used for 10 days or longer, intraocular pressure should be monitored even though it may be difficult in children and uncooperative patients (see WARNINGS).

Fungal infections of the cornea are particularly prone to develop coincidentally with long-term local steroid application. Fungus invasion must be considered in any persistent corneal ulceration where a steroid has been used or is in use. Fungal cultures should be taken when appropriate.

Information for Patients: This product is sterile when packaged. Patients should be advised not to allow the dropper tip to touch any surface, as this may contaminate the suspension. If pain develops, redness, itching or inflammation becomes aggravated, the patient should be advised to consult a physician. As with all ophthalmic preparations containing benzalkonium chloride, patients should be advised not to wear soft contact lenses when using LOTEMAX®.

Carcinogenesis, mutagenesis, impairment of fertility: Long-term animal studies have not been conducted to evaluate the carcinogenic potential of loteprednol etabonate. Loteprednol etabonate was not genotoxic *in vitro* in the Ames test, the mouse lymphoma tk assay, or in a chromosome aberration test in human lymphocytes, or *in vivo* in the single dose mouse micronucleus assay. Treatment of male and female rats with up to 50 mg/kg/day and 25 mg/kg/day of loteprednol etabonate, respectively, (600 and 300 times the maximum clinical dose, respectively) prior to and during mating did not impair fertility in either gender.

Pregnancy: Teratogenic effects: Pregnancy Category C. Loteprednol etabonate has been shown to be embryotoxic (delayed ossification) and teratogenic (increased incidence of meningocele, abnormal left common carotid artery, and limb flexures) when administered orally to rabbits during organogenesis at a dose of 3 mg/kg/day (35 times the maximum daily clinical dose), a dose which caused no maternal toxicity. The no-observed-effect-level (NOEL) for these effects was 0.5 mg/kg/day (6 times the maximum daily clinical dose). Oral treatment of rats during organogenesis resulted in teratogenicity (absent innominate artery at ≥ 5mg/kg/day doses, and cleft palate and umbilical hernia at ≥ 50 mg/kg/day) and embryotoxicity (increased post-implantation losses at 100 mg/kg/day and decreased fetal body weight and skeletal ossification with ≥ 50 mg/kg/day). Treatment of rats with 0.5 mg/kg/day (6 times the maximum clinical dose) during organogenesis did not result in any reproductive toxicity. Loteprednol etabonate was maternally toxic (significantly reduced body weight gain during treatment) when administered to pregnant rats during organogenesis at doses of ≥ 5 mg/kg/day.

Oral exposure of female rats to 50 mg/kg/day of loteprednol etabonate from the start of the fetal period through the end of lactation, a maternally toxic treatment regimen (significantly decreased body weight gain), gave rise to decreased growth and survival, and retarded development in the offspring during lactation; the NOEL for these effects was 5 mg/kg/day. Loteprednol etabonate had no effect on the duration of gestation or parturition when administered orally to pregnant rats at doses up to 50 mg/kg/day during the fetal period.

Nursing Mothers: It is not known whether topical ophthalmic administration of corticosteroids could result in sufficient systemic absorption to produce detectable quantities in human milk. Systemic steroids appear in human milk and could suppress growth, interfere with endogenous corticosteroid production, or cause other untoward effects. Caution should be exercised when LOTEMAX is administered to a nursing woman.

Pediatric Use: Safety and effectiveness in pediatric patients have not been established.

Adverse Reactions: Reactions associated with ophthalmic steroids include elevated intraocular pressure, which may be associated with optic nerve damage, visual acuity and field defects, posterior subcapsular cataract formation, secondary ocular infection from pathogens including herpes simplex, and perforation of the globe where there is thinning of the cornea or sclera.

Ocular adverse reactions occurring in 5–15% of patients treated with loteprednol etabonate ophthalmic suspension (0.2%–0.5%) in clinical studies included abnormal vision/blurring, burning on instillation, chemosis, discharge, dry eyes, epiphora, foreign body sensation, itching, injection, and photophobia. Other ocular adverse reactions occurring in less than 5% of patients include conjunctivitis, corneal abnormalities, eyelid erythema, keratoconjunctivitis, ocular irritation/pain/discomfort, papillae, and uveitis. Some of these events were similar to the underlying ocular disease being studied.

Non-ocular adverse reactions occurred in less than 15% of patients. These include headache, rhinitis and pharyngitis.

In a summation of controlled, randomized studies of individuals treated for 28 days or longer with loteprednol etabonate, the incidence of significant elevation of intraocular pressure (≥ 10 mmHg) was 2% (15/901) among patients receiving loteprednol etabonate, 7% (11/164) among patients receiving 1% prednisolone acetate and 0.5% (3/583) among patients receiving placebo.

Dosage and Administration: SHAKE VIGOROUSLY BEFORE USING.

Steroid Responsive Disease Treatment: Apply one to two drops of LOTEMAX into the conjunctival sac of the affected eye(s) four times daily. During the initial treatment within the first week, the dosing may be increased, up to 1 drop every hour, if necessary. Care should be taken not to discontinue therapy prematurely. If signs and symptoms fail to improve after two days, the patient should be re-evaluated (See PRECAUTIONS).

Post-Operative Inflammation: Apply one to two drops of LOTEMAX into the conjunctival sac of the operated eye(s) four times daily beginning 24 hours after surgery and continuing throughout the first 2 weeks of the post-operative period.

How Supplied: LOTEMAX® (loteprednol etabonate ophthalmic suspension) is supplied in a plastic bottle with a controlled drop tip in the following sizes:
2.5 mL (NDC 24208-299-25)-AB29904
5 mL (NDC 24208-299-05)-AB29907
10 mL (NDC 24208-299-10)-AB29909
15 mL (NDC 24208-299-15)-AB29911

DO NOT USE IF NECKBAND IMPRINTED WITH "Protective Seal" AND YELLOW IS NOT INTACT.

Storage: Store upright between 15°–25°C (59°–77°F). DO NOT FREEZE.
KEEP OUT OF REACH OF CHILDREN.
Bausch & Lomb Incorporated
Tampa, Florida 33637
U.S. Patent No. 4,996,335
U.S. Patent No. 5,540,930
©Bausch & Lomb Incorporated
Lotemax® are trademarks of Bausch & Lomb Incorporated.

Rev. 11/03-83
Shown in Product Identification Guide, page 104

MURO® 128® 2% OTC
[mū 'rō 128]
Sodium Chloride Hypertonicity Ophthalmic Solution, 2%
MURO® 128® 5% OTC
Sodium Chloride Hypertonicity Ophthalmic Solution, 5%
STERILE OPHTHALMIC SOLUTION

Description: Muro® 128® 2% Solution is a sterile ophthalmic solution used to draw water out of the cornea of the eye.

Each mL Contains: ACTIVE: Sodium Chloride 2%; INACTIVES: Boric Acid, Hypromellose, Propylene Glycol, Purified Water, Sodium Borate. Sodium Hydroxide and/or Hydrochloric Acid may be added to adjust pH.
PRESERVATIVES: Methylparaben 0.028%, Propylparaben 0.012%
Description: Muro® 128® 5% Solution is a sterile ophthalmic solution used to draw water out of the cornea of the eye.
Each mL Contains: ACTIVE: Sodium Chloride 5%; INACTIVES: Boric Acid, Hypromellose, Propylene Glycol, Purified Water, Sodium Borate. Sodium Hydroxide and/or Hydrochloric Acid may be added to adjust pH.
PRESERVATIVES: Methylparaben 0.023%, Propylparaben 0.01%
Uses: For the temporary relief of corneal edema.
Warnings: Do not use this product except under the advice and supervision of a doctor.
If you experience eye pain, changes in vision, continued redness or irritation of the eye, or if the condition worsens or persists, consult a doctor.
To avoid contamination of the product, do not touch the tip of the container to any surface.
Replace cap after using.
This product may cause temporary burning and irritation on being instilled into the eye.
If the solution changes color or becomes cloudy, do not use.
In case of accidental ingestion, seek professional assistance or contact a Poison Control Center immediately.
Directions: Instill 1 or 2 drops in the affected eye(s) every 3 or 4 hours, or as directed by a doctor.
FOR OPHTHALMIC USE ONLY
How Supplied: Muro® 128® 2% Solution is supplied in a plastic controlled drop tip bottle in the following size:
1/2 Fl. Oz. (15 mL) (NDC 24208-276-15)—Prod. No. AB15511
How Supplied: Muro® 128® 5% Solution is supplied in 1/2 Fl. Oz. (15 mL) or 1 Fl. Oz. (30 mL) plastic controlled dropper tip bottles.
15 mL [NDC 24208-277-15]—Prod. No. AB15611
30 mL [NDC 24208-277-30]—Prod. No. AB15616

DO NOT USE IF IMPRINTED NECKBAND IS NOT INTACT

Storage: Store between 15°–30°C [59°–86°F]. KEEP TIGHTLY CLOSED. **STORE UPRIGHT AND IMMEDIATELY REPLACE CAP AFTER USE.**
KEEP OUT OF REACH OF CHILDREN.
Bausch & Lomb Incorporated
Tampa, FL 33637
MURO is a trademark of MURO Pharmaceutical, Inc.
128 is a registered trademark of Bausch & Lomb Incorporated
2/04-03
Shown in Product Identification Guide, page 104

MURO® 128® 5% OINTMENT OTC
[mŭ 'rō 128]
Sodium Chloride Hypertonicity Ophthalmic Ointment, 5%
FOR TEMPORARY RELIEF OF CORNEAL EDEMA
STERILE OPHTHALMIC OINTMENT

Description: Muro® 128® 5% Ointment is a sterile ophthalmic ointment used to draw water out of the cornea of the eye.

Each Gram Contains: ACTIVE: Sodium Chloride 5% INACTIVES: Lanolin, Mineral Oil, Purified Water, White Petrolatum.
Uses: For the temporary relief of corneal edema.
Warnings: Do not use this product except under the advice and supervision of a doctor.
If you experience eye pain, changes in vision, continued redness or irritation of the eye, or if the condition worsens or persists, consult a doctor.
To avoid contamination of the product, do not touch the tip of the container to any surface.
Replace cap after using.
This product may cause temporary burning and irritation on being instilled into the eye.
In case of accidental ingestion, seek professional assistance or contact a Poison Control Center immediately.
Directions: Pull down lower lid of the affected eye(s) and apply a small amount (approximately 1/4 inch) of the ointment to the inside of the eyelid every 3 or 4 hours, or as directed by a doctor.
FOR OPHTHALMIC USE ONLY
How Supplied: Muro 128® 5% Ointment is supplied in 1/8 oz (3.5 g) tube.
[NDC 24208-385-55]—Prod. No. AB15834
TWIN PACK: 2 x 1/8 oz (2 x 3.5 g)
[NDC 24208-385-56]—Prod. No. AB15899
NOTE: Tubes are filled by weight (1/8 oz/3.5g) not volume.
See Crimp of tube for Lot Number and Expiration Date.

DO NOT USE IF BOTTOM RIDGE OF TUBE CAP IS EXPOSED AND IMPRINTED SEAL ON BOX IS BROKEN OR MISSING.

KEEP OUT OF REACH OF CHILDREN.
Storage: Store between 15°–30°C (59°–86°F).
DO NOT FREEZE.
KEEP TIGHTLY CLOSED.
Bausch & Lomb Incorporated
Tampa, FL 33637
MURO is a trademark of MURO Pharmaceutical, Inc.
128 is a registered trademark of Bausch & Lomb Incorporated
11/03-72
Shown in Product Identification Guide, page 104

OCUVITE® OTC
Antioxidant Vitamin and Mineral Supplement

Description: Each tablet contains:
[See table above]
Other Ingredients: Dibasic calcium phosphate, microcrystalline cellulose, calcium carbonate, crospovidone, hypromellose, titanium dioxide, silicon dioxide, magnesium stearate, stearic acid, FD&C Yellow No. 6, triethyl citrate, polysorbate 80 and sodium lauryl sulfate.

	Source	Amount	% Daily Value
Vitamin A	beta carotene	1000 IU	20%
Vitamin C	ascorbic acid	200 mg	333%
Vitamin E	dl-alpha tocopheryl acetate	60 IU	200%
Zinc	zinc oxide*	40 mg	267%
Selenium	sodium selenate	55 mcg	79%
Copper	cupric oxide	2 mg	100%
Lutein		2 mg	†

* Zinc oxide is the most concentrated form of zinc and contains more elemental zinc than any other zinc salt (ie: zinc sulfate or zinc acetate).
† Daily value not established.

Indications: OCUVITE is specifically formulated to provide nutritional support for the eye.*
Recommended Intake: Adults. One tablet, one or two times daily or as directed by their doctor.
How Supplied: Peach, eye shaped, film coated tablet engraved with "Ocuvite" on one side and 02 on the other side divided by a 90° bisect.
NDC 24208-387-60—Bottle of 60
NDC 24208-387-62—Bottle of 120
Store at Room Temperature.
MADE IN U.S.A.
Marketed by
Bausch & Lomb Incorporated
Rochester, NY
Shown in Product Identification Guide, page 104

* This statement has not been evaluated by the Food and Drug Administration. This product is not intended to diagnose, treat, cure, or prevent any disease.

OCUVITE® EXTRA® OTC
Vitamin and Mineral Supplement

Description: Each tablet contains:
[See first table at top of next page]
Other Inactive Ingredients: dibasic calcium phosphate, microcrystalline cellulose, calcium carbonate, crospovidone, hypromellose, titanium dioxide, silicon dioxide, magnesium stearate, stearic acid, FD&C yellow No. 6, triethyl citrate, polysorbate 80 and sodium lauryl sulfate.
Indications: OCUVITE EXTRA is specifically formulated to provide nutritional support for the eye.*
Recommended Intake: Adults: One tablet, one or two times daily or as directed by their doctor.
How Supplied: Orange, eye shaped, film coated tablet engraved OCUVITE on one side, 03 on the other side divided by a 90° bisect.
NDC 24208-388-19—Bottle of 50
Store at Room Temperature
MADE IN U.S.A.
Marketed by
Bausch & Lomb Incorporated
Rochester, NY
Shown in Product Identification Guide, page 104

* This statement has not been evaluated by the Food and Drug Administration. This product is not intended to diagnose, treat, cure or prevent any disease.

Continued on next page

	Source	Amount	% Daily Value
Vitamin A	beta carotene	1000 IU	20%
Vitamin C	ascorbic acid	300 mg	500%
Vitamin E	dl-alpha tocopheryl acetate	100 IU	333%
Riboflavin		3 mg	176%
Niacin		40 mg	200%
Zinc	zinc oxide*	40 mg	266%
Selenium	sodium selenate	55 mcg	79%
Copper	cupric oxide	2 mg	100%
Manganese		5 mg	250%
L-Glutathione		5 mg	†
Lutein		2 mg	†

* Zinc oxide is the most concentrated form of zinc and contains more elemental zinc than any other zinc salt (ie: zinc sulfate or zinc acetate).
† Daily value not established.

	Source	Amount	% Daily Value
Vitamin C	ascorbic acid	60 mg	100%
Vitamin E	dl-alpha tocopheryl acetate	30 IU	100%
Zinc	zinc oxide*	15 mg	100%
Copper	cupric oxide	2 mg	100%
Lutein		6 mg	†

*Zinc oxide is the most concentrated form of zinc and contains more elemental zinc than any other zinc salt (ie:zinc sulfate or zinc acetate)
† Daily value not established

OCUVITE® LUTEIN   OTC
[lu "teen]
Vitamin and Mineral Supplement

Description: Each capsule contains:
[See second table above]
Other Ingredients: Lactose monohydrate, Crospovidone, Magnesium Stearate, Silicon dioxide.
Indications: Ocuvite Lutein is an advanced new antioxidant supplement formulated to provide nutritional support for the eye.* The Ocuvite Lutein formulation contains essential antioxidant vitamins, minerals and 6 mg of Lutein.
Recommended Intake: Adults: One capsule, one or two times daily or as directed by their physician.
How Supplied: Yellow capsule with Ocuvite Lutein printed in black.
NDC 24208-403-19—Bottle of 36
Store at Room Temperature
MADE IN U.S.A.
Marketed by
Bausch & Lomb Incorporated
Rochester, NY
Shown in Product Identification Guide, page 104

---

* This statement has not been evaluated by the Food and Drug Administration. This product is not intended to diagnose, treat, cure, or prevent any disease.

OCUVITE® PRESERVISION™   OTC
Uniquely Formulated Eye Vitamin and Mineral Supplement

VITAMINS for the EYES
- Your eyesight is among your most valuable of assets. As the leader in ocular nutritional research and vitamin supplements for the eye, Bausch & Lomb is committed to helping you preserve the health of your eyes with our new **Ocuvite PreserVision** supplements.*
- **Ocuvite PreserVision** is a unique antioxidant vitamin and mineral formula which was specifically developed for use in the National Eye Institute age related eye study (AREDS).
- **Ocuvite PreserVision** is a high-potency antioxidant supplement with the antioxidant vitamins A, C, E and select minerals in amounts well above 100% of the US Government recommended daily value.

RECOMMENDED INTAKE: Adults, take two tablets, two times daily or as directed by your doctor. May be used with other vitamin supplements following consultation with your doctor or pharmacist.
SMOKERS: Please consult your eye care professional about the risks associated with smoking and using Beta-Carotene.
Ocuvite® is the #1 recommended eye vitamin and mineral supplement brand among eye care professionals.[1]

---

* This statement has not been evaluated by the Food and Drug Administration. This product is not intended to diagnose, treat, cure or prevent any disease.

References: 1. Data on file, Bausch & Lomb, Inc.
© Bausch & Lomb Incorporated. All Rights Reserved.
Bausch & Lomb, Ocuvite and PreserVision are trademarks of Bausch & Lomb Incorporated or its affiliates. Other brand names are trademarks of their respective owners.
Shown in Product Identification Guide, page 104

OFLOXACIN   ℞
[ō-flŏks-ă-sĭn]
Ophthalmic Solution 0.3%
STERILE
Rx only

Description: Ofloxacin Ophthalmic Solution 0.3% is a sterile ophthalmic solution. It is a fluorinated carboxyquinolone anti-infective for topical ophthalmic use.

$C_{18}H_{20}FN_3O_4$ Mol. Wt. 361.37

Chemical Name:
($\pm$)-9-Fluoro-2,3-dihydro-3-methyl-10-(4-methyl-1-piperazinyl)-7-oxo-7H-pyrido[1,2,3-de]-1,4 benzoxazine-6-carboxylic acid.
Each mL Contains: Active:
ofloxacin 0.3% (3 mg/mL)
Preservative Added:
benzalkonium chloride (0.005%)
Inactives: sodium chloride and purified water. Hydrochloric Acid and/or Sodium Hydroxide may be added to adjust pH. Ofloxacin ophthalmic solution is unbuffered and formulated with a pH of 6.4 (range - 6.0 to 6.8). It has an osmolality of 300 mOsm/kg. Ofloxacin is a fluorinated 4-quinolone which differs from other fluorinated 4-quinolones in that there is a six member (pyridobenzoxazine) ring from positions 1 to 8 of the basic ring structure.
How Supplied: Ofloxacin Ophthalmic Solution 0.3% is supplied sterile in plastic dropper bottles in the following sizes:
5 mL   NDC 24208-434-05   AB43407
10 mL   NDC 24208-434-10   AB43409
Storage: Store at 15°–25°C (59°–77°F)
KEEP OUT OF REACH OF CHILDREN.
FOR OPHTHALMIC USE ONLY.
Bausch & Lomb Incorporated
Tampa, FL 33637
©Bausch & Lomb Incorporated
X051054 **(FOLDED)**
XM10124 **(FLAT)**
R.2/04-01

OPTIPRANOLOL®   ℞
(metipranolol ophthalmic solution) 0.3%
Rx only

Description: OPTIPRANOLOL® (metipranolol ophthalmic solution) 0.3% contains metipranolol, a non-selective beta-adrenergic receptor blocking agent. Metipranolol is a white, odorless, crystalline powder.
The chemical name of metipranolol is ($\pm$)-1-(4-Hydroxy-2,3,5-trimethylphenoxy)-3-(isopropylamino)-2-propanol-4-acetate.
The chemical structure of metipranolol is:

$C_{17}H_{27}NO_4$ Mol. Wt. 309.40
Each mL of OPTIPRANOLOL® contains 3 mg metipranolol. INACTIVES: Povidone, Glycerin, Hydrochloric Acid, Sodium Chloride, Edetate Disodium, and Purified Water. Sodium Hydroxide and/or Hydrochloric Acid may be added to adjust pH. PRESERVATIVE: Benzalkonium Chloride 0.004%.
Clinical Pharmacology: Metipranolol blocks beta$_1$ and beta$_2$ (non-selective) adrenergic receptors. It does not have significant intrinsic sympathomimetic activity, and has only weak local anesthetic (membrane-stabilizing) and myocardial depressant activity.
Orally administered beta-adrenergic blocking agents reduce cardiac output in both healthy subjects and patients with heart disease. In

patients with severe impairment of myocardial function, beta-adrenergic receptor antagonists may inhibit the sympathetic stimulatory effect necessary to maintain adequate cardiac output.

Beta-adrenergic receptor blockade in the bronchi and bronchioles may result in significantly increased airway resistance from unopposed para-sympathetic activity. Such an effect is potentially dangerous in patients with asthma or other bronchospastic conditions (see CONTRAINDICATIONS and WARNINGS).

OPTIPRANOLOL® Ophthalmic Solution, when applied topically in the eye, has the action of reducing elevated as well as normal intraocular pressure (IOP), whether or not accompanied by glaucoma. Elevated intraocular pressure is a major risk factor in the pathogenesis of glaucomatous visual field loss. The higher the level of intraocular pressure, the greater the likelihood of glaucomatous visual field loss and optic nerve damage.

The primary mechanism of the ocular hypotensive action of metipranolol is most likely due to a reduction in aqueous humor production. A slight increase in outflow may be an additional mechanism. OPTIPRANOLOL Ophthalmic Solution reduces IOP with little or no effect on pupil size or accommodation.

In controlled studies of patients with intraocular pressure greater than 24 mmHg at baseline, OPTIPRANOLOL Ophthalmic Solution reduced the average intraocular pressure approximately 20–26%.

The onset of action of OPTIPRANOLOL Ophthalmic Solution, as measured by a reduction in intraocular pressure, occurs within 30 minutes after a single administration. The maximum effect occurs at about 2 hours. A reduction in intraocular pressure can be demonstrated 24 hours after a single dose. Clinical studies in patients with glaucoma treated for up to two years indicate that an intraocular pressure lowering effect is maintained.

Animal Pharmacology: In rabbits administered metipranolol in one eye at 2 to 4 fold increased concentrations, multi-focal interstitial nephritis was observed in male animals, and lympho-hystiocytic and heterophilic interstitial pneumonia was observed in female animals. The clinical relevance of these findings in unknown.

Indications and Usage: OPTIPRANOLOL Ophthalmic Solution is indicated in the treatment of elevated intraocular pressure in patients with ocular hypertension or open angle glaucoma.

Contraindications: Hypersensitivity to any component of this product.

OPTIPRANOLOL Ophthalmic Solution is contraindicated in patients with bronchial asthma or a history of bronchial asthma, or severe chronic obstructive pulmonary disease; symptomatic sinus bradycardia; greater than a first degree atrioventricular block; cardiogenic shock; or overt cardiac failure.

Warnings: As with other topically applied ophthalmic drugs, this drug may be absorbed systemically. Thus, the same adverse reactions found with systemic administration of beta-adrenergic blocking agents may occur with topical administration. For example, severe respiratory reactions and cardiac reactions, including death due to bronchospasm in patients with asthma, and rarely, death in association with cardiac failure, have been reported following topical application of beta-adrenergic blocking agents (see CONTRAINDICATIONS).

Since OPTIPRANOLOL Ophthalmic Solution had a minor effect on heart rate and blood pressure in clinical studies, caution should be observed in treating patients with a istory of cardiac failure. Treatment with OPTIPRANOLOL Ophthalmic Solution should be discontinued at the first evidence of cardiac failure.

OPTIPRANOLOL Ophthalmic Solution, or other beta-blockers, should not, in general, be administered to patients with chronic obstructive pulmonary disease (e.g., chronic bronchitis, emphysema) of mild or moderate severity (see CONTRAINDICATIONS). However, if the drug is necessary in such patients, then it should be administered with caution since it may block bronchodilation produced by endogenous and exogenous catecholamine stimulation of beta$_2$ receptors.

Precautions: General: Because of potential effects of beta-adrenergic receptor blocking agents relative to blood pressure and pulse, these should be used with caution in patients with cerebrovascular insufficiency. If signs or symptoms suggesting reduced cerebral blood flow develop following initiation of therapy with OPTIPRANOLOL Ophthalmic Solution, alternative therapy shoulld be considered.

Some authorities recommend gradual withdrawal of beta-adrenergic receptor blocking agents in patients undergoing elective surgery. If necessary during surgery, the effects of beta-adrenergic receptor blocking agents may be reversed by sufficient doses of such agonists as isoproterenol, dopamine, dobutamine or levarterenol.

While OPTIPRANOLOL Ophthalmic Solution has demonstrated a low potential for systemic effect, it should be used with caution in patients with diabetes (especially labile diabetes,) because of possible masking of signs and symptoms of acute hypoglycemia.

Beta-adrenergic receptor blocking agents may mask certain signs and symptoms of hyperthyroidism, and their abrupt withdrawal might precipitate a thyroid storm.

Beta-adrenergic blockade has been reported to potentiate muscle weakness consistent with certain myasthenic symptoms (e.g., diplopia, ptosis, and generalized weakness).

Risk of anaphylactic reaction: While taking beta-blockers, patients with a history of severe anaphylactic reaction to a variety of allergens may be more reactive to repeated challenge, either accidental, diagnostic, or therapeutic. Such patients may be unresponsive to the usual doses of epinephrine used to treat allergic reaction.

Information for Patients:
Patients should be instructed to avoid allowing the tip of the dispensing container to contact the eye or surrounding structures.

Patients should be advised that OPTIPRANOLOL contains benzalkonium chloride which may be absorbed by soft contact lenses. Contact lenses should be removed prior to administration of the solution. Lenses may be reinserted 15 minutes following OPTIPRANOLOL administration.

Drug Interactions:
OPTIPRANOLOL Ophthalmic Solution should be used with caution in patients who are receiving a beta-adrenergic blocking agent orally, because of the potential for additive effects on systemic beta-blockade.

Close observation of the patient is recommended when a beta-blocker is administered to patients receiving catecholamine-depleting drugs such as reserpine, because of possible additive effects and the production of hypotension and/or bradycardia.

Caution should be used in the coadministration of beta-adrenergic receptor blocking agents, such as metipranolol, and oral or intravenous calcium channel antagonists, because of possible precipitation of left ventricular failure, and hypotension. In patients with impaired cardiac function, who are receiving calcium channel antagonists, coadministration should be avoided. The concomitant use of beta-adrenergic receptor blocking agents with digitalis and calcium channel antagonists may have additive effecets, prolonging atrioventricular conduction time.

Caution should be used in patients using concomitant adrenergic psychotropic drugs.
Ocular:
In patients with angle-closure glaucoma, the immediate treatment objective is to re-open the angle by constriction of the pupil with a miotic agent. OPTIPRANOLOL Ophthalmic Solution has little or no effect on the pupil, therefore, when it is used to reduce intraocular pressure in angle-closure glaucoma, it should be used only with concomitant administration of a miotic agent.

Carcinogenesis, Mutagensis, Impairment of Fertility:
Lifetime studies with metipranolol have heen conducted in mice at oral doses of 5, 50, and 100 mg/kg/day and in rats at oral doses of up to 70 mg/kg/day. Metipranolol demonstrated no carcinogenic effect. In the mouse study, female animals receiving the low, but not the intermediate or high dose, had an increased number of pulmonary adenomas. The significance of this observation is unknown. In a variety of *in vitro* and *in vivo* bacterial and mammalian cell assays, metipranolol was nonmutagenic.

Reproduction and fertility studies of metipranolol in rats and mice showed no adverse effect on male fertility at oral doses of up to 50 mg/kg/day, and female fertility at oral doses of up to 25 mg/kg/day.

Pregnancy: Teratogenic effects:
Pregnancy Category C: No drug related effects were reported for the segment II teratology study in fetal rats after administration, during organogenesis, to dams of up to 50 mg/kg/day. OPTIPRANOLOL Ophthalmic Solution has been shown to increase fetal resorption, fetal death, and delayed development when administered orally to rabbits at 50 mg/kg/day during organogenesis.

There are no adequate and well-controlled studies in pregnant women. OPTIPRANOLOL Ophthalmic Solution should be used during pregnancy only if the potential benefit justifies the potential risk to the fetus.

Nursing Mothers:
It is not known whether OPTIPRANOLOL Ophthalmic Solution is excreted in human milk. Because many drugs are excreted in human milk, caution should be exercised when OPTIPRANOLOL Ophthalmic Solution is administered to nursing women.

Pediatric Use:
Safety and effectiveness in children have not been established.

Geriatric Use: No overall differences in safety or effectiveness have been observed between elderly and younger patients.

Adverse Reactions: In clinical trials, the use of OPTIPRANOLOL Ophthalmic Solution has been associated with transient local discomfort.

Other ocular adverse reactions, such as abnormal vision, blepharitis, blurred vision, browache, conjunctivitis, edema, eyelid dermatitis, photophobia, tearing, and uveitis have been reported in small numbers of patients.

Other systemic adverse reactions, such as allergic reaction, angina, anxiety, arthritis, asthenia, atrial fibrillation, bradycardia, bronchitis, coughing, depression, dizziness, dyspnea, epistaxis, headache, hypertension, myalgia, myocardial infarct, nausea nervousness, palpitation, rash, rhinitis and somnolence have also been reported in small numbers of patients.

Overdosage: No information is available on overdosage of OPTIPRANOLOL Ophthalmic Solution in humans. The symptoms which

Continued on next page

Optipranolol—Cont.

might be expected with an overdose of a systemically administered beta-adrenergic receptor blocking agent are bradycardia, hypotension and accute cardiac failure.

Dosage and Administration: The recommended dose is one drop of OPTIPRANOLOL Ophthalmic Solution in the affected eye(s) twice a day.

If the patients's IOP is not at a satisfactory level on this regimen, use of more frequent administration or a larger dose of OPTIPRANOLOL Ophthalmic Solution is not known to be of benefit. Concomitant therapy to lower intraocular pressure can be instituted.

In clinical trials, OPTIPRANOLOL Ophthalmic Solution was safely used during concomitant therapy with pilocarpine, epinephrine or acetazolamide.

How Supplied: OPTIPRANOLOL® (metipranolol ophthalmic solution) 0.3% is supplied in a plastic with a controlled drop tip and a yellow plastic screw-top cap as follows:
5 mL: NDC 24208-275-07-AB40207
10 mL: NDC 24208-275-09-AB40209

Storage: Store between, 15°–30°C (59°–86°F). Replace cap immediately after use.
[See figure at top of next column]

```
DO NOT USE IF IMPRINTED
NECKBAND IS NOT INTACT.
```

FOR OPHTHALMIC USE ONLY
Bausch & Lomb
Incorporated, Inc.
Tampa, FL 33637   Rev. 11/03-91
©Bausch & Lomb Incorporated, Inc.
Shown in Product Identification Guide, page 104

RĒV-EYES™   ℞
[reev-eyes]
(dapirazole hydrochloride ophthalmic solution)
Ophthalmic Eyedrops, 0.5%—Sterile

Description: For ophthalmic use only.
Dapiprazole hydrochloride is an alpha-adrenergic blocking agent.
Dapiprazole hydrochloride is 5,6,7,8-tetrahydro-3-[2-(4-o.tolyl-1-piperazinyl)ethyl]-s-triazolo[4,3-a]pyridine hydrochloride.
Dapiprazole hydrochloride has the empirical formula $C_{19}H_{27}N_5 \bullet HCl$ and a molecular weight of 361.93.
Dapiprazole hydrochloride is a sterile, white, lyophilized powder soluble in water.
RĒV-EYES™ (dapiprazole hydrochloride ophthalmic solution) Ophthalmic Eyedrops is a clear, colorless, slightly viscous solution for topical application. Each mL (when reconstituted as directed) contains 5 mg of dapiprazole hydrochloride as the active ingredient.
The reconstituted solution has a pH of approximately 6.6 and an osmolarity of approximately 415 mOsm.
The inactive ingredients include: mannitol (2%), sodium chloride, hydroxypropyl methylcellulose (0.4%), edetate sodium (0.01%), sodium phosphate dibasic, sodium phosphate monobasic, water for injection, and benzalkonium chloride (0.01%) as a preservative.
RĒV-EYES™ Ophthalmic Eyedrops, 0.5% is supplied in a kit consisting of one vial of dapiprazole hydrochloride (25 mg), one vial of diluent (5 mL) and one dropper for dispensing.

Clinical Pharmacology: Dapiprazole hydrochloride ophthalmic solution acts through blocking the alpha-adrenergic receptors in smooth muscle. Dapiprazole hydrochloride ophthalmic solution produces miosis through an effect on the dilator muscle of the iris.
Dapiprazole hydrochloride ophthalmic solution does not have any significant activity on ciliary muscle contraction and, therefore does not induce a significant change in the anterior chamber depth or the thickness of the lens.
Dapiprazole hydrochloride ophthalmic solution has demonstrated safe and rapid reversal of mydriasis produced by phenylephrine and to a lesser degree tropicamide. In patients with decreased accommodative amplitude due to treatment with tropicamide, dapiprazole hydrochloride ophthalmic solution partially restores the accommodative amplitude. This activity is not only due to its miotic effect but also to a direct effect on accommodation.
Eye color affects the rate of pupillary constriction. In individuals with brown irides, the rate of pupillary constriction may be slightly slower than in individuals with blue or green irides. Eye color does not appear to affect the final pupil size.
Dapiprazole hydrochloride ophthalmic solution does not significantly alter intraocular pressure in normotensive eyes or in eyes with elevated intraocular pressure.

Indications and Usage: Dapiprazole hydrochloride ophthalmic solution is indicated in the treatment of iatrogenically induced mydriasis produced by adrenergic (phenylephrine) or parasympatholytic (tropicamide) agents. Dapiprazole hydrochloride ophthalmic solution is not indicated for the reduction of intraocular pressure or in the treatment of open angle glaucoma.

Contraindications: Miotics are contraindicated where constriction is undesirable; such as acute iritis, and in those subjects showing hypersensitivity to any component of this preparation.

Warning: For Topical Ophthalmic Use Only. NOT FOR INJECTION. Do not touch the dropper up to lids or any surface, as this may contaminate the solution. Dapiprazole hydrochloride ophthalmic solution should not be used in the same patient more frequently than once a week.

Precautions:
Information to Patients: Miosis may cause difficulty in dark adaptation and may reduce the field of vision. Patients should exercise caution when involved in night driving or other activities in poor illumination.

Carcinogenesis, Mutagenesis, Impairment of Fertility: Dapiprazole has been shown to significantly increase the incidence of liver tumors in rats after continuous dietary administration for 104 weeks. This effect was found only in male rats treated with the highest dose administered in the study, i.e., 300 mg/kg/day, (80,000 times the human dose) and was not observed in male and female rats at doses of 30 and 100 mg/kg/day and female rats at doses of 300 mg/kg/day.
Negative results have been reported on the mutagenicity and impairment of fertility studies with dapiprazole hydrochloride.

Pregnancy: Pregnancy Category B. Reproduction studies have been performed in rats and rabbits at doses up to 128,000 (rat) and 27,000 (rabbit) times the human ophthalmic dose and revealed no evidence of impaired fertility or harm to the fetus due to dapiprazole hydrochloride. There are, however, no adequate and well-controlled studies in pregnant women. Because animal reproduction studies are not always predictive of human response, this drug should be used during pregnancy only if clearly needed.

Nursing Mothers: It is not known whether this drug is excreted in human milk. Because many drugs are excreted in human milk, caution should be exercised when dapiprazole hydrochloride ophthalmic solution is administered to a nursing woman.

Pediatric Use: Safety and effectiveness in pediatric patients below the age of 4 have not been established.

Adverse Reactions: In controlled studies the most frequent reaction to dapiprazole was conjunctival injection lasting 20 minutes in over 80% of patients. Burning on instillation of dapiprazole hydrochloride ophthalmic solution was reported in approximately half of all patients. Reactions occurring in 10% to 40% of patients included ptosis, lid erythema, lid edema, chemosis, itching, punctate keratitis, corneal edema, browache, photophobia and headaches. Other reactions reported less frequently included dryness of eyes, tearing and blurring of vision.

Dosage and Administration: Two drops followed 5 minutes later by an additional 2 drops applied topically to the conjunctiva of each eye should be administered after the ophthalmic examination to reverse the diagnostic mydriasis. Dapiprazole hydrochloride ophthalmic solution should not be used in the same patient more frequently than once per week.

Directions for Preparing Eyedrops:
1. Use aseptic technique.
2. Tear off aluminum seals, remove and discard rubber plugs from both drug and diluent vials.
3. Pour diluent into drug vial.
4. Remove dropper assembly from its sterile wrapping and attach to the drug vial.
5. Shake container for several minutes to ensure mixing.

How Supplied: RĒV-EYES™ Ophthalmic Eyedrops, 0.5% Sterile (NDC 24208-394-07) Each package contains one vial of dapiprazole hydrochloride (25 mg) lyophilized powder, one vial of diluent (5 mL) and dropper for dispensing.

Storage and Stability of Eyedrops: Once the ophthalmic solution has been reconstituted it may be stored at room temperature 15°–30°C (59°–86°F) for 21 days. Discard any solution that is not clear and colorless.
Patented U.S. Patent No. 4,252,721
Revised: July, 1998

Manufactured by
Abbott Laboratories
North Chicago, IL 60064
For
Angelini Pharmaceuticals Inc.
River Edge, NJ 07661
Marketed by
Bausch & Lomb Incorporated
Tampa, FL 33637
Rx only
Shown in Product Identification Guide, page 104

Refer to Section 8
for information on
Intraocular Products.

Duramed Pharmaceuticals, Inc.
Subsidiary of Barr Pharmaceuticals, Inc.
2 QUAKER RD.
POMONA, NY 10970

Direct Inquiries to:
877-405-0369

DIAMOX® ℞
[dī 'ă-mŏks]
(Acetazolamide)
SEQUELS®
Sustained-Release Capsules
℞ only

Description: DIAMOX® (acetazolamide) is an inhibitor of the enzyme carbonic anhydrase. DIAMOX is a white to faintly yellowish white crystalline, odorless powder, weakly acidic, very slightly soluble in water, and slightly soluble in alcohol. The chemical name for DIAMOX is N-(5-Sulfamoyl-1,3,4-thiadiazol-2-yl) acetamide and has the following chemical structure:

MW 222.24 $C_4H_6N_4O_3S_2$

DIAMOX SEQUELS are sustained-release capsules, for oral administration, each containing 500 mg of acetazolamide and the following inactive ingredients: Ethyl Vanillin, FD&C Blue No. 1, FD&C Yellow No. 6, Gelatin, Glycerin, Microcrystalline Cellulose, Methylparaben, Propylene Glycol, Propylparaben, Silicon Dioxide, and Sodium Lauryl Sulfate.

Clinical Pharmacology: DIAMOX is a potent carbonic anhydrase inhibitor, effective in the control of fluid secretion (eg, some types of glaucoma), in the treatment of certain convulsive disorders (eg, epilepsy), and in the promotion of diuresis in instances of abnormal fluid retention (eg, cardiac edema).

DIAMOX is not a mercurial diuretic. Rather, it is a nonbacteriostatic sulfonamide possessing a chemical structure and pharmacological activity distinctly different from the bacteriostatic sulfonamides.

DIAMOX is an enzyme inhibitor that acts specifically on carbonic anhydrase, the enzyme which catalyzes the reversible reaction involving the hydration of carbon dioxide and the dehydration of carbonic acid. In the eye, this inhibitory action of acetazolamide decreases the secretion of aqueous humor and results in a drop in intraocular pressure, a reaction considered desirable in cases of glaucoma and even in certain nonglaucomatous conditions. Evidence seems to indicate that DIAMOX has utility as an adjuvant in the treatment of certain dysfunctions of the central nervous system (eg, epilepsy). Inhibition of carbonic anhydrase in this area appears to retard abnormal, paroxysmal, excessive discharge from central nervous system neurons. The diuretic effect of DIAMOX is due to its action in the kidney on the reversible reaction involving hydration of carbon dioxide and dehydration of carbonic acid. The result is renal loss of HCO_3 ion, which carries out sodium, water, and potassium. Alkalinization of the urine and promotion of diuresis are thus affected. Alteration in ammonia metabolism occurs due to increased reabsorption of ammonia by the renal tubules as a result of urinary alkalinization.

DIAMOX SEQUELS sustained-release capsules provide prolonged action to inhibit aqueous humor secretion for 18 to 24 hours after each dose, whereas tablets act for only eight to 12 hours. The prolonged continuous effect of SEQUELS permits a reduction in dosage frequency.

Plasma concentrations of acetazolamide peak from three to six hours after administration of DIAMOX SEQUELS, compared to one to four hours with tablets. Food does not affect bioavailability of DIAMOX SEQUELS.

Placebo-controlled clinical trials have shown that prophylactic administration of DIAMOX at a dose of 250 mg every eight to 12 hours (or a 500 mg controlled-release capsule once daily) before and during rapid ascent to altitude results in fewer and/or less severe symptoms of acute mountain sickness (AMS) such as headache, nausea, shortness of breath, dizziness, drowsiness, and fatigue. Pulmonary function (eg, minute ventilation, expired vital capacity, and peak flow) is greater in the DIAMOX treated group, both in subjects with AMS and asymptomatic subjects. The DIAMOX treated climbers also had less difficulty in sleeping.

Indications and Usage: For adjunctive treatment of: chronic simple (open-angle) glaucoma, secondary glaucoma, and preoperatively in acute angle-closure glaucoma where delay of surgery is desired in order to lower intraocular pressure. DIAMOX is also indicated for the prevention or amelioration of symptoms associated with acute mountain sickness in climbers attempting rapid ascent and in those who are very susceptible to acute mountain sickness despite gradual ascent.

Contraindications: Hypersensitivity to acetazolamide or to any excipients in the formulation. Since acetazolamide is a sulfonamide derivative, cross-sensitivity between acetazolamide, sulfonamides, and other sulfonamide derivatives is possible.

Acetazolamide therapy is contraindicated in situations in which sodium and/or potassium blood serum levels are depressed, in cases of marked kidney and liver disease or dysfunction, in suprarenal gland failure, and in hyperchloremic acidosis. It is contraindicated in patients with cirrhosis because of the risk of development of hepatic encephalopathy.

Long-term administration of DIAMOX is contraindicated in patients with chronic noncongestive angle-closure glaucoma since it may permit organic closure of the angle to occur while the worsening glaucoma is masked by lowered intraocular pressure.

Warnings: Fatalities have occurred, although rarely, due to severe reactions to sulfonamides including Stevens-Johnson syndrome, toxic epidermal necrolysis, fulminant hepatic necrosis, agranulocytosis, aplastic anemia, and other blood dyscrasias. Sensitizations may recur when a sulfonamide is readministered irrespective of the route of administration. If signs of hypersensitivity or other serious reactions occur, discontinue use of this drug.

Caution is advised for patients receiving concomitant high-dose aspirin and DIAMOX, as anorexia, tachypnea, lethargy, metabolic acidosis, coma, and death have been reported.

Precautions:
General
Increasing the dose does not increase the diuresis and may increase the incidence of drowsiness and/or paresthesia. Increasing the dose often results in a decrease in diuresis. Under certain circumstances, however, very large doses have been given in conjunction with other diuretics in order to secure diuresis in complete refractory failure.

Information for Patients
Adverse reactions common to all sulfonamide derivatives may occur: anaphylaxis, fever, rash (including erythema multiforme, Stevens-Johnson syndrome, toxic epidermal necrolysis), crystalluria, renal calculus, bone marrow depression, thrombocytopenic purpura, hemolytic anemia, leukopenia, pancytopenia, and agranulocytosis. Precaution is advised for early detection of such reactions, and the drug should be discontinued and appropriate therapy instituted.

In patients with pulmonary obstruction or emphysema where alveolar ventilation may be impaired, DIAMOX, which may aggravate acidosis, should be used with caution.

Gradual ascent is desirable to try to avoid acute mountain sickness. If rapid ascent is undertaken and DIAMOX® is used, it should be noted that such use does not obviate the need for prompt descent if severe forms of high altitude sickness occur, ie, high altitude pulmonary edema (HAPE) or high altitude cerebral edema.

Caution is advised for patients receiving concomitant high-dose aspirin and DIAMOX, as anorexia, tachypnea, lethargy, metabolic acidosis, coma, and death have been reported (see **WARNINGS**).

Both increases and decreases in blood glucose levels have been described in patients treated with acetazolamide. This should be taken into consideration in patients with impaired glucose tolerance or diabetes mellitus.

Laboratory Tests
To monitor for hematologic reactions common to all sulfonamides, it is recommended that a baseline CBC and platelet count be obtained on patients prior to initiating DIAMOX therapy and at regular intervals during therapy. If significant changes occur, early discontinuance and institution of appropriate therapy are important. Periodic monitoring of serum electrolytes is recommended.

Carcinogenesis, Mutagenesis, Impairment of Fertility
Long-term studies in animals to evaluate the carcinogenic potential of DIAMOX have not been conducted. In a bacterial mutagenicity assay, DIAMOX was not mutagenic when evaluated with and without metabolic activation. The drug had no effect on fertility when administered in the diet to male and female rats at a daily intake of up to 4 times the maximum recommended human dose of 1000 mg in a 50 kg individual.

Pregnancy Category C
Acetazolamide, administered orally or parenterally, has been shown to be teratogenic (defects of the limbs) in mice, rats, hamsters, and rabbits. There are no adequate and well-controlled studies in pregnant women. Acetazolamide should be used in pregnancy only if the potential benefit justifies the potential risk to the fetus.

Nursing Mothers
Because of the potential for serious adverse reactions in nursing infants from DIAMOX, a decision should be made whether to discontinue nursing or to discontinue the drug, taking into account the importance of the drug to the mother. Acetazolamide should only be used by nursing women if the potential benefit justifies the potential risk to the child.

Pediatric Use
The safety and effectiveness of DIAMOX in pediatric patients have not been established.
Growth retardation has been reported in children receiving long-term therapy, believed secondary to chronic acidosis.

Geriatric Use
Metabolic acidosis, which can be severe, may occur in the elderly with reduced renal function.

Adverse Reactions: Body as a whole: Headache, malaise, fatigue, flushing, growth retardation in children, flaccid paralysis, anaphylaxis

Continued on next page

Diamox Sequels—Cont.

Digestive: Gastrointestinal disturbances such as nausea, vomiting, diarrhea
Hematological/Lymphatic: Blood dyscrasias such as aplastic anemia, agranulocytosis, leukopenia, thrombocytopenia, thrombocytopenic purpura, melena
Hepato-biliary disorders: Abnormal liver function, cholestatic jaundice, hepatic insufficiency, fulminant hepatic necrosis
Metabolic/Nutritional: Metabolic acidosis, electrolyte imbalance, including hypokalemia, hyponatremia, osteomalacia with long-term phenytoin therapy, loss of appetite, taste alteration, hyperglycemia, hypoglycemia
Nervous: Drowsiness, paraesthesia (including numbness and tingling of extremities and face), depression, excitement, ataxia, confusion, convulsions, dizziness
Skin: Allergic skin reactions including urticaria, photosensitivity, Stevens-Johnson syndrome, toxic epidermal necrolysis
Special senses: Hearing disturbances, tinnitus, myopia
Urogenital: Crystalluria, increased risk of nephrolithiasis with long-term therapy, hematuria, glycosuria, renal failure, polyuria

DRUG INTERACTIONS
Aspirin—See **WARNINGS**.
DIAMOX modifies phenytoin metabolism with increased serum levels of phenytoin. This may increase or enhance the occurrence of osteomalacia in some patients receiving chronic phenytoin therapy. Caution is advised in patients receiving chronic concomitant therapy. By decreasing the gastrointestinal absorption of primidone, DIAMOX may decrease serum concentrations of primidone and its metabolites, with a consequent possible decrease in anticonvulsant effect. Caution is advised when beginning, discontinuing, or changing the dose of DIAMOX in patients receiving primidone.
Because of possible additive effects with other carbonic anhydrase inhibitors, concomitant use is not advisable.
Acetazolamide may increase the effects of other folic acid antagonists.
Acetazolamide may increase or decrease blood glucose levels. Consideration should be taken in patients being treated with antidiabetic agents.
Acetazolamide decreases urinary excretion of amphetamine and may enhance the magnitude and duration of their effect.
Acetazolamide reduces urinary excretion of quinidine and may enhance its effect.
Acetazolamide may prevent the urinary antiseptic effect of methenamine.
Acetazolamide increases lithium excretion and the lithium may be decreased.
Acetazolamide and sodium bicarbonate used concurrently increase the risk of renal calculus formation.
Acetazolamide may elevate cyclosporine levels.

Overdosage: No specific antidote is known. Treatment should be symptomatic and supportive.
Electrolyte imbalance, development of an acidotic state, and central nervous system effects might be expected to occur. Serum electrolyte levels (particularly potassium) and blood pH levels should be monitored.
Supportive measures are required to restore electrolyte and pH balance. The acidotic state can usually be corrected by the administration of bicarbonate.
Despite its high intraerythrocytic distribution and plasma protein binding properties, DIAMOX is dialyzable. This may be particularly important in the management of DIAMOX overdosage when complicated by the presence of renal failure.

Dosage and Administration:
Glaucoma
The recommended dosage is 1 capsule (500 mg) two times a day. Usually 1 capsule is administered in the morning and 1 capsule in the evening. It may be necessary to adjust the dose, but it has usually been found that dosage in excess of 2 capsules (1 g) does not produce an increased effect. The dosage should be adjusted with careful individual attention both to symptomatology and intraocular tension. In all cases, continuous supervision by a physician is advisable.
In those unusual instances where adequate control is not obtained by the twice-a-day administration of DIAMOX acetazolamide SEQUELS sustained-release capsules, the desired control may be established by means of DIAMOX (tablets or parenteral). Use tablets or parenteral in accordance with the more frequent dosage schedules recommended for these dosage forms, such as 250 mg every four hours, or an initial dose of 500 mg followed by 250 mg or 125 mg every four hours, depending on the case in question.

Acute Mountain Sickness
Dosage is 500 mg to 1000 mg daily, in divided doses using tablets or sustained-release capsules as appropriate. In circumstances of rapid ascent, such as in rescue or military operations, the higher dose level of 1000 mg is recommended. It is preferable to initiate dosing 24 to 48 hours before ascent and to continue for 48 hours while at high altitude, or longer as necessary to control symptoms.

Interference with Laboratory Tests
Sulfonamides may give false negative or decreased values for urinary phenolsulfonphthalein and phenol red elimination values for urinary protein, serum non-protein and for serum uric acid. Acetazolamide may produce an increased level of crystals in the urine.
Acetazolamide interferes with the HPLC method of assay for theophylline. Interference with the theophylline assay by acetazolamide depends on the solvent used in the extraction; acetazolamide may not interfere with other assay methods for theophylline.

How Supplied: DIAMOX® acetazolamide SEQUELS®, 500 mg orange capsules printed with DIAMOX over D3 are supplied as follows:
NDC 51285-754-02 – Bottle of 100
Store at controlled room temperature 20°–25°C (68°–77°F).
Manufactured By:
WYETH PHARMACEUTICALS INC.
Philadelphia, PA 19101
Manufactured For:
DURAMED PHARMACEUTICALS, INC.
Subsidiary of Barr Laboratories, Inc.
Pomona, NY 10970

1007542501
CI 7865-1
Revised March 2003

Refer to Section 8
for information on
Intraocular Products.

Falcon Pharmaceuticals, Ltd.
6201 SOUTH FREEWAY
FORT WORTH, TX 76134

Direct Inquiries to:
Falcon Pharmaceuticals, Ltd.
(800) 343-2133

TIMOLOL GFS ℞
(timolol maleate ophthalmic gel forming solution)
0.25% and 0.5%
Sterile

Description: Timolol GFS (timolol maleate ophthalmic gel forming solution) is a non-selective beta-adrenergic receptor blocking agent. Its chemical name is (-)-1-(*tert*-butylamino)-3-[(4-morpholino-1,2,5-thiadiazol-3-yl)oxy]-2-propanol maleate (1:1) (salt). Timolol maleate possesses an asymmetric carbon atom in its structure and is provided as the levo-isomer. The nominal optical rotation of timolol maleate is:
$[\alpha]$ 25° in 0.1N HCl (C=5%) = $-12.2°$.
405 nm
Its molecular formula is $C_{13}H_{24}N_4O_3S \cdot C_4H_4O_4$ and its structural formula is:

Timolol maleate has a molecular weight of 432.50. It is a white, odorless, crystalline powder which is soluble in water, methanol, and alcohol.
Timolol GFS is supplied as a sterile, isotonic, buffered, aqueous solution of timolol maleate in two dosage strengths. Each mL of Timolol GFS 0.25% contains 2.5 mg of timolol (3.4 mg of timolol maleate). Each mL of Timolol GFS 0.5% contains 5.0 mg of timolol (6.8 mg of timolol maleate). Inactive ingredients: xanthan gum, trometamine, boric acid, mannitol, polysorbate-80, and purified water. Preservative: benzododecinium bromide 0.012%.

DM-00
Xanthan gum is a purified high molecular weight polysaccharide gum produced from the fermentation by bacterium *Xathomonas campestris*. An aqueous solution of xanthan gum, in the presence of tear protein (lysozyme), forms a gel. Upon contact with the precorneal tear film, Timolol GFS forms a gel that is subsequently removed by the flow of tears.

Clinical Pharmacology:
Mechanism of Action
Timolol maleate is a $beta_1$ and $beta_2$ (non-selective) adrenergic receptor-blocking agent that does not have significant intrinsic sympathomimetic, direct myocardial depressant, or local anesthetic (membrane-stabilizing) activity. Timolol GFS, when applied topically to the eye, has the action of reducing elevated, as well as normal, intraocular pressure, whether or not accompanied by glaucoma. Elevated intraocular pressure is a major risk factor in the pathogenesis of glaucomatous visual field loss and optic nerve damage. The precise mechanism of the ocular hypotensive action of Timolol GFS is not clearly established at this time. Tonography and fluorophotometry studies of Timolol GFS in man suggest that its predominant action may be related to reduced aqueous formation. However, in some studies, a slight increase in outflow facility was also observed. Beta-adrenergic receptor blockade reduces cardiac output in both healthy subjects and patients with heart disease. In patients with severe impairment of myocardial function

beta-adrenergic receptor blockade may inhibit the stimulatory effect of the sympathetic nervous system necessary to maintain adequate cardiac function. Beta-adrenergic receptor blockade in the bronchi and bronchioles results in increased airway resistance from unopposed parasympathetic activities. Such an effect in patients with asthma or other bronchospastic conditions is potentially dangerous.

Pharmacokinetics
Following topical ocular administration of timolol to humans, low concentrations of drug are found in plasma. After bilateral administration of a 0.5% timolol maleate solution to healthy volunteers, maximum plasma concentrations were generally below 5 ng/mL. Pharmacokinetic studies in humans using this gel forming solution formulation were not performed. However, systemic uptake from a gel matrix is expected to be slower than from a non-gel forming solution based on studies using other gel forming solutions. The maximum plasma timolol concentration from the gel forming drop is not expected to exceed those of the 0.5% timolol maleate solution.

Clinical Studies
In controlled, double-masked, multicenter clinical studies, Timolol GFS administered once daily was compared to equivalent concentrations of TIMOPTIC* (timolol maleate ophthalmic solution) [Merck and Co., Inc.] administered twice daily. Timolol GFS once daily was shown to be equally effective in lowering intraocular pressure as the equivalent concentration of TIMOPTIC administered twice daily.

The effect of timolol in lowering intraocular pressure was evident for 24 hours with a single dose of Timolol GFS. Repeated observations over a three-month study period indicate that the intraocular pressure-lowering effect of Timolol GFS was consistent. The results from the clinical trials are shown in the following figures.
[See graphic at right]

Timolol GFS administered once daily had a safety profile similar to that of an equivalent concentration of TIMOPTIC administered twice daily. Due to the physical characteristics of the formulation, transient blurred vision was reported more frequently in patients administered Timolol GFS. (See **Adverse Reactions**.) Timolol GFS has not been studied in patients wearing contact lenses.

Indications and Usage: Timolol GFS 0.25% and 0.5% are indicated in the treatment of elevated intraocular pressure in patients with ocular hypertension or open-angle glaucoma.

Contraindications: Timolol GFS is contraindicated in patients with (1) bronchial asthma; (2) a history of bronchial asthma; (3) severe chronic obstructive pulmonary disease (see **Warnings**); (4) sinus bradycardia; (5) second or third degree atrioventricular block; (6) overt cardiac failure (see **Warnings**); (7) cardiogenic shock; or (8) hypersensitivity to any component of this product.

Warnings: As with many topically applied ophthalmic drugs, this drug is absorbed systemically.

The same adverse reactions found with systemic administration of beta-adrenergic blocking agents may occur with topical ophthalmic administration. For example, severe respiratory reactions and cardiac reactions, including death due to bronchospasm in patients with asthma, and, rarely death in association with cardiac failure, have been reported following systemic or ophthalmic administration of timolol maleate. (See Contraindications.)

Cardiac Failure
Sympathetic stimulation may be essential for support of the circulation in individuals with diminished myocardial contractility, and its inhibition by beta-adrenergic receptor blockade may precipitate more severe failure.

Mean IOP and Std Dev (mmHg) by Treatment Group

Timolol GFS 0.25% Study

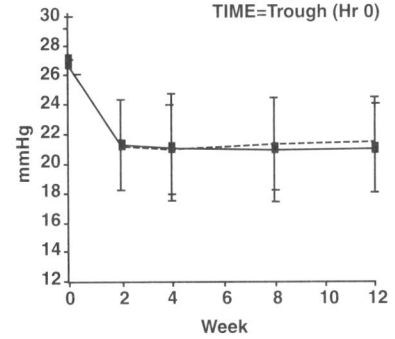
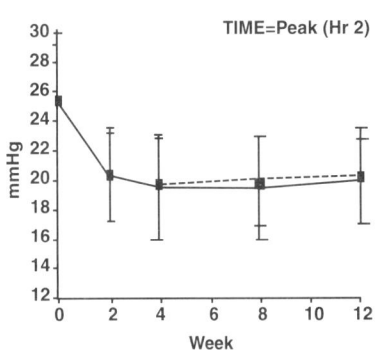

Timolol GFS 0.5% Study

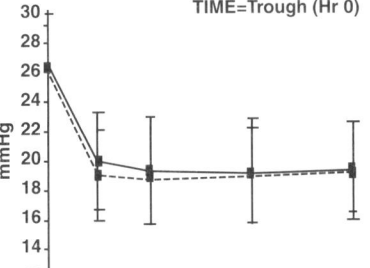
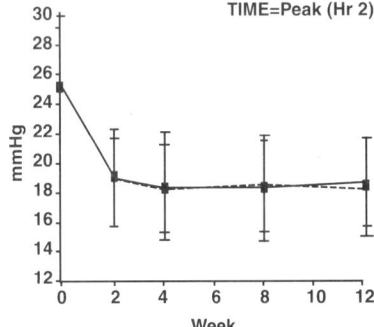

In Patients Without a History of Cardiac Failure, continued depression of the myocardium with beta-blocking agents over a period of time can, in some cases, lead to cardiac failure. At the first sign or symptom of cardiac failure, Timolol GFS should be discontinued.

Obstructive Pulmonary Disease
Patients with chronic obstructive pulmonary disease (e.g., chronic bronchitis, emphysema) of mild or moderate severity, bronchospastic disease, or a history of bronchospastic disease (other than bronchial asthma or a history of bronchial asthma, in which Timolol GFS is contraindicated [see **Contraindications**]) should, in general, not receive beta-blockers, including Timolol GFS.

Major Surgery
The necessity or desirability of withdrawal of beta-adrenergic blocking agents prior to major surgery is controversial. Beta-adrenergic receptor blockade impairs the ability of the heart to respond to beta-adrenergically mediated reflex stimuli. This may augment the risk of general anesthesia in surgical procedures. Some patients receiving beta-adrenergic receptor blocking agents have experienced protracted, severe hypotension during anesthesia. Difficulty in restarting and maintaining the heartbeat has also been reported. For these reasons, in patients undergoing elective surgery, some authorities recommend gradual withdrawal of beta-adrenergic receptor blocking agents. If necessary during surgery, the effects of beta-adrenergic blocking agents may be reversed by sufficient doses of adrenergic agonists.

Diabetes Mellitus
Beta-adrenergic blocking agents should be administered with caution in patients subject to spontaneous hypoglycemia or to diabetic patients (especially those with labile diabetes) who are receiving insulin or oral hypoglycemic agents. Beta-adrenergic receptor blocking agents may mask the signs and symptoms of acute hypoglycemia.

Thyrotoxicosis
Beta-adrenergic blocking agents may mask certain clinical signs (e.g., tachycardia) of hyperthyroidism. Patients suspected of developing thyrotoxicosis should be managed carefully to avoid abrupt withdrawal of beta-adrenergic blocking agents that might precipitate a thyroid storm.

Precautions:
General
Because of potential effects of beta-adrenergic blocking agents on blood pressure and pulse, these agents should be used with caution in patients with cerebrovascular insufficiency. If signs or symptoms suggesting reduced cerebral blood flow develop following initiation of therapy with Timolol GFS, alternative therapy should be considered. There have been reports of bacterial keratitis associated with the use of multiple dose containers of topical ophthalmic

Continued on next page

Timolol GFS—Cont.

products. These containers had been inadvertently contaminated by patients who, in most cases, had a concurrent corneal disease or a disruption of the ocular epithelial surface. (see **Precautions**, Information for Patients.) Choroidal detachment after filtration procedures has been reported with the administration of aqueous suppressant (e.g., timolol) therapy.

Angle-closure glaucoma: In patients with angle-closure glaucoma, the immediate objective of treatment is to reopen the angle. This may require constricting the pupil. Timolol GFS has little or no effect on the pupil and should not be used alone in the treatment of angle-closure glaucoma.

Anaphylaxis: While taking beta-blockers, patients with a history of atopy or a history of severe anaphylactic reactions to a variety of allergens may be more reactive to repeated accidental, diagnostic, or therapeutic challenge with such allergens. Such patients may be unresponsive to the usual doses of epinephrine used to treat anaphylactic reactions.

Muscle Weakness: Beta-adrenergic blockade has been reported to potentiate muscle weakness consistent with certain myasthenic symptoms (e.g., diplopia, ptosis, and generalized weakness). Timolol has been reported rarely to increase muscle weakness in some patients with myasthenia gravis or myasthenic symptoms.

Information for Patients
Patients should be instructed to avoid allowing the tip of the dispensing container to contact the eye or surrounding structures. Patients should also be instructed that ocular solutions, if handled improperly, could become contaminated by common bacteria known to cause ocular infections. Serious damage to the eye and subsequent loss of vision may result from using contaminated solutions. (See **Precautions**, General.)

Patients should also be advised that if they have ocular surgery or develop an intercurrent ocular condition (e.g., trauma or infection), they should immediately seek their physician's advice concerning the continued use of the present multidose container. Patients should be instructed to invert the closed container and shake once before each use. It is not necessary to shake the container more than once. Patients requiring concomitant topical ophthalmic medications should be instructed to administer these at least 10 minutes before instilling Timolol GFS. Patients with bronchial asthma, a history of bronchial asthma, severe chronic obstructive pulmonary disease, sinus bradycardia, second or third degree atrioventricular block, or cardiac failure should be advised not to take this product. (See **Contraindications**.) Transient blurred vision or visual disturbance, generally lasting from 30 seconds to 5 minutes, following instillation may impair the ability to perform hazardous tasks such as operating machinery or driving a motor vehicle.

Drug Interactions
Beta-adrenergic blocking agents: Patients who are receiving a beta-adrenergic blocking agent orally and Timolol GFS should be observed for potential additive effects of beta-blockade, both systemic and on intraocular pressure. Patients should not usually receive two topical ophthalmic beta-adrenergic blocking agents concurrently.
Calcium antagonists: Caution should be used in the co-administration of beta-adrenergic blocking agents, such as Timolol GFS, and oral or intravenous calcium antagonists because of possible atrioventricular conduction disturbances, left ventricular failure, or hypotension. In patients with impaired cardiac function, co-administration should be avoided.

Catecholamine-depleting drugs: Close observation of the patient is recommended when a beta blocker is administered to patients receiving catecholamine-depleting drugs such as reserpine, because of possible additive effects and the production of hypotension and/or marked bradycardia, which may result in vertigo, syncope, or postural hypotension.
Digitalis and calcium antagonists: The concomitant use of beta-adrenergic blocking agents with digitalis and calcium antagonists may have additive effects in prolonging atrioventricular conduction time.
Quinidine: Potentiated systemic beta-blockade (e.g., decreased heart rate) has been reported during combined treatment with quinidine and timolol, possibly because quinidine inhibits the metabolism of timolol via the P-450 enzyme, CYP2D6.
Injectable Epinephrine: (See **Precautions**, General, Anaphylaxis)
Carcinogenesis, Mutagenesis, Impairment of Fertility
In a two-year study of timolol maleate administered orally to rats, there was a statistically significant increase in the incidence of adrenal pheochromocytomas in male rats administered 300 mg/kg/day (approximately 42,000 times the systemic exposure following the maximum recommended human ophthalmic dose). Similar differences were not observed in rats administered oral doses equivalent to approximately 14,000 times the maximum recommended human ophthalmic dose. In a lifetime oral study in mice, there were statistically significant increases in the incidence of benign and malignant pulmonary tumors, benign uterine polyps, and mammary adenocarcinomas in female mice at 500 mg/kg/day (approximately 71,000 times the systemic exposure following the maximum recommended human ophthalmic dose), but not at 5 or 50 mg/kg/day (approximately 700 or 7,000, respectively, times the systemic exposure following the maximum recommended human ophthalmic dose). In a subsequent study in female mice, in which postmortem examinations were limited to the uterus and the lungs, a statistically significant increase in the incidence of pulmonary tumors was again observed at 500 mg/kg/day. The increased occurrence of mammary adenocarcinomas was associated with elevations in serum prolactin, which occurred in female mice administered oral timolol at 500 mg/kg/day, but not at oral doses of 5 or 50 mg/kg/day. An increased incidence of mammary adenocarcinomas in rodents has been associated with administration of several other therapeutic agents that elevate serum prolactin, but no correlation between serum prolactin levels and mammary tumors has been established in humans. Furthermore, in adult human female subjects who received oral dosages of up to 60 mg of timolol maleate (the maximum recommended human oral dosage), there were no clinically meaningful changes in serum prolactin. Timolol maleate was devoid of mutagenic potential when tested *in vivo* (mouse) in the micronucleus test and cytogenetic assay (doses up to 800 mg) and *in vitro* in a neoplastic cell transformation assay (up to 100 µg/mL). In Ames tests, the highest concentrations of timolol employed, 5,000 or 10,000 µg/plate, were associated with statistically significant elevations of revertants observed with tester strain TA 100 (in seven replicate assays), but not in the remaining three strains. In the assays with tester strain TA 100, no consistent dose response relationship was observed, and the ratio of test to control revertants did not reach 2. A ratio of 2 is usually considered the criterion for a positive Ames test. Reproduction and fertility studies in rats demonstrated no adverse effect on male

or female fertility at doses up to 21,000 times the systemic exposure following the maximum recommended human ophthalmic dose.
Pregnancy
— Teratogenic effects:
Pregnancy Category C. Teratogenicity studies with timolol in mice, rats, and rabbits at oral doses up to 50 mg/kg/day (7,000 times the systemic exposure following the maximum recommended human ophthalmic dose) demonstrated no evidence of fetal malformations. Although delayed fetal ossification was observed at this dose in rats, there were no adverse effects on postnatal development of offspring. Doses of 1000 mg/kg/day (142,000 times the systemic exposure following the maximum recommended human ophthalmic dose) were maternotoxic in mice and resulted in an increased number of fetal resorptions. Increased fetal resorptions were also seen in rabbits at doses of 14,000 times the systemic exposure following the maximum recommended human ophthalmic dose, in this case without apparent maternotoxicity. There are no adequate and well-controlled studies in pregnant women. Timolol GFS should be used during pregnancy only if the potential benefit justifies the potential risk to the fetus.
Nursing Mothers
Timolol maleate has been detected in human milk following oral and ophthalmic drug administration. Because of the potential for serious adverse reactions from Timolol GFS in nursing infants, a decision should be made whether to discontinue nursing or to discontinue the drug, taking into account the importance of the drug to the mother.
Pediatric Use
Safety and effectiveness in pediatric patients have not been established.
Adverse Reactions: In clinical trials with Timolol GFS, transient blurred vision upon instillation of the drop was reported in approximately one in three patients but was rarely the cause of discontinuation. The frequency of patients reporting burning and stinging upon instillation was approximately one in eight patients which was comparable to that observed for TIMOPTIC*.
Adverse experiences reported in 1–5% of patients were:
Ocular: Blepharitis, conjunctivitis, crusting, discomfort, foreign body sensation, hyperemia, pruritus and tearing;
Systemic: Headache, hypertension, and upper respiratory infections.
The following additional adverse experiences have been reported with the ocular administration of this or other timolol maleate formulations:
BODY AS A WHOLE
Asthenia/fatigue and chest pain.
CARDIOVASCULAR
Bradycardia, arrhythmia, hypotension, hypertension, syncope, heart block, cerebral vascular accident, cerebral ischemia, cardiac failure, worsening of angina pectoris, palpitation, cardiac arrest, pulmonary edema, dizziness, edema, claudication, Raynaud's phenomenon, and cold hands and feet.
DIGESTIVE
Nausea, diarrhea, dyspepsia, anorexia, and dry mouth.
IMMUNOLOGIC
Systemic lupus erythematosus.
NERVOUS SYSTEM/PSYCHIATRIC
Depression, increase in signs and symptoms of myasthenia gravis, paresthesia, somnolence, insomnia, nightmares, behavioral changes and psychic disturbances including confusion, hallucinations, anxiety, disorientation, nervousness, and memory loss.
SKIN
Alopecia and psoriasiform rash or exacerbation of psoriasis.

HYPERSENSITIVITY
Signs and symptoms of systemic allergic reactions, including angioedema, urticaria and localized and generalized rash.
RESPIRATORY
Bronchospasm (predominantly in patients with pre-existing bronchospastic disease), respiratory failure, dyspnea, nasal congestion, and cough.
ENDOCRINE
Masked symptoms of hypoglycemia in diabetic patients (see **Warnings**).
SPECIAL SENSES
Signs and symptoms of ocular irritation including blepharitis, keratitis, and dry eyes; ptosis; decreased corneal sensitivity; cystoid macular edema; visual disturbances including refractive changes and diplopia; pseudopemphigoid; tinnitus and choroidal detachment following filtration surgery (see **Precautions**, General).
UROGENITAL
Retroperitoneal fibrosis, decreased libido, impotence and Peyronie's disease.

The following additional adverse effects have been reported in clinical experience with ORAL timolol maleate or other ORAL beta-blocking agents and may be considered potential effects of ophthalmic timolol maleate: *Allergic*: Erythematous rash, fever combined with aching and sore throat, laryngospasm with respiratory distress; *Body as a Whole*: Extremity pain, decreased exercise tolerance, weight loss; *Cardiovascular*: Worsening of arterial insufficiency, vasodilatation; *Digestive*: Gastrointestinal pain, hepatomegaly, vomiting, mesenteric arterial thrombosis, ischemic colitis; *Hematologic*: Nonthrombocytopenic purpura, thrombocytopenic purpura, agranulocytosis; *Endocrine*: Hyperglycemia, hypoglycemia; *Skin*: Pruritus, skin irritation, increased pigmentation, sweating; *Musculoskeletal*: Arthralgia; *Nervous System / Psychiatric*: Vertigo, local weakness, diminished concentration, reversible mental depression progressing to catatonia, an acute reversible syndrome characterized by disorientation for time and place, emotional lability, slightly clouded sensorium, and decreased performance on neuropsychometric tests; *Respiratory*: Rales, bronchial obstruction; *Urogenital*: Urination difficulties.

Overdosage: No data are available in regard to human overdose with, or accidental oral ingestion of Timolol GFS. There have been reports of inadvertent overdose with Timolol maleate ophthalmic solution resulting in systemic effects similar to those seen with systemic beta-adrenergic blocking agents such as dizziness, headache, shortness of breath, bradycardia, bronchospasm, and cardiac arrest (see also **Adverse Reactions**).

Overdosage has been reported with Tablets BLOCADREN* (timolol maleate tablets). A 30 year old female ingested 650 mg of BLOCADREN (maximum recommended oral daily dose is 60 mg) and experienced second and third degree heart block. She recovered without treatment but approximately two months later developed irregular heartbeat, hypertension, dizziness, tinnitus, faintness, increased pulse rate, and borderline first degree heart block.

An *in vitro* hemodialysis study, using ^{14}C timolol added to human plasma or whole blood, showed that timolol was readily dialyzed from these fluids; however, a study of patients with renal failure showed that timolol did not dialyze readily.

Dosage and Administration: Patients should be instructed to invert the closed container and shake once before each use. It is not necessary to shake the container more than once. Other topically applied ophthalmic medications should be administered at least 10 minutes before Timolol GFS (See **Precau-** tions, *Information for Patients*). Timolol GFS is available in concentrations of 0.25%, and 0.5%. The dose is one drop of Timolol GFS (either 0.25% or 0.5%) in the affected eye(s) once daily. Because in some patients the intraocular pressure-lowering response to Timolol GFS may require a few weeks to stabilize, evaluation should include a determination of intraocular pressure after approximately 4 weeks of treatment with Timolol GFS. Dosages higher than one drop of 0.5% Timolol GFS once daily have not been studied. If the patient's intraocular pressure is still not at a satisfactory level on this regimen, concomitant therapy can be considered. Other topically applied ophthalmic medications should be administered at least 10 minutes before Timolol GFS. (See **Precautions**, *Information for Patients*.)

How Supplied: Timolol GFS is a colorless to nearly colorless, slightly opalescent, and slightly viscous solution supplied in a DROP-TAINER® package system.
Timolol GFS, 0.25% timolol equivalent and 0.5% timolol equivalent, are both supplied as either a 2.5 mL or 5 mL solution in a 5 mL white polyethylene bottle with a natural polyethylene dropper tip and a yellow polypropylene overcap. Tamper evidence is provided with a shrink band around the closure and neck area of the package.

0.25% NDC 61314-224-25, 2.5 mL fill
       NDC 61314-224-05, 5 mL fill
0.5%   NDC 61314-225-25, 2.5 mL fill
       NDC 61314-225-05, 5 mL fill

Storage
Store between 2° and 25°C (36° and 77°F). Protect from light.
Rx Only

*TIMOPTIC and BLOCADREN are Registered trademarks of Merck & Co., Inc.
Revised: March 2001

King Pharmaceuticals, Inc.
501 FIFTH STREET
BRISTOL, TN 37620

Direct Inquiries:
Telephone: 1 (800) 776-3637
Fax: 1 (423) 989-8786

CORTISPORIN® Ophthalmic Suspension Sterile ℞
[cŏrtĭ-spōrĭn]
(neomycin and polymyxin B sulfates and hydrocortisone ophthalmic suspension, USP)

Description: CORTISPORIN Ophthalmic Suspension (neomycin and polymyxin B sulfates and hydrocortisone ophthalmic suspension) is a sterile antimicrobial and anti-inflammatory suspension for ophthalmic use. Each mL contains: neomycin sulfate equivalent to 3.5 mg neomycin base, polymyxin B sulfate equivalent to 10,000 polymyxin B units, and hydrocortisone 10 mg (1%). The vehicle contains thimerosal 0.001% (added as a preservative) and the inactive ingredients cetyl alcohol, glyceryl monostearate, mineral oil, polyoxyl 40 stearate, propylene glycol, and Water for Injection. Sulfuric acid may be added to adjust pH.
Neomycin sulfate is the sulfate salt of neomycin B and C, which are produced by the growth of *Streptomyces fradiae* Waksman (Fam. Streptomycetaceae). It has a potency equivalent of not less than 600 μg of neomycin standard per mg, calculated on an anhydrous basis. The structural formulae are:
[See chemical structure at top of next column]
Polymyxin B sulfate is the sulfate salt of polymyxin B_1 and B_2, which are produced by the growth of *Bacillus polymyxa* (Prazmowski) Migula (Fam. Bacillaceae). It has a potency of not less than 6,000 polymyxin B units per mg, calculated on an anhydrous basis. The structural formulae are:

Neomycin B (R_1=H, R_2=CH_2NH_2)
Neomycin C (R_1=CH_2NH_2, R_2=H)

Polymyxin B_1 (R=CH_3)
Polymyxin B_2 (R=H)
DAB=α, γ-diaminobutyric acid

Hydrocortisone, 11β,17,21-trihydroxypregn-4-ene-3,20-dione, is an antiinflammatory hormone. Its structural formula is:

Clinical Pharmacology: Corticosteroids suppress the inflammatory response to a variety of agents, and they probably delay or slow healing. Since corticosteroids may inhibit the body's defense mechanism against infection, concomitant antimicrobial drugs may be used when this inhibition is considered to be clinically significant in a particular case.

When a decision to administer both a corticosteroid and antimicrobials is made, the administration of such drugs in combination has the advantage of greater patient compliance and convenience, with the added assurance that the appropriate dosage of all drugs is administered. When each type of drug is in the same formulation, compatibility of ingredients is assured and the correct volume of drug is delivered and retained.

The relative potency of corticosteroids depends on the molecular structure, concentration, and release from the vehicle.

Microbiology: The anti-infective components in CORTISPORIN Ophthalmic Suspension are included to provide action against specific organisms susceptible to it. Neomycin sulfate and polymyxin B sulfate are active in vitro against susceptible strains of the following microorganisms: *Staphylococcus aureus, Escherichia coli, Haemophilus influenzae, Klebsiella / Enterobacter* species, *Neisseria* species, and *Pseudomonas aeruginosa*. The product does not provide adequate coverage against *Serratia marcescens* and streptococci, including *Streptococcus pneumoniae* (see **Indications And Usage**).

Indications and Usage: CORTISPORIN Ophthalmic Suspension is indicated for steroid-responsive inflammatory ocular conditions for which a corticosteroid is indicated and where bacterial infection or a risk of bacterial infection exists.

Ocular corticosteroids are indicated in inflammatory conditions of the palpebral and bulbar conjunctiva, cornea, and anterior segment of

Continued on next page

Cortisporin—Cont.

the globe where the inherent risk of corticosteroid use in certain infective conjunctivitides is accepted to obtain a diminution in edema and inflammation. They are also indicated in chronic anterior uveitis and corneal injury from chemical, radiation, or thermal burns, or penetration of foreign bodies.

The use of a combination drug with an anti-infective component is indicated where the risk of infection is high or where there is an expectation that potentially dangerous numbers of bacteria will be present in the eye (see **Clinical Pharmacology: Microbiology**).

The particular anti-infective drugs in this product are active against the following common bacterial eye pathogens: *Staphylococcus aureus*, *Escherichia coli*, *Haemophilus influenzae*, *Klebsiella/Enterobacter* species, *Neisseria* species, and *Pseudomonas aeruginosa*.

The product does not provide adequate coverage against *Serratia marcescens* and streptococci, including *Streptococcus pneumoniae*.

Contraindications: CORTISPORIN Ophthalmic Suspension is contraindicated in most viral diseases of the cornea and conjunctiva including: epithelial herpes simplex keratitis (dendritic keratitis), vaccinia and varicella, and also in mycobacterial infection of the eye and fungal diseases of ocular structures. CORTISPORIN Ophthalmic Suspension is also contraindicated in individuals who have shown hypersensitivity to any of its components. Hypersensitivity to the antibiotic component occurs at a higher rate than for other components.

Warnings: NOT FOR INJECTION INTO THE EYE. CORTISPORIN Ophthalmic Suspension should never be directly introduced into the anterior chamber of the eye.

Prolonged use of corticosteroids may result in ocular hypertension and/or glaucoma, with damage to the optic nerve, defects in visual acuity and fields of vision, and in posterior subcapsular cataract formation.

Prolonged use may suppress the host response and thus increase the hazard of secondary ocular infections. In those diseases causing thinning of the cornea or sclera, perforations have been known to occur with the use of topical corticosteroids. In acute purulent conditions of the eye, corticosteroids may mask infection or enhance existing infection.

If these products are used for 10 days or longer, intraocular pressure should be routinely monitored even though it may be difficult in uncooperative patients. Corticosteroids should be used with caution in the presence of glaucoma.

The use of corticosteroids after cataract surgery may delay healing and increase the incidence of filtering blebs.

Use of ocular corticosteroids may prolong the course and may exacerbate the severity of many viral infections of the eye (including herpes simplex). Employment of corticosteroid medication in the treatment of herpes simplex requires great caution.

Topical antibiotics, particularly neomycin sulfate, may cause cutaneous sensitization. A precise incidence of hypersensitivity reactions (primarily skin rash) due to topical antibiotics is not known. The manifestations of sensitization to topical antibiotics are usually itching, reddening, and edema of the conjunctiva and eyelid. A sensitization reaction may manifest simply as a failure to heal. During long-term use of topical antibiotic products, periodic examination for such signs is advisable, and the patient should be told to discontinue the product if they are observed. Symptoms usually subside quickly on withdrawing the medication. Application of products containing these ingredients should be avoided for the patient thereafter (see **Precautions: General**).

Precautions:
General: The initial prescription and renewal of the medication order beyond 20 milliliters should be made by a physician only after examination of the patient with the aid of magnification, such as slit lamp biomicroscopy and, where appropriate, fluorescein staining. If signs and symptoms fail to improve after 2 days, the patient should be re-evaluated.

The possibility of fungal infections of the cornea should be considered after prolonged corticosteroid dosing. Fungal cultures should be taken when appropriate.

If this product is used for 10 days or longer, intraocular pressure should be monitored (see **Warnings**).

There have been reports of bacterial keratitis associated with the use of topical ophthalmic products in multiple-dose containers which have been inadvertently contaminated by patients, most of whom had a concurrent corneal disease or a disruption of the ocular epithelial surface (see **Precautions: Information for Patients**).

Allergic cross-reactions may occur which could prevent the use of any or all of the following antibiotics for the treatment of future infections: kanamycin, paromomycin, streptomycin, and possibly gentamicin.

Information for Patients: Patients should be instructed to avoid allowing the tip of the dispensing container to contact the eye, eyelid, fingers, or any other surface. The use of this product by more than one person may spread infection.

Patients should also be instructed that ocular products, if handled improperly, can become contaminated by common bacteria known to cause ocular infections. Serious damage to the eye and subsequent loss of vision may result from using contaminated products (see **Precautions: General**).

If the condition persists or gets worse, or if a rash or allergic reaction develops, the patient should be advised to stop use and consult a physician. Do not use this product if you are allergic to any of the listed ingredients.

Keep tightly closed when not in use. Keep out of reach of children.

Carcinogenesis, Mutagenesis, Impairment of Fertility: Long-term studies in animals to evaluate carcinogenic or mutagenic potential have not been conducted with polymyxin B sulfate. Treatment of cultured human lymphocytes in vitro with neomycin increased the frequency of chromosome aberrations at the highest concentrations (80 μg/mL) tested; however, the effects of neomycin on carcinogenesis and mutagenesis in humans are unknown.

Long-term studies in animals (rats, rabbits, mice) showed no evidence of carcinogenicity or mutagenicity attributable to oral administration of corticosteroids. Long-term animal studies have not been performed to evaluate the carcinogenic potential of topical corticosteroids. Studies to determine mutagenicity with hydrocortisone have revealed negative results. Polymyxin B has been reported to impair the motility of equine sperm, but its effects on male or female fertility are unknown. Long-term animal studies have not been performed to evaluate the effect on fertility of topical corticosteroids.

Pregnancy: *Teratogenic Effects:* Pregnancy Category C. Corticosteroids have been found to be teratogenic in rabbits when applied topically at concentrations of 0.5% on days 6 to 18 of gestation and in mice when applied topically at a concentration of 15% on days 10 to 13 of gestation. There are no adequate and well-controlled studies in pregnant women. CORTISPORIN Ophthalmic Suspension should be used during pregnancy only if the potential benefit justifies the potential risk to the fetus.

Nursing Mothers: It is not known whether topical administration of corticosteroids could result in sufficient systemic absorption to produce detectable quantities in human milk. Systemically administered corticosteroids appear in human milk and could suppress growth, interfere with endogenous corticosteroid production, or cause other untoward effects. Because of the potential for serious adverse reactions in nursing infants from CORTISPORIN Ophthalmic Suspension, a decision should be made whether to discontinue nursing or to discontinue the drug, taking into account the importance of the drug to the mother.

Pediatric Use: Safety and effectiveness in pediatric patients have not been established.

Adverse Reactions: Adverse reactions have occurred with corticosteroid/anti-infective combination drugs which can be attributed to the corticosteroid component, the anti-infective component, or the combination. The exact incidence is not known.

Reactions occurring most often from the presence of the anti-infective ingredient are allergic sensitization reactions including itching, swelling, and conjunctival erythema (see **Warnings**). More serious hypersensitivity reactions, including anaphylaxis, have been reported rarely.

The reactions due to the corticosteroid component in decreasing order of frequency are: elevation of intraocular pressure (IOP) with possible development of glaucoma, and infrequent optic nerve damage; posterior subcapsular cataract formation; and delayed wound healing.

Secondary Infection: The development of secondary infection has occurred after use of combinations containing corticosteroids and antimicrobials. Fungal and viral infections of the cornea are particularly prone to develop coincidentally with long-term applications of a corticosteroid. The possibility of fungal invasion must be considered in any persistent corneal ulceration where corticosteroid treatment has been used.

Local irritation on instillation has also been reported.

Dosage and Administration: One or two drops in the affected eye every 3 or 4 hours, depending on the severity of the condition. The suspension may be used more frequently if necessary.

Not more than 20 milliliters should be prescribed initially and the prescription should not be refilled without further evaluation as outlined in **Precautions** above.

SHAKE WELL BEFORE USING.

How Supplied: Plastic DROP DOSE® dispenser bottle of 7.5 mL (NDC 61570-036-75).

Rx only.

Store at 15° to 25°C (59° to 77°F).

Prescribing Information as of October 2003.

Monarch Pharmaceuticals®

Distributed by: Monarch Pharmaceuticals, Inc., Bristol, TN 37620
(A wholly owned subsidiary of King Pharmaceuticals, Inc.)
Manufactured by: DSM Pharmaceuticals, Inc., Greenville, NC 27834
455232

Shown in Product Identification Guide, page 104

NEOSPORIN® OPHTHALMIC SOLUTION STERILE ℞

[nē″ō-spor-ĭn]

(neomycin and polymyxin B sulfates and gramicidin ophthalmic solution, USP)

Description: NEOSPORIN Ophthalmic Solution (neomycin and polymyxin B sulfates and gramicidin ophthalmic solution) is a sterile antimicrobial solution for ophthalmic use. Each mL contains: neomycin sulfate equivalent to 1.75 mg neomycin base, polymyxin B sulfate equivalent to 10,000 polymyxin B units, and gramicidin 0.025 mg. The vehicle contains alcohol 0.5%, thimerosal 0.001% (added as a preservative), and the inactive ingredients propylene glycol, polyoxyethylene polyoxypropylene compound, sodium chloride, and Water for Injection.

Neomycin sulfate is the sulfate salt of neomycin B and C, which are produced by the growth of *Streptomyces fradiae* Waksman (Fam. Streptomycetaceae). It has a potency equivalent of not less than 600 μg of neomycin standard per mg, calculated on an anhydrous basis. The structural formulae are:

[Chemical structure diagram]

Neomycin B (R_1=H, R_2=CH_2NH_2)
Neomycin C (R_1=CH_2NH_2, R_2=H)

Polymyxin B sulfate is the sulfate salt of polymyxin B_1 and B_2 which are produced by the growth of *Bacillus polymyxa* (Prazmowski) Migula (Fam. Bacillaceae). It has a potency of not less than 6,000 polymyxin B units per mg, calculated on an anhydrous basis. The structural formulae are:

[Chemical structure diagram]

Polymyxin B_1 (R=CH_3)
Polymyxin B_2 (R=H)
DAB=α, γ-diaminobutyric acid

Gramicidin (also called Gramicidin D) is a mixture of three pairs of antibacterial substances (Gramicidin A, B, and C) produced by the growth of *Bacillus brevis* Dubos (Fam. Bacillaceae). It has a potency of not less than 900 μg of standard gramicidin per mg. The structural formulae are:

Gramicidin D

HC-X-Gly-Ala-D-Leu-Ala-D-Val-Val-D-Val-Trp-D-Leu-Y-D-Leu-Trp-D-Leu-Trp-NHCH$_2$CH$_2$OH

	X	Y
Valine-gramicidin A	Val	Trp
Isoleucine-gramicidin A	Ile	Trp
Valine-gramicidin B	Val	Phe
Isoleucine-gramicidin B	Ile	Phe
Valine-gramicidin C	Val	Tyr
Isoleucine-gramicidin C	Ile	Tyr

Clinical Pharmacology: A wide range of antibacterial action is provided by the overlapping spectra of neomycin, polymyxin B sulfate, and gramicidin.

Neomycin is bactericidal for many gram-positive and gram-negative organisms. It is an aminoglycoside antibiotic which inhibits protein synthesis by binding with ribosomal RNA and causing misreading of the bacterial genetic code.

Polymyxin B is bactericidal for a variety of gram-negative organisms. It increases the permeability of the bacterial cell membrane by interacting with the phospholipid components of the membrane.

Gramicidin is bactericidal for a variety of gram-positive organisms. It increases the permeability of the bacterial cell membrane to inorganic cations by forming a network of channels through the normal lipid bilayer of the membrane.

Microbiology: Neomycin sulfate, polymyxin B sulfate, and gramicidin together are considered active against the following microorganisms: *Staphylococcus aureus,* streptococci, including *Streptococcus pneumoniae, Escherichia coli, Haemophilus influenzae, Klebsiella/Enterobacter* species, *Neisseria* species, and *Pseudomonas aeruginosa.* The product does not provide adequate coverage against *Serratia marcescens.*

Indications and Usage: NEOSPORIN Ophthalmic Solution is indicated for the topical treatment of superficial infections of the external eye and its adnexa caused by susceptible bacteria. Such infections encompass conjunctivitis, keratitis and keratoconjunctivitis, blepharitis and blepharoconjunctivitis.

Contraindications: NEOSPORIN Ophthalmic Solution is contraindicated in individuals who have shown hypersensitivity to any of its components.

Warnings: NOT FOR INJECTION INTO THE EYE. NEOSPORIN Ophthalmic Solution should never be directly introduced into the anterior chamber of the eye or injected subconjunctivally.

Topical antibiotics, particularly neomycin sulfate, may cause cutaneous sensitization. A precise incidence of hypersensitivity reactions (primarily skin rash) due to topical antibiotics is not known. The manifestations of sensitization to topical antibiotics are usually itching, reddening, and edema of the conjunctiva and eyelid. A sensitization reaction may manifest simply as a failure to heal. During long-term use of topical antibiotic products, periodic examination for such signs is advisable, and the patient should be told to discontinue the product if they are observed. Symptoms usually subside quickly on withdrawing the medication. Application of products containing these ingredients should be avoided for the patient thereafter (see **PRECAUTIONS: General**).

Precautions:
General: As with other antibiotic preparations, prolonged use of NEOSPORIN Ophthalmic Solution may result in overgrowth of non-susceptible organisms including fungi. If superinfection occurs, appropriate measures should be initiated.

Bacterial resistance to NEOSPORIN Ophthalmic Solution may also develop. If purulent discharge, inflammation, or pain becomes aggravated, the patient should discontinue use of the medication and consult a physician.

There have been reports of bacterial keratitis associated with the use of topical ophthalmic products in multiple-dose containers which have been inadvertently contaminated by patients, most of whom had a concurrent corneal disease or a disruption of the ocular epithelial surface (see **PRECAUTIONS: Information for Patients**).

Allergic cross-reactions may occur which could prevent the use of any or all of the following antibiotics for the treatment of future infections: kanamycin, paromomycin, streptomycin, and possibly gentamicin.

Information for Patients: Patients should be instructed to avoid allowing the tip of the dispensing container to contact the eye, eyelid, fingers, or any other surface. The use of this product by more than one person may spread infection.

Patients should also be instructed that ocular products, if handled improperly, can become contaminated by common bacteria known to cause ocular infections. Serious damage to the eye and subsequent loss of vision may result from using contaminated products (see **PRECAUTIONS: General**).

If the condition persists or gets worse, or if a rash or other allergic reaction develops, the patient should be advised to stop use and consult a physician. Do not use this product if you are allergic to any of the listed ingredients.

Keep tightly closed when not in use. Keep out of reach of children.

Carcinogenesis, Mutagenesis, Impairment of Fertility: Long-term studies in animals to evaluate carcinogenic or mutagenic potential have not been conducted with polymyxin B sulfate or gramicidin. Treatment of cultured human lymphocytes in vitro with neomycin increased the frequency of chromosome aberrations at the highest concentration (80 μg/mL) tested. However, the effects of neomycin on carcinogenesis and mutagenesis in humans are unknown.

Polymyxin B has been reported to impair the motility of equine sperm, but its effects on male or female fertility are unknown.

Pregnancy: *Teratogenic Effects:* Pregnancy Category C. Animal reproduction studies have not been conducted with neomycin sulfate, polymyxin B sulfate, or gramicidin. It is also not known whether NEOSPORIN Ophthalmic Solution can cause fetal harm when administered to a pregnant woman or can affect reproduction capacity. NEOSPORIN Ophthalmic Solution should be given to a pregnant woman only if clearly needed.

Nursing Mothers: It is not known whether this drug is excreted in human milk. Because many drugs are excreted in human milk, caution should be exercised when NEOSPORIN Ophthalmic Solution is administered to a nursing woman.

Pediatric Use: Safety and effectiveness in pediatric patients have not been established.

Adverse Reactions: Adverse reactions have occurred with the anti-infective components of NEOSPORIN Ophthalmic Solution. The exact incidence is not known. Reactions occurring most often are allergic sensitization reactions including itching, swelling, and conjunctival erythema (see **WARNINGS**). More serious hypersensitivity reactions, including anaphylaxis, have been reported rarely.

Local irritation on instillation has also been reported.

Dosage and Administration: Instill one or two drops into the affected eye every 4 hours for 7 to 10 days. In severe infections, dosage may be increased to as much as two drops every hour.

How Supplied: Drop Dose® of 10 mL (plastic dispenser bottle) (NDC 61570-045-10).

Rx only.

Store at 15° to 25°C (59° to 77°F) and protect from light.

Prescribing Information as of April 2003.
Monarch Pharmaceuticals®
Distributed by: Monarch Pharmaceuticals, Inc., Bristol, TN 37620
Manufactured by: DSM Pharmaceuticals, Inc., Greenville, NC 27834

561913

Refer to Section 8
for information on
Intraocular Products.

Merck & Co., Inc.
PO BOX 4 WP39-206
WEST POINT, PA 19486-0004

For Medical Information Contact:
Generally:
Product and service information:
Call the Merck National Service Center, 8:00 AM to 7:00 PM (ET), Monday through Friday:
(800) NSC-MERCK
(800) 672-6372
FAX: (800) MERCK-68
FAX: (800) 637-2568
Adverse Drug Experiences:
Call the Merck National Service Center, 8:00 AM to 7:00 PM (ET), Monday through Friday:
(800) NSC-MERCK
(800) 672-6372
Pregnancy Registries
(800) 986-8999
In Emergencies:
24-hour emergency information for healthcare professionals:
(800) NSC-MERCK
(800) 672-6372

Sales and Ordering:
For product orders and direct account inquiries only, call the Order Management Center, 8:00 AM to 7:00 PM (ET), Monday through Friday:
(800) MERCK RX
(800) 637-2579

COSOPT® ℞
(dorzolamide hydrochloride-timolol maleate ophthalmic solution)
Sterile Ophthalmic Solution

Description
COSOPT* (dorzolamide hydrochloride-timolol maleate ophthalmic solution) is the combination of a topical carbonic anhydrase inhibitor and a topical beta-adrenergic receptor blocking agent.
Dorzolamide hydrochloride is described chemically as: (4S-trans)-4-(ethylamino)-5,6-dihydro-6-methyl-4H-thieno[2,3-b]thiopyran-2-sulfonamide 7,7-dioxide monohydrochloride. Dorzolamide hydrochloride is optically active. The specific rotation is:

$[\alpha]_{405 \text{ nm}}^{25°C}$ (C=1, water) = $\sim -17°$.

Its empirical formula is $C_{10}H_{16}N_2O_4S_3 \cdot HCl$ and its structural formula is:

Dorzolamide hydrochloride has a molecular weight of 360.91. It is a white to off-white, crystalline powder, which is soluble in water and slightly soluble in methanol and ethanol.
Timolol maleate is described chemically as: (-)-1-(tert-butylamino)-3-[(4-morpholino-1,2,5-thiadiazol-3-yl)oxy]-2-propanol maleate (1:1) (salt). Timolol maleate possesses an asymmetric carbon atom in its structure and is provided as the levo-isomer. The nominal optical rotation of timolol maleate is:

$[\alpha]_{405 \text{ nm}}^{25°C}$ in 1N HCl (C=5) = $-12.2°$
($-11.7°$ to $-12.5°$).

Its molecular formula is $C_{13}H_{24}N_4O_3S \cdot C_4H_4O_4$ and its structural formula is:

Timolol maleate has a molecular weight of 432.50. It is a white, odorless, crystalline powder which is soluble in water, methanol, and alcohol. Timolol maleate is stable at room temperature.
COSOPT is supplied as a sterile, isotonic, buffered, slightly viscous, aqueous solution. The pH of the solution is approximately 5.65, and the osmolarity is 242-323 mOsM. Each mL of COSOPT contains 20 mg dorzolamide (22.26 mg of dorzolamide hydrochloride) and 5 mg timolol (6.83 mg timolol maleate). Inactive ingredients are sodium citrate, hydroxyethyl cellulose, sodium hydroxide, mannitol, and water for injection. Benzalkonium chloride 0.0075% is added as a preservative.

---

*Registered trademark of MERCK & CO., Inc.

Clinical Pharmacology
Mechanism of Action
COSOPT is comprised of two components: dorzolamide hydrochloride and timolol maleate. Each of these two components decreases elevated intraocular pressure, whether or not associated with glaucoma, by reducing aqueous humor secretion. Elevated intraocular pressure is a major risk factor in the pathogenesis of optic nerve damage and glaucomatous visual field loss. The higher the level of intraocular pressure, the greater the likelihood of glaucomatous field loss and optic nerve damage.
Dorzolamide hydrochloride is an inhibitor of human carbonic anhydrase II. Inhibition of carbonic anhydrase in the ciliary processes of the eye decreases aqueous humor secretion, presumably by slowing the formation of bicarbonate ions with subsequent reduction in sodium and fluid transport. Timolol maleate is a beta$_1$ and beta$_2$ (non-selective) adrenergic receptor blocking agent that does not have significant intrinsic sympathomimetic, direct myocardial depressant, or local anesthetic (membrane-stabilizing) activity. The combined effect of these two agents administered as COSOPT b.i.d. results in additional intraocular pressure reduction compared to either component administered alone, but the reduction is not as much as when dorzolamide t.i.d. and timolol b.i.d. are administered concomitantly (see *Clinical Studies*).
Pharmacokinetics/Pharmacodynamics
Dorzolamide Hydrochloride
When topically applied, dorzolamide reaches the systemic circulation. To assess the potential for systemic carbonic anhydrase inhibition following topical administration, drug and metabolite concentrations in RBCs and plasma and carbonic anhydrase inhibition in RBCs were measured. Dorzolamide accumulates in RBCs during chronic dosing as a result of binding to CA-II. The parent drug forms a single N-desethyl metabolite, which inhibits CA-II less potently than the parent drug but also inhibits CA-I. The metabolite also accumulates in RBCs where it binds primarily to CA-I. Plasma concentrations of dorzolamide and metabolite are generally below the assay limit of quantitation (15nM). Dorzolamide binds moderately to plasma proteins (approximately 33%).
Dorzolamide is primarily excreted unchanged in the urine; the metabolite also is excreted in urine. After dosing is stopped, dorzolamide washes out of RBCs nonlinearly, resulting in a rapid decline of drug concentration initially, followed by a slower elimination phase with a half-life of about four months.

To simulate the systemic exposure after long-term topical ocular administration, dorzolamide was given orally to eight healthy subjects for up to 20 weeks. The oral dose of 2 mg b.i.d. closely approximates the amount of drug delivered by topical ocular administration of dorzolamide 2% t.i.d. Steady state was reached within 8 weeks. The inhibition of CA-II and total carbonic anhydrase activities was below the degree of inhibition anticipated to be necessary for a pharmacological effect on renal function and respiration in healthy individuals.
Timolol Maleate
In a study of plasma drug concentrations in six subjects, the systemic exposure to timolol was determined following twice daily topical administration of timolol maleate ophthalmic solution 0.5%. The mean peak plasma concentration following morning dosing was 0.46 ng/mL.
Clinical Studies
Clinical studies of 3 to 15 months duration were conducted to compare the IOP-lowering effect over the course of the day of COSOPT b.i.d. (dosed morning and bedtime) to individually- and concomitantly-administered 0.5% timolol (b.i.d.) and 2.0% dorzolamide (b.i.d. and t.i.d.). The IOP-lowering effect of COSOPT b.i.d. was greater (1-3 mmHg) than that of monotherapy with either 2.0% dorzolamide t.i.d. or 0.5% timolol b.i.d. The IOP-lowering effect of COSOPT b.i.d. was approximately 1 mmHg less than that of concomitant therapy with 2.0% dorzolamide t.i.d. and 0.5% timolol b.i.d.
Open-label extensions of two studies were conducted for up to 12 months. During this period, the IOP-lowering effect of COSOPT b.i.d. was consistent during the 12 month follow-up period.

Indications and Usage
COSOPT is indicated for the reduction of elevated intraocular pressure in patients with open-angle glaucoma or ocular hypertension who are insufficiently responsive to beta-blockers (failed to achieve target IOP determined after multiple measurements over time). The IOP-lowering of COSOPT b.i.d. was slightly less than that seen with the concomitant administration of 0.5% timolol b.i.d. and 2.0% dorzolamide t.i.d. (see CLINICAL PHARMACOLOGY, *Clinical Studies*).

Contraindications
COSOPT is contraindicated in patients with (1) bronchial asthma; (2) a history of bronchial asthma; (3) severe chronic obstructive pulmonary disease (see WARNINGS); (4) sinus bradycardia; (5) second or third degree atrioventricular block; (6) overt cardiac failure (see WARNINGS); (7) cardiogenic shock; or (8) hypersensitivity to any component of this product.

Warnings
Systemic Exposure
COSOPT contains dorzolamide, a sulfonamide, and timolol maleate, a beta-adrenergic blocking agent; and although administered topically, is absorbed systemically. Therefore, the same types of adverse reactions that are attributable to sulfonamides and/or systemic administration of beta-adrenergic blocking agents may occur with topical administration. For example, severe respiratory reactions and cardiac reactions, including death due to bronchospasm in patients with asthma, and rarely death in association with cardiac failure, have been reported following systemic or ophthalmic administration of timolol maleate (see CONTRAINDICATIONS). Fatalities have occurred, although rarely, due to severe reactions to sulfonamides including Stevens-Johnson syndrome, toxic epidermal necrolysis, fulminant hepatic necrosis, agranulocytosis, aplastic anemia, and other blood dyscrasias. Sensitization may recur when a sulfonamide is readministered irrespective of the route of ad-

ministration. If signs of serious reactions or hypersensitivity occur, discontinue the use of this preparation.
Cardiac Failure
Sympathetic stimulation may be essential for support of the circulation in individuals with diminished myocardial contractility, and its inhibition by beta-adrenergic receptor blockade may precipitate more severe failure.
In Patients Without a History of Cardiac Failure continued depression of the myocardium with beta-blocking agents over a period of time can, in some cases, lead to cardiac failure. At the first sign or symptom of cardiac failure, COSOPT should be discontinued.
Obstructive Pulmonary Disease
Patients with chronic obstructive pulmonary disease (e.g., chronic bronchitis, emphysema) of mild or moderate severity, bronchospastic disease, or a history of bronchospastic disease (other than bronchial asthma or a history of bronchial asthma, in which COSOPT is contraindicated [see CONTRAINDICATIONS]) should, in general, not receive beta-blocking agents, including COSOPT.
Major Surgery
The necessity or desirability of withdrawal of beta-adrenergic blocking agents prior to major surgery is controversial. Beta-adrenergic receptor blockade impairs the ability of the heart to respond to beta-adrenergically mediated reflex stimuli. This may augment the risk of general anesthesia in surgical procedures. Some patients receiving beta-adrenergic receptor blocking agents have experienced protracted severe hypotension during anesthesia. Difficulty in restarting and maintaining the heartbeat has also been reported. For these reasons, in patients undergoing elective surgery, some authorities recommend gradual withdrawal of beta-adrenergic receptor blocking agents.
If necessary during surgery, the effects of beta-adrenergic blocking agents may be reversed by sufficient doses of adrenergic agonists.
Diabetes Mellitus
Beta-adrenergic blocking agents should be administered with caution in patients subject to spontaneous hypoglycemia or to diabetic patients (especially those with labile diabetes) who are receiving insulin or oral hypoglycemic agents. Beta-adrenergic receptor blocking agents may mask the signs and symptoms of acute hypoglycemia.
Thyrotoxicosis
Beta-adrenergic blocking agents may mask certain clinical signs (e.g., tachycardia) of hyperthyroidism. Patients suspected of developing thyrotoxicosis should be managed carefully to avoid abrupt withdrawal of beta-adrenergic blocking agents that might precipitate a thyroid storm.
Precautions
General
Dorzolamide has not been studied in patients with severe renal impairment (CrCl <30 mL/min). Because dorzolamide and its metabolite are excreted predominantly by the kidney, COSOPT is not recommended in such patients. Dorzolamide has not been studied in patients with hepatic impairment and should therefore be used with caution in such patients.
While taking beta-blockers, patients with a history of atopy or a history of severe anaphylactic reactions to a variety of allergens may be more reactive to repeated accidental, diagnostic, or therapeutic challenge with such allergens. Such patients may be unresponsive to the usual doses of epinephrine used to treat anaphylactic reactions.
In clinical studies, local ocular adverse effects, primarily conjunctivitis and lid reactions, were reported with chronic administration of COSOPT. Many of these reactions had the clinical appearance and course of an allergic-type reaction that resolved upon discontinuation of drug therapy. If such reactions are observed,

COSOPT should be discontinued and the patient evaluated before considering restarting the drug. (See ADVERSE REACTIONS.)
The management of patients with acute angle-closure glaucoma requires therapeutic interventions in addition to ocular hypotensive agents. COSOPT has not been studied in patients with acute angle-closure glaucoma.
Choroidal detachment after filtration procedures has been reported with the administration of aqueous suppressant therapy (e.g., timolol).
Beta-adrenergic blockade has been reported to potentiate muscle weakness consistent with certain myasthenic symptoms (e.g., diplopia, ptosis, and generalized weakness). Timolol has been reported rarely to increase muscle weakness in some patients with myasthenia gravis or myasthenic symptoms.
There have been reports of bacterial keratitis associated with the use of multiple dose containers of topical ophthalmic products. These containers had been inadvertently contaminated by patients who, in most cases, had a concurrent corneal disease or a disruption of the ocular epithelial surface. (See PRECAUTIONS, *Information for Patients*.)
Information for Patients
Patients with bronchial asthma, a history of bronchial asthma, severe chronic obstructive pulmonary disease, sinus bradycardia, second or third degree atrioventricular block, or cardiac failure should be advised not to take this product. (See CONTRAINDICATIONS.)
COSOPT contains dorzolamide (which is a sulfonamide) and although administered topically is absorbed systemically. Therefore the same types of adverse reactions that are attributable to sulfonamides may occur with topical administration. Patients should be advised that if serious or unusual reactions or signs of hypersensitivity occur, they should discontinue the use of the product (see WARNINGS).
Patients should be advised that if they develop any ocular reactions, particularly conjunctivitis and lid reactions, they should discontinue use and seek their physician's advice.
Patients should be instructed to avoid allowing the tip of the dispensing container to contact the eye or surrounding structures.
Patients should also be instructed that ocular solutions, if handled improperly or if the tip of the dispensing container contacts the eye or surrounding structures, can become contaminated by common bacteria known to cause ocular infections. Serious damage to the eye and subsequent loss of vision may result from using contaminated solutions. (See PRECAUTIONS, *General*.)
Patients also should be advised that if they have ocular surgery or develop an intercurrent ocular condition (e.g., trauma or infection), they should immediately seek their physician's advice concerning the continued use of the present multidose container.
If more than one topical ophthalmic drug is being used, the drugs should be administered at least ten minutes apart.
Patients should be advised that COSOPT contains benzalkonium chloride which may be absorbed by soft contact lenses. Contact lenses should be removed prior to administration of the solution. Lenses may be reinserted 15 minutes following administration of COSOPT.
Drug Interactions
Carbonic anhydrase inhibitors: There is a potential for an additive effect on the known systemic effects of carbonic anhydrase inhibition in patients receiving an oral carbonic anhydrase inhibitor and COSOPT. The concomitant administration of COSOPT and oral carbonic anhydrase inhibitors is not recommended.
Acid-base disturbances: Although acid-base and electrolyte disturbances were not reported in the clinical trials with dorzolamide hydro-

chloride ophthalmic solution, these disturbances have been reported with oral carbonic anhydrase inhibitors and have, in some instances, resulted in drug interactions (e.g., toxicity associated with high-dose salicylate therapy). Therefore, the potential for such drug interactions should be considered in patients receiving COSOPT.
Beta-adrenergic blocking agents: Patients who are receiving a beta-adrenergic blocking agent orally and COSOPT should be observed for potential additive effects of beta-blockade, both systemic and on intraocular pressure. The concomitant use of two topical beta-adrenergic blocking agents is not recommended.
Calcium antagonists: Caution should be used in the coadministration of beta-adrenergic blocking agents, such as COSOPT, and oral or intravenous calcium antagonists because of possible atrioventricular conduction disturbances, left ventricular failure, and hypotension. In patients with impaired cardiac function, coadministration should be avoided.
Catecholamine-depleting drugs: Close observation of the patient is recommended when a beta-blocker is administered to patients receiving catecholamine-depleting drugs such as reserpine, because of possible additive effects and the production of hypotension and/or marked bradycardia, which may result in vertigo, syncope, or postural hypotension.
Digitalis and calcium antagonists: The concomitant use of beta-adrenergic blocking agents with digitalis and calcium antagonists may have additive effects in prolonging atrioventricular conduction time.
Quinidine: Potentiated systemic beta-blockade (e.g., decreased heart rate) has been reported during combined treatment with quinidine and timolol, possibly because quinidine inhibits the metabolism of timolol via the P-450 enzyme, CYP2D6.
Clonidine: Oral beta-adrenergic blocking agents may exacerbate the rebound hypertension which can follow the withdrawal of clonidine. There have been no reports of exacerbation of rebound hypertension with ophthalmic timolol maleate.
Injectable Epinephrine: (See PRECAUTIONS, *General, Anaphylaxis*.)
Carcinogenesis, Mutagenesis, Impairment of Fertility
In a two-year study of dorzolamide hydrochloride administered orally to male and female Sprague-Dawley rats, urinary bladder papillomas were seen in male rats in the highest dosage group of 20 mg/kg/day (250 times the recommended human ophthalmic dose). Papillomas were not seen in rats given oral doses equivalent to approximately 12 times the recommended human ophthalmic dose. No treatment-related tumors were seen in a 21-month study in female and male mice given oral doses up to 75 mg/kg/day (~900 times the recommended human ophthalmic dose).
The increased incidence of urinary bladder papillomas seen in the high-dose male rats is a class-effect of carbonic anhydrase inhibitors in rats. Rats are particularly prone to developing papillomas in response to foreign bodies, compounds causing crystalluria, and diverse sodium salts.
No changes in bladder urothelium were seen in dogs given oral dorzolamide hydrochloride for one year at 2 mg/kg/day (25 times the recommended human ophthalmic dose) or mon-

Continued on next page

Information on the Merck & Co., Inc., products listed on these pages is from the prescribing information in use August 31, 2004.

Cosopt—Cont.

keys dosed topically to the eye at 0.4 mg/kg/day (~5 times the recommended human ophthalmic dose) for one year.

In a two-year study of timolol maleate administered orally to rats, there was a statistically significant increase in the incidence of adrenal pheochromocytomas in male rats administered 300 mg/kg/day (approximately 42,000 times the systemic exposure following the maximum recommended human ophthalmic dose). Similar differences were not observed in rats administered oral doses equivalent to approximately 14,000 times the maximum recommended human ophthalmic dose.

In a lifetime oral study of timolol maleate in mice, there were statistically significant increases in the incidence of benign and malignant pulmonary tumors, benign uterine polyps and mammary adenocarcinomas in female mice at 500 mg/kg/day, (approximately 71,000 times the systemic exposure following the maximum recommended human ophthalmic dose), but not at 5 or 50 mg/kg/day (approximately 700 or 7,000, respectively, times the systemic exposure following the maximum recommended human ophthalmic dose). In a subsequent study in female mice, in which post-mortem examinations were limited to the uterus and the lungs, a statistically significant increase in the incidence of pulmonary tumors was again observed at 500 mg/kg/day.

The increased occurrence of mammary adenocarcinomas was associated with elevations in serum prolactin which occurred in female mice administered oral timolol at 500 mg/kg/day, but not at doses of 5 or 50 mg/kg/day. An increased incidence of mammary adenocarcinomas in rodents has been associated with administration of several other therapeutic agents that elevate serum prolactin, but no correlation between serum prolactin levels and mammary tumors has been established in humans. Furthermore, in adult human female subjects who received oral dosages of up to 60 mg of timolol maleate (the maximum recommended human oral dosage), there were no clinically meaningful changes in serum prolactin.

The following tests for mutagenic potential were negative for dorzolamide: (1) *in vivo* (mouse) cytogenetic assay; (2) *in vitro* chromosomal aberration assay; (3) alkaline elution assay; (4) V-79 assay; and (5) Ames test.

Timolol maleate was devoid of mutagenic potential when tested *in vivo* (mouse) in the micronucleus test and cytogenetic assay (doses up to 800 mg/kg) and *in vitro* in a neoplastic cell transformation assay (up to 100 µg/mL). In Ames tests the highest concentrations of timolol employed, 5,000 or 10,000 µg/plate, were associated with statistically significant elevations of revertants observed with tester strain TA100 (in seven replicate assays), but not in the remaining three strains. In the assays with tester strain TA100, no consistent dose response relationship was observed, and the ratio of test to control revertants did not reach 2. A ratio of 2 is usually considered the criterion for a positive Ames test.

Reproduction and fertility studies in rats with either timolol maleate or dorzolamide hydrochloride demonstrated no adverse effect on male or female fertility at doses up to approximately 100 times the systemic exposure following the maximum recommended human ophthalmic dose.

Pregnancy
Teratogenic Effects. Pregnancy Category C. Developmental toxicity studies with dorzolamide hydrochloride in rabbits at oral doses of ≥2.5 mg/kg/day (31 times the recommended human ophthalmic dose) revealed malformations of the vertebral bodies. These malformations occurred at doses that caused metabolic acidosis with decreased body weight gain in dams and decreased fetal weights. No treatment-related malformations were seen at 1.0 mg/kg/day (13 times the recommended human ophthalmic dose).

Teratogenicity studies with timolol in mice, rats, and rabbits at oral doses up to 50 mg/kg/day (7,000 times the systemic exposure following the maximum recommended human ophthalmic dose) demonstrated no evidence of fetal malformations. Although delayed fetal ossification was observed at this dose in rats, there were no adverse effects on postnatal development of offspring. Doses of 1000 mg/kg/day (142,000 times the systemic exposure following the maximum recommended human ophthalmic dose) were maternotoxic in mice and resulted in an increased number of fetal resorptions. Increased fetal resorptions were also seen in rabbits at doses of 14,000 times the systemic exposure following the maximum recommended human ophthalmic dose, in this case without apparent maternotoxicity.

There are no adequate and well-controlled studies in pregnant women. COSOPT should be used during pregnancy only if the potential benefit justifies the potential risk to the fetus.

Nursing Mothers
It is not known whether dorzolamide is excreted in human milk. Timolol maleate has been detected in human milk following oral and ophthalmic drug administration. Because of the potential for serious adverse reactions from COSOPT in nursing infants, a decision should be made whether to discontinue nursing or to discontinue the drug, taking into account the importance of the drug to the mother.

Pediatric Use
Safety and effectiveness in pediatric patients have not been established.

Geriatric Use
No overall differences in safety or effectiveness have been observed between elderly and younger patients.

Adverse Reactions
COSOPT was evaluated for safety in 1035 patients with elevated intraocular pressure treated for open-angle-glaucoma or ocular hypertension. Approximately 5% of all patients discontinued therapy with COSOPT because of adverse reactions. The most frequently reported adverse events were taste perversion (bitter, sour, or unusual taste) or ocular burning and/or stinging in up to 30% of patients. Conjunctival hyperemia, blurred vision, superficial punctate keratitis or eye itching were reported between 5-15% of patients. The following adverse events were reported in 1-5% of patients: abdominal pain, back pain, blepharitis, bronchitis, cloudy vision, conjunctival discharge, conjunctival edema, conjunctival follicles, conjunctival injection, conjunctivitis, corneal erosion, corneal staining, cortical lens opacity, cough, dizziness, dryness of eyes, dyspepsia, eye debris, eye discharge, eye pain, eye tearing, eyelid edema, eyelid erythema, eyelid exudate/scales, eyelid pain or discomfort, foreign body sensation, glaucomatous cupping, headache, hypertension, influenza, lens nucleus coloration, lens opacity, nausea, nuclear lens opacity, pharyngitis, post-subcapsular cataract, sinusitis, upper respiratory infection, urinary tract infection, visual field defect, vitreous detachment.

The following adverse events have occurred either at low incidence (<1%) during clinical trials or have been reported during the use of COSOPT in clinical practice where these events were reported voluntarily from a population of unknown size and frequency of occurrence cannot be determined precisely. They have been chosen for inclusion based on factors such as seriousness, frequency of reporting, possible causal connection to COSOPT, or a combination of these factors: bradycardia, cardiac failure, cerebral vascular accident, chest pain, choroidal detachment following filtration surgery (see PRECAUTIONS, *General*), depression, diarrhea, dry mouth, dyspnea, heart block, hypotension, iridocyclitis, myocardial infarction, nasal congestion, paresthesia, photophobia, respiratory failure, skin rashes, urolithiasis, and vomiting.

Other adverse reactions that have been reported with the individual components are listed below:

Dorzolamide — *Allergic/Hypersensitivity:* Signs and symptoms of local reactions including palpebral reactions and systemic allergic reactions including angioedema, bronchospasm, pruritus, urticaria; *Body as a Whole:* Asthenia/fatigue; *Skin/Mucous Membranes:* Contact dermatitis, epistaxis, throat irritation; *Special Senses:* Eyelid crusting, signs and symptoms of ocular allergic reaction, and transient myopia.

Timolol (ocular administration) — *Body as a Whole:* Asthenia/fatigue; *Cardiovascular:* Arrhythmia, syncope, cerebral ischemia, worsening of angina pectoris, palpitation, cardiac arrest, pulmonary edema, edema, claudication, Raynaud's phenomenon, and cold hands and feet; *Digestive:* Anorexia; *Immunologic:* Systemic lupus erythematosus; *Nervous System/Psychiatric:* Increase in signs and symptoms of myasthenia gravis, somnolence, insomnia, nightmares, behavioral changes and psychic disturbances including confusion, hallucinations, anxiety, disorientation, nervousness, and memory loss; *Skin:* Alopecia, psoriasiform rash or exacerbation of psoriasis; *Hypersensitivity:* Signs and symptoms of systemic allergic reactions, including anaphylaxis, angioedema, urticaria, and localized and generalized rash; *Respiratory:* Bronchospasm (predominantly in patients with pre-existing bronchospastic disease); *Endocrine:* Masked symptoms of hypoglycemia in diabetic patients (see WARNINGS); *Special Senses:* Ptosis; decreased corneal sensitivity; cystoid macular edema; visual disturbances including refractive changes and diplopia; pseudopemphigoid; and tinnitus; *Urogenital:* Retroperitoneal fibrosis, decreased libido, impotence, and Peyronie's disease.

The following additional adverse effects have been reported in clinical experience with ORAL timolol maleate or other ORAL beta-blocking agents and may be considered potential effects of ophthalmic timolol maleate: *Allergic:* Erythematous rash, fever combined with aching and sore throat, laryngospasm with respiratory distress; *Body as a Whole:* Extremity pain, decreased exercise tolerance, weight loss; *Cardiovascular:* Worsening of arterial insufficiency, vasodilatation; *Digestive:* Gastrointestinal pain, hepatomegaly, mesenteric arterial thrombosis, ischemic colitis; *Hematologic:* Nonthrombocytopenic purpura; thrombocytopenic purpura, agranulocytosis; *Endocrine:* Hyperglycemia, hypoglycemia; *Skin:* Pruritus, skin irritation, increased pigmentation, sweating; *Musculoskeletal:* Arthralgia; *Nervous System/Psychiatric:* Vertigo, local weakness, diminished concentration, reversible mental depression progressing to catatonia, an acute reversible syndrome characterized by disorientation for time and place, emotional lability, slightly clouded sensorium, and decreased performance on neuropsychometrics; *Respiratory:* Rales, bronchial obstruction; *Urogenital:* Urination difficulties.

Overdosage
There are no human data available on overdosage with COSOPT.

Symptoms consistent with systemic administration of beta-blockers or carbonic anhydrase inhibitors may occur, including electrolyte imbalance, development of an acidotic state, dizziness, headache, shortness of breath, bradycardia, bronchospasm, cardiac arrest and possible central nervous system effects. Serum electrolyte levels (particularly potassium) and blood pH levels should be monitored (see also ADVERSE REACTIONS).

A study of patients with renal failure showed that timolol did not dialyze readily.

Dosage and Administration
The dose is one drop of COSOPT in the affected eye(s) two times daily.
If more than one topical ophthalmic drug is being used, the drugs should be administered at least ten minutes apart (see also PRECAUTIONS, *Drug Interactions*).

How Supplied
COSOPT Ophthalmic Solution is a clear, colorless to nearly colorless, slightly viscous solution.
No. 3628 — COSOPT Ophthalmic Solution is supplied in an OCUMETER®* PLUS container, a white, translucent, HDPE plastic ophthalmic dispenser with a controlled drop tip and a white polystyrene cap with dark blue label as follows:
NDC 0006-3628-35, 5 mL in a 7.5 mL bottle
NDC 0006-3628-36, 10 mL in an 18 mL bottle.
Storage
Store COSOPT at 25°C (77°F), excursions permitted to 15–30°C (59–86°F) [see USP Controlled Room Temperature]. Protect from light.

INSTRUCTIONS FOR USE
Please follow these instructions carefully when using COSOPT*. Use COSOPT as prescribed by your doctor.
1. If you use other topically applied ophthalmic medications, they should be administered at least 10 minutes before or after COSOPT.
2. Wash hands before each use.
3. Before using the medication for the first time, be sure the Safety Strip on the front of the bottle is unbroken. A gap between the bottle and the cap is normal for an unopened bottle.

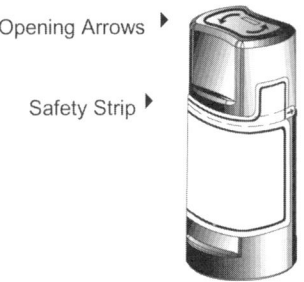

4. Tear off the Safety Strip to break the seal. [See first graphic above]
5. To open the bottle, unscrew the cap by turning as indicated by the arrows.

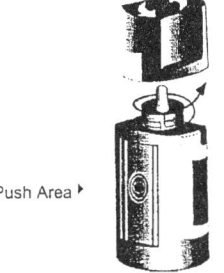

6. Tilt your head back and pull your lower eyelid down slightly to form a pocket between your eyelid and your eye.

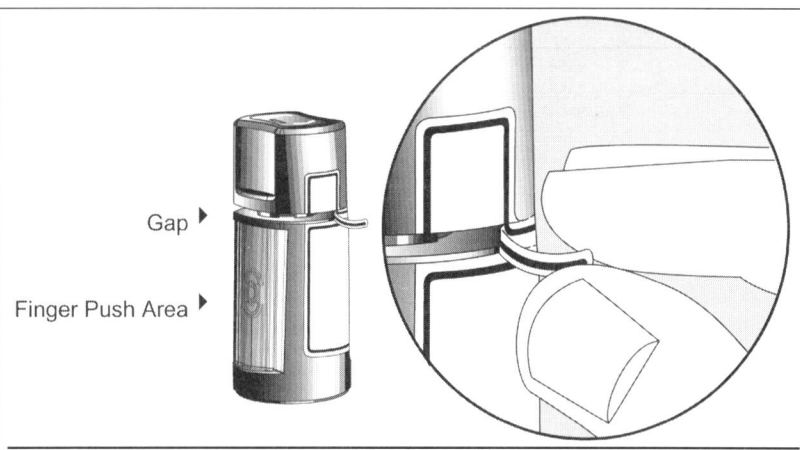

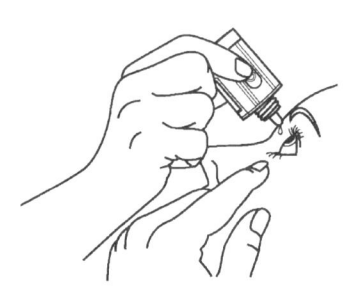
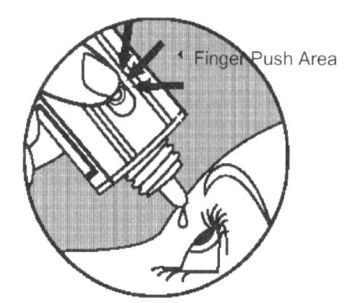

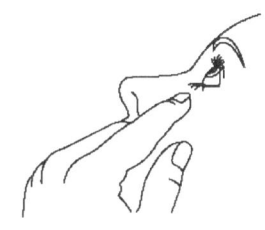

7. Invert the bottle, and press lightly with the thumb or index finger over the "Finger Push Area" (as shown) until a single drop is dispensed into the eye as directed by your doctor.
[See second graphic above]
   DO NOT TOUCH YOUR EYE OR EYELID WITH THE DROPPER TIP.
   Ophthalmic medications, if handled improperly, can become contaminated by common bacteria known to cause eye infections. Serious damage to the eye and subsequent loss of vision may result from using contaminated ophthalmic medications. If you think your medication may be contaminated, or if you develop an eye infection, contact your doctor immediately concerning continued use of this bottle.
8. Repeat steps 6 & 7 with the other eye if instructed to do so by your doctor.
9. Replace the cap by turning until it is firmly touching the bottle. Do not overtighten the cap.
10. The dispenser tip is designed to provide a pre-measured drop; therefore, do NOT enlarge the hole of the dispenser tip.
11. After you have used all doses, there will be some COSOPT left in the bottle. You should not be concerned since an extra amount of COSOPT has been added and you will get the full amount of COSOPT that your doctor prescribed. Do not attempt to remove the excess medicine from the bottle.

WARNING: Keep out of reach of children.
If you have any questions about the use of COSOPT, please consult your doctor.

* Registered trademark of MERCK & CO., Inc.
Manuf. for:
Merck & Co., Inc., Whitehouse Station, NJ 08889, USA
By: Laboratories Merck Sharp & Dohme-Chibret
  63963 Clermont-Ferrand Cedex 9, France
  9359302   Issued January 2004
COPYRIGHT © MERCK & CO., Inc., 1998
All rights reserved
Shown in Product Identification Guide, page 104

DARANIDE® ℞
(Dichlorphenamide)
Tablets

Description
DARANIDE* (Dichlorphenamide) is an oral carbonic anhydrase inhibitor. Dichlorphenamide, a dichlorinated benzenedisulfonamide, is known chemically as 4,5-dichloro-1,3-benzenedisulfonamide. Its empirical formula is $C_6H_6Cl_2N_2O_4S_2$ and its structural formula is:
[See chemical structure at top of next column]
Dichlorphenamide is a white or practically white, crystalline compound with a molecular weight of 305.16. It is very slightly soluble in water but soluble in dilute solutions of sodium

Continued on next page

Information on the Merck & Co., Inc., products listed on these pages is from the prescribing information in use August 31, 2004.

Daranide—Cont.

carbonate and sodium hydroxide. Dilute alkaline solutions of dichlorphenamide are stable at room temperature.
DARANIDE is supplied as tablets, for oral administration, each containing 50 mg dichlorphenamide. Inactive ingredients are D&C Yellow 10, lactose, magnesium stearate, and starch.

---

*Registered trademark of MERCK & CO., Inc.

Clinical Pharmacology
Carbonic anhydrase inhibitors reduce intraocular pressure by partially suppressing the secretion of aqueous humor (inflow), although the mechanism by which they do this is not fully understood. Evidence suggests that HCO_3^- ions are produced in the ciliary body by hydration of carbon dioxide under the influence of carbonic anhydrase and diffuse into the posterior chamber with Na+ ions. The aqueous fluid contains more Na+ and HCO_3^- ions than does plasma and consequently is hypertonic. Water is attracted to the posterior chamber by osmosis. Systemic administration of a carbonic anhydrase inhibitor has been shown to inactivate carbonic anhydrase in the ciliary body of the rabbit's eye and to reduce the high concentration of HCO_3^- ions in ocular fluids. As is the case with all carbonic anhydrase inhibitors, DARANIDE in high doses causes some decrease in renal blood flow and glomerular filtration rate.
In man, DARANIDE begins to act within an hour and maximal effect is observed in two to four hours. The lowered intraocular tension may be maintained for approximately 6 to 12 hours.

Indications and Usage
For adjunctive treatment of: chronic simple (open-angle) glaucoma, secondary glaucoma, and preoperatively in acute angle-closure glaucoma where delay of surgery is desired in order to lower intraocular pressure.

Contraindications
DARANIDE is contraindicated in hepatic insufficiency, renal failure, adrenocortical insufficiency, hyperchloremic acidosis, or in conditions in which serum levels of sodium or potassium are depressed. DARANIDE should not be used in patients with severe pulmonary obstruction who are unable to increase their alveolar ventilation since their acidosis may be increased.
DARANIDE is contraindicated in patients who are hypersensitive to this product.

Precautions
General
Potassium excretion is increased by DARANIDE and hypokalemia may develop with brisk diuresis, when severe cirrhosis is present, or during concomitant use of steroids or ACTH.
Interference with adequate oral electrolyte intake will also contribute to hypokalemia. Hypokalemia can sensitize or exaggerate the response of the heart to the toxic effects of digitalis (e.g., increased ventricular irritability). Hypokalemia may be avoided or treated by use of potassium supplements such as foods with a high potassium content. DARANIDE should be used with caution in patients with respiratory acidosis.

Drug Interactions
Caution is advised in patients receiving concomitant high-dose aspirin and carbonic anhydrase inhibitors, as anorexia, tachypnea, lethargy and coma have been rarely reported due to a possible drug interaction.
Carcinogenesis, Mutagenesis, Impairment of Fertility
Long-term studies in animals have not been performed to evaluate the effects upon fertility or carcinogenic potential of DARANIDE.
Pregnancy
Pregnancy Category C. Dichlorphenamide has been shown to be teratogenic in the rat (skeletal anomalies) when given in doses 100 times the human dose. There are no adequate and well-controlled studies in pregnant women. DARANIDE should not be used in women of childbearing age or in pregnancy, especially during the first trimester, unless the potential benefits outweigh the potential risks.
Nursing Mothers
It is not known whether dichlorphenamide is excreted in human milk. Because many drugs are excreted in human milk, caution should be exercised when dichlorphenamide is administered to a nursing woman.
Pediatric Use
Safety and effectiveness in pediatric patients have not been established.

Adverse Reactions
Certain side effects characteristic of carbonic anhydrase inhibitors may occur with DARANIDE, particularly with increasing doses.
The most common effects include gastrointestinal disturbances (anorexia, nausea, and vomiting), drowsiness and paresthesias.
Included in the listing which follows are some adverse reactions which have not been reported with DARANIDE. However, pharmacological similarities among the carbonic anhydrase inhibitors make it advisable to consider the following reactions when dichlorphenamide is administered.
Central Nervous System/Psychiatric: ataxia, tremor, tinnitus, headache, weakness, nervousness, globus hystericus, lassitude, depression, confusion, disorientation, dizziness;
Gastrointestinal: constipation, hepatic insufficiency;
Metabolic: loss of weight, metabolic acidosis, electrolyte imbalance (hypokalemia, hyperchloremia), hyperuricemia;
Hypersensitivity: skin eruptions, pruritus, fever;
Hematologic: leukopenia, agranulocytosis, thrombocytopenia;
Genitourinary: urinary frequency, renal colic, renal calculi, phosphaturia.

Overdosage
The oral LD_{50} of DARANIDE is 1710 and 2600 mg/kg in the mouse and rat respectively. Symptoms of overdosage or toxicity may include drowsiness, anorexia, nausea, vomiting, dizziness, paresthesias, ataxia, tremor and tinnitus.
In the event of overdosage, induce emesis or perform gastric lavage. The electrolyte disturbance most likely to be encountered from overdosage is hyperchloremic acidosis that may respond to bicarbonate administration. Potassium supplementation may be required. The patient should be carefully observed and given supportive treatment.

Dosage and Administration
DARANIDE is usually given in conjunction with topical ocular hypotensive agents. In acute angle-closure glaucoma, it may be used together with miotics and osmotic agents in an attempt to reduce intraocular tension rapidly. If this is not quickly relieved, surgery may be mandatory.
Dosage must be adjusted carefully to meet the requirements of the individual patient. A priming dose of 100 to 200 mg of DARANIDE (2 to 4 tablets) is suggested for adults, followed by 100 mg (2 tablets) every 12 hours until the desired response has been obtained. The recommended maintenance dosage for adults is 25 to 50 mg ($^1/_2$ to 1 tablet) once to three times daily.

How Supplied
No. 3256—Tablets DARANIDE, 50 mg each, are yellow, round, scored, compressed tablets, coded MSD 49 on one side and DARANIDE on the other. They are supplied as follows:
NDC 0006-0049-68 bottles of 100.
7870319   Issued October 1996
COPYRIGHT © MERCK & CO., Inc., 1985
All rights reserved
Shown in Product Identification Guide, page 104

LACRISERT® Sterile Ophthalmic Insert ℞
(Hydroxypropyl Cellulose Ophthalmic Insert)

Description
LACRISERT* (hydroxypropyl cellulose ophthalmic insert) is a sterile, translucent, rod-shaped, water soluble, ophthalmic insert made of hydroxypropyl cellulose, for administration into the inferior cul-de-sac of the eye.
The chemical name for hydroxypropyl cellulose is cellulose, 2-hydroxypropyl ether. It is an ether of cellulose in which hydroxypropyl groups ($-CH_2CHOHCH_3$) are attached to the hydroxyls present in the anhydroglucose rings of cellulose by ether linkages. A representative structure of the monomer is:

The molecular weight is typically 1×10^6.
Hydroxypropyl cellulose is an off-white, odorless, tasteless powder. It is soluble in water below 38°C, and in many polar organic solvents such as ethanol, propylene glycol, dioxane, methanol, isopropyl alcohol (95%), dimethyl sulfoxide, and dimethyl formamide.
Each LACRISERT is 5 mg of hydroxypropyl cellulose. LACRISERT contains no preservatives or other ingredients. It is about 1.27 mm in diameter by about 3.5 mm long.
LACRISERT is supplied in packages of 60 units, together with illustrated instructions and a special applicator for removing LACRISERT from the unit dose blister and inserting it into the eye. A spare applicator is included in each package.

---

*Registered trademark of MERCK & CO., Inc.

Clinical Pharmacology
Pharmacodynamics
LACRISERT acts to stabilize and thicken the precorneal tear film and prolong the tear film breakup time which is usually accelerated in patients with dry eye states. LACRISERT also acts to lubricate and protect the eye.
LACRISERT usually reduces the signs and symptoms resulting from moderate to severe dry eye syndromes, such as conjunctival hyperemia, exudation, itching, burning, foreign body sensation, smarting, photophobia, dryness and blurred or cloudy vision. Progressive visual deterioration which occurs in some patients may be retarded, halted, or sometimes reversed.
In a multicenter crossover study the 5 mg LACRISERT administered once a day during

the waking hours was compared to artificial tears used four or more times daily. There was a prolongation of tear film breakup time and a decrease in foreign body sensation associated with dry eye syndrome in patients during treatment with inserts as compared to artificial tears; these findings were statistically significantly different between the treatment groups. Improvement, as measured by amelioration of symptoms, by slit lamp examination and by rose bengal staining of the cornea and conjunctiva, was greater in most patients with moderate to severe symptoms during treatment with LACRISERT. Patient comfort was usually better with LACRISERT than with artificial tears solution, and most patients preferred LACRISERT.

In most patients treated with LACRISERT for over one year, improvement was observed as evidenced by amelioration of symptoms generally associated with keratoconjunctivitis sicca such as burning, tearing, foreign body sensation, itching, photophobia and blurred or cloudy vision.

During studies in healthy volunteers, a thickened precorneal tear film was visually observed through the slit-lamp while LACRISERT was present in the conjunctival sac.

Pharmacokinetics and Metabolism
Hydroxypropyl cellulose is a physiologically inert substance. In a study of rats fed hydroxypropyl cellulose or unmodified cellulose at levels up to 5% of their diet, it was found that the two were biologically equivalent in that neither was metabolized.

Studies conducted in rats fed ^{14}C-labeled hydroxypropyl cellulose demonstrated that when orally administered, hydroxypropyl cellulose is not absorbed from the gastrointestinal tract and is quantitatively excreted in the feces.

Dissolution studies in rabbits showed that hydroxypropyl cellulose inserts became softer within 1 hour after they were placed in the conjunctival sac. Most of the inserts dissolved completely in 14 to 18 hours; with a single exception, all had disappeared by 24 hours after insertion. Similar dissolution of the inserts was observed during prolonged administration (up to 54 weeks).

Indications and Usage
LACRISERT is indicated in patients with moderate to severe dry eye syndromes, including keratoconjunctivitis sicca. LACRISERT is indicated especially in patients who remain symptomatic after an adequate trial of therapy with artifical tear solutions.
LACRISERT is also indicated for patients with:
  Exposure keratitis
  Decreased corneal sensitivity
  Recurrent corneal erosions

Contraindications
LACRISERT is contraindicated in patients who are hypersensitive to hydroxypropyl cellulose.

Warnings
Instructions for inserting and removing LACRISERT should be carefully followed.

Precautions
General
If improperly placed, LACRISERT may result in corneal abrasion (see DOSAGE AND ADMINISTRATION).
Information for Patients
Patients should be advised to follow the instructions for using LACRISERT which accompany the package.
Because this product may produce transient blurring of vision, patients should be instructed to exercise caution when operating hazardous machinery or driving a motor vehicle.
Drug Interactions
Application of hydroxypropyl cellulose ophthalmic inserts to the eyes of unanesthetized rabbits immediately prior to or two hours before instilling pilocarpine, proparacaine HCl (0.5%), or phenylephrine (5%) did not markedly alter the magnitude and/or duration of the miotic, local corneal anesthetic, or mydriatic activity, respectively, of these agents.
Under various treatment schedules, the anti-inflammatory effect of ocularly instilled dexamethasone (0.1%) in unanesthetized rabbits with primary uveitis was not affected by the presence of hydroxypropyl cellulose inserts.
Carcinogenesis, Mutagenesis, Impairment of Fertility
Feeding of hydroxypropyl cellulose to rats at levels up to 5% of their diet produced no gross or histopathologic changes or other deleterious effects.
Pediatric Use
Safety and effectiveness in pediatric patients have not been established.
Geriatric Use
No overall differences in safety or effectiveness have been observed between elderly and younger patients.

Adverse Reactions
The following adverse reactions have been reported in patients treated with LACRISERT, but were in most instances mild and transient:
Transient blurring of vision
(See PRECAUTIONS)
Ocular discomfort or irritation
Matting or stickiness of eyelashes
Photophobia
Hypersensitivity
Edema of the eyelids
Hyperemia

Dosage and Administration
One LACRISERT ophthalmic insert in each eye once daily is usually sufficient to relieve the symptoms associated with moderate to severe dry eye syndromes. Individual patients may require more flexibility in the use of LACRISERT; some patients may require twice daily use for optimal results.
Clinical experience with LACRISERT indicates that in some patients several weeks may be required before satisfactory improvement of symptoms is achieved.
LACRISERT is inserted into the inferior cul-de-sac of the eye beneath the base of the tarsus, not in apposition to the cornea, nor beneath the eyelid at the level of the tarsal plate. If not properly positioned, it will be expelled into the interpalpebral fissure, and may cause symptoms of a foreign body. Illustrated instructions are included in each package. While in the licensed practitioner's office, the patient should read the instructions, then practice insertion and removal of LACRISERT until proficiency is achieved.
NOTE: Occasionally LACRISERT is inadvertently expelled from the eye, especially in patients with shallow conjunctival fornices. The patient should be cautioned against rubbing the eye(s) containing LACRISERT, especially upon awakening, so as not to dislodge or expel the insert. If required, another LACRISERT ophthalmic insert may be inserted. If experience indicates that transient blurred vision develops in an individual patient, the patient may want to remove LACRISERT a few hours after insertion to avoid this. Another LACRISERT ophthalmic insert may be inserted if needed.
If LACRISERT causes worsening of symptoms, the patient should be instructed to inspect the conjunctival sac to make certain LACRISERT is in the proper location, deep in the inferior cul-de-sac of the eye beneath the base of the tarsus. If these symptoms persist, LACRISERT should be removed and the patient should contact the practitioner.

How Supplied
No. 3380—LACRISERT, a sterile, translucent, rod-shaped, water soluble, ophthalmic insert made of hydroxypropyl cellulose, 5 mg, is supplied as follows:
NDC 0006-3380-60 in packages containing 60 unit doses (each wrapped in an aluminum blister), two reusable applicators, and a plastic storage container to store the applicators after use.
Storage
Store below 30°C (86°F).
  9246112 Issued June 2002
COPYRIGHT © MERCK & CO., Inc., 1988
All rights reserved
Shown in Product Identification Guide, page 105

TIMOPTIC® ℞
0.25% and 0.5%
(Timolol Maleate Ophthalmic Solution)
Sterile Ophthalmic Solution

Description
TIMOPTIC* (timolol maleate ophthalmic solution) is a non-selective beta-adrenergic receptor blocking agent. Its chemical name is (-)-1-(*tert*-butylamino)-3-[(4-morpholino-1,2,5-thiadiazol-3-yl)oxy]-2-propanol maleate (1:1) (salt). Timolol maleate possesses an asymmetric carbon atom in its structure and is provided as the levo-isomer. The nominal optical rotation of timolol maleate is:

$[\alpha]_{405\ nm}^{25°}$ in 1.0N HCl (C = 5%) = $-12.2°$
($-11.7°$ to $-12.5°$).

Its molecular formula is $C_{13}H_{24}N_4O_3S \cdot C_4H_4O_4$ and its structural formula is:

Timolol maleate has a molecular weight of 432.50. It is a white, odorless, crystalline powder which is soluble in water, methanol, and alcohol. TIMOPTIC is stable at room temperature.
TIMOPTIC Ophthalmic Solution is supplied as a sterile, isotonic, buffered, aqueous solution of timolol maleate in two dosage strengths: Each mL of TIMOPTIC 0.25% contains 2.5 mg of timolol (3.4 mg of timolol maleate). The pH of the solution is approximately 7.0, and the osmolarity is 274-328 mOsm. Each mL of TIMOPTIC 0.5% contains 5 mg of timolol (6.8 mg of timolol maleate). Inactive ingredients: monobasic and dibasic sodium phosphate, sodium hydroxide to adjust pH, and water for injection. Benzalkonium chloride 0.01% is added as preservative.

---
*Registered trademark of MERCK & CO., Inc.

Clinical Pharmacology
Mechanism of Action
Timolol maleate is a beta$_1$ and beta$_2$ (non-selective) adrenergic receptor blocking agent that does not have significant intrinsic sympathomimetic, direct myocardial depressant, or local anesthetic (membrane-stabilizing) activity.
Beta-adrenergic receptor blockade reduces cardiac output in both healthy subjects and patients with heart disease. In patients with severe impairment of myocardial function, beta-adrenergic receptor blockade may inhibit the

Continued on next page

Information on the Merck & Co., Inc., products listed on these pages is from the prescribing information in use August 31, 2004.

Timoptic—Cont.

stimulatory effect of the sympathetic nervous system necessary to maintain adequate cardiac function.

Beta-adrenergic receptor blockade in the bronchi and bronchioles results in increased airway resistance from unopposed parasympathetic activity. Such an effect in patients with asthma or other bronchospastic conditions is potentially dangerous.

TIMOPTIC Ophthalmic Solution, when applied topically on the eye, has the action of reducing elevated as well as normal intraocular pressure, whether or not accompanied by glaucoma. Elevated intraocular pressure is a major risk factor in the pathogenesis of glaucomatous visual field loss. The higher the level of intraocular pressure, the greater the likelihood of glaucomatous visual field loss and optic nerve damage.

The onset of reduction in intraocular pressure following administration of TIMOPTIC can usually be detected within one-half hour after a single dose. The maximum effect usually occurs in one to two hours and significant lowering of intraocular pressure can be maintained for periods as long as 24 hours with a single dose. Repeated observations over a period of one year indicate that the intraocular pressure-lowering effect of TIMOPTIC is well maintained.

The precise mechanism of the ocular hypotensive action of TIMOPTIC is not clearly established at this time. Tonography and fluorophotometry studies in man suggest that its predominant action may be related to reduced aqueous formation. However, in some studies a slight increase in outflow facility was also observed.

Pharmacokinetics
In a study of plasma drug concentration in six subjects, the systemic exposure to timolol was determined following twice daily administration of TIMOPTIC 0.5%. The mean peak plasma concentration following morning dosing was 0.46 ng/mL and following afternoon dosing was 0.35 ng/mL.

Clinical Studies
In controlled multiclinic studies in patients with untreated intraocular pressures of 22 mmHg or greater, TIMOPTIC 0.25 percent or 0.5 percent administered twice a day produced a greater reduction in intraocular pressure than 1, 2, 3, or 4 percent pilocarpine solution administered four times a day or 0.5, 1, or 2 percent epinephrine hydrochloride solution administered twice a day.

In these studies, TIMOPTIC was generally well tolerated and produced fewer and less severe side effects than either pilocarpine or epinephrine. A slight reduction of resting heart rate in some patients receiving TIMOPTIC (mean reduction 2.9 beats/minute standard deviation 10.2) was observed.

Indications and Usage
Timoptic Ophthalmic Solution is indicated in the treatment of elevated intraocular pressure in patients with ocular hypertension or open-angle glaucoma.

Contraindications
TIMOPTIC is contraindicated in patients with (1) bronchial asthma; (2) a history of bronchial asthma; (3) severe chronic obstructive pulmonary disease (see **WARNINGS**); (4) sinus bradycardia; (5) second or third degree atrioventricular block; (6) overt cardiac failure (see **WARNINGS**); (7) cardiogenic shock; or (8) hypersensitivity to any component of this product.

Warnings
As with many topically applied ophthalmic drugs, this drug is absorbed systemically.

The same adverse reactions found with systemic administration of beta-adrenergic blocking agents may occur with topical administration. For example, severe respiratory reactions and cardiac reactions, including death due to bronchospasm in patients with asthma, and rarely death in association with cardiac failure, have been reported following systemic or ophthalmic administration of timolol maleate (see CONTRAINDICATIONS).

Cardiac Failure
Sympathetic stimulation may be essential for support of the circulation in individuals with diminished myocardial contractility, and its inhibition by beta-adrenergic receptor blockade may precipitate more severe failure.

In Patients Without a History of Cardiac Failure continued depression of the myocardium with beta-blocking agents over a period of time can, in some cases, lead to cardiac failure. At the first sign or symptom of cardiac failure TIMOPTIC should be discontinued.

Obstructive Pulmonary Disease
Patients with chronic obstructive pulmonary disease (e.g., chronic bronchitis, emphysema) of mild or moderate severity, bronchospastic disease, or a history of bronchospastic disease (other than bronchial asthma or a history of bronchial asthma, in which TIMOPTIC is contraindicated [see **CONTRAINDICATIONS**]) should, in general, not receive beta-blockers, including TIMOPTIC.

Major Surgery
The necessity or desirability of withdrawal of beta-adrenergic blocking agents prior to major surgery is controversial. Beta-adrenergic receptor blockade impairs the ability of the heart to respond to beta-adrenergically mediated reflex stimuli. This may augment the risk of general anesthesia in surgical procedures. Some patients receiving beta-adrenergic receptor blocking agents have experienced protracted severe hypotension during anesthesia. Difficulty in restarting and maintaining the heartbeat has also been reported. For these reasons, in patients undergoing elective surgery, some authorities recommend gradual withdrawal of beta-adrenergic receptor blocking agents.

If necessary during surgery, the effects of beta-adrenergic blocking agents may be reversed by sufficient doses of adrenergic agonists.

Diabetes Mellitus
Beta-adrenergic blocking agents should be administered with caution in patients subject to spontaneous hypoglycemia or to diabetic patients (especially those with labile diabetes) who are receiving insulin or oral hypoglycemic agents. Beta-adrenergic receptor blocking agents may mask the signs and symptoms of acute hypoglycemia.

Thyrotoxicosis
Beta-adrenergic blocking agents may mask certain clinical signs (e.g., tachycardia) of hyperthyroidism. Patients suspected of developing thyrotoxicosis should be managed carefully to avoid abrupt withdrawal of beta-adrenergic blocking agents that might precipitate a thyroid storm.

Precautions
General
Because of potential effects of beta-adrenergic blocking agents on blood pressure and pulse, these agents should be used with caution in patients with cerebrovascular insufficiency. If signs or symptoms suggesting reduced cerebral blood flow develop following initiation of therapy with TIMOPTIC, alternative therapy should be considered.

There have been reports of bacterial keratitis associated with the use of multiple dose containers of topical ophthalmic products. These containers had been inadvertently contaminated by patients who, in most cases, had a concurrent corneal disease or a disruption of the ocular epithelial surface. (See **PRECAUTIONS**, *Information for Patients*.)

Choroidal detachment after filtration procedures has been reported with the administration of aqueous suppressant therapy (e.g. timolol).

Angle-closure glaucoma: In patients with angle-closure glaucoma, the immediate objective of treatment is to reopen the angle. This requires constricting the pupil. Timolol maleate has little or no effect on the pupil. TIMOPTIC should not be used alone in the treatment of angle-closure glaucoma.

Anaphylaxis: While taking beta-blockers, patients with a history of atopy or a history of severe anaphylactic reactions to a variety of allergens may be more reactive to repeated accidental, diagnostic, or therapeutic challenge with such allergens. Such patients may be unresponsive to the usual doses of epinephrine used to treat anaphylactic reactions.

Muscle Weakness: Beta-adrenergic blockade has been reported to potentiate muscle weakness consistent with certain myasthenic symptoms (e.g., diplopia, ptosis, and generalized weakness). Timolol has been reported rarely to increase muscle weakness in some patients with myasthenia gravis or myasthenic symptoms.

Information for Patients
Patients should be instructed to avoid allowing the tip of the dispensing container to contact the eye or surrounding structures.

Patients should also be instructed that ocular solutions, if handled improperly, can become contaminated by common bacteria known to cause ocular infections. Serious damage to the eye and subsequent loss of vision may result from using contaminated solutions. (See **PRECAUTIONS**, *General*.)

Patients should also be advised that if they have ocular surgery or develop an intercurrent ocular condition (e.g., trauma or infection), they should immediately seek their physician's advice concerning the continued use of the present multidose container.

Patients with bronchial asthma, a history of bronchial asthma, severe chronic obstructive pulmonary disease, sinus bradycardia, second or third degree atrioventricular block, or cardiac failure should be advised not to take this product. (See **CONTRAINDICATIONS**.)

Patients should be advised that TIMOPTIC contains benzalkonium chloride which may be absorbed by soft contact lenses. Contact lenses should be removed prior to administration of the solution. Lenses may be reinserted 15 minutes following TIMOPTIC administration.

Drug Interactions
Although TIMOPTIC used alone has little or no effect on pupil size, mydriasis resulting from concomitant therapy with TIMOPTIC and epinephrine has been reported occasionally.

Beta-adrenergic blocking agents: Patients who are receiving a beta-adrenergic blocking agent orally and TIMOPTIC should be observed for potential additive effects of beta-blockade, both systemic and on intraocular pressure. The concomitant use of two topical beta-adrenergic blocking agents is not recommended.

Calcium antagonists: Caution should be used in the coadministration of beta-adrenergic blocking agents, such as TIMOPTIC, and oral or intravenous calcium antagonists because of possible atrioventricular conduction disturbances, left ventricular failure, and hypotension. In patients with impaired cardiac function, coadministration should be avoided.

Catecholamine-depleting drugs: Close observation of the patient is recommended when a beta blocker is administered to patients receiving catecholamine-depleting drugs such as reserpine, because of possible additive effects and the production of hypotension and/or marked bradycardia, which may result in vertigo, syncope, or postural hypotension.

Digitalis and calcium antagonists: The concomitant use of beta-adrenergic blocking agents with digitalis and calcium antagonists may have additive effects in prolonging atrioventricular conduction time.
Quinidine: Potentiated systemic beta-blockade (e.g., decreased heart rate) has been reported during combined treatment with quinidine and timolol, possibly because quinidine inhibits the metabolism of timolol via the P-450 enzyme, CYP2D6.
Clonidine: Oral beta-adrenergic blocking agents may exacerbate the rebound hypertension which can follow the withdrawal of clonidine. There have been no reports of exacerbation of rebound hypertension with ophthalmic timolol maleate.
Injectable epinephrine: (See **PRECAUTIONS**, *General, Anaphylaxis*)
Carcinogenesis, Mutagenesis, Impairment of Fertility
In a two-year oral study of timolol maleate administered orally to rats, there was a statistically significant increase in the incidence of adrenal pheochromocytomas in male rats administered 300 mg/kg/day (approximately 42,000 times the systemic exposure following the maximum recommended human ophthalmic dose). Similar difference were not observed in rats administered oral doses equivalent to approximately 14,000 times the maximum recommended human ophthalmic dose.
In a lifetime oral study in mice, there were statistically significant increases in the incidence of benign and malignant pulmonary tumors, benign uterine polyps and mammary adenocarcinomas in female mice at 500 mg/kg/day, (approximately 71,000 times the systemic exposure following the maximum recommended human ophthalmic dose), but not at 5 or 50 mg/kg/day (approximately 700 or 7,000, respectively, times the systemic exposure following the maximum recommended human ophthalmic dose). In a subsequent study in female mice, in which post-mortem examinations were limited to the uterus and the lungs, a statistically significant increase in the incidence of pulmonary tumors was again observed at 500 mg/kg/day.
The increased occurrence of mammary adenocarcinomas was associated with elevations in serum prolactin which occurred in female mice administered oral timolol at 500 mg/kg/day, but not at doses of 5 or 50 mg/kg/day. An increased incidence of mammary adenocarcinomas in rodents has been associated with administration of several other therapeutic agents that elevate serum prolactin, but no correlation between serum prolactin levels and mammary tumors has been established in humans. Furthermore, in adult human female subjects who received oral dosages of up to 60 mg of timolol maleate (the maximum recommended human oral dosage), there were no clinically meaningful changes in serum prolactin.
Timolol maleate was devoid of mutagenic potential when tested *in vivo* (mouse) in the micronucleus test and cytogenetic assay (doses up to 800 mg/kg) and *in vitro* in a neoplastic cell transformation assay (up to 100 mcg/mL). In Ames tests the highest concentrations of timolol employed, 5000 or 10,000 mcg/plate, were associated with statistically significant elevations of revertants observed with tester strain TA100 (in seven replicate assays), but not in the remaining three strains. In the assays with tester strain TA100, no consistent dose response relationship was observed, and the ratio of test to control revertants did not reach 2. A ratio of 2 is usually considered the criterion for a positive Ames test.
Reproduction and fertility studies in rats demonstrated no adverse effect on male or female fertility at doses up to 21,000 times the systemic exposure following the maximum recommended human ophthalmic dose.
Pregnancy:
Teratogenic Effects—Pregnancy Category C. Teratogenicity studies with timolol in mice, rats, and rabbits at oral doses up to 50 mg/kg/day (7,000 times the systemic exposure following the maximum recommended human ophthalmic dose) demonstrated no evidence of fetal malformations. Although delayed fetal ossification was observed at this dose in rats, there were no adverse effects on postnatal development of offspring. Doses of 1000 mg/kg/day (142,000 times the systemic exposure following the maximum recommended human ophthalmic dose) were maternotoxic in mice and resulted in an increased number of fetal resorptions. Increased fetal resorptions were also seen in rabbits at doses of 14,000 times the systemic exposure following the maximum recommended human ophthalmic dose, in this case without apparent maternotoxicity.
There are no adequate and well-controlled studies in pregnant women. TIMOPTIC should be used during pregnancy only if the potential benefit justifies the potential risk to the fetus.
Nursing Mothers
Timolol maleate has been detected in human milk following oral and ophthalmic drug administration. Because of the potential for serious adverse reactions from TIMOPTIC in nursing infants, a decision should be made whether to discontinue nursing or to discontinue the drug, taking into account the importance of the drug to the mother.
Pediatric Use
Safety and effectiveness in pediatric patients have not been established.
Geriatric Use
No overall differences in safety or effectiveness have been observed between elderly and younger patients.
Adverse Reactions
The most frequently reported adverse experiences have been burning and stinging upon instillation (approximately one in eight patients).
The following additional adverse experiences have been reported less frequently with ocular administration of this or other timolol maleate formulations:
BODY AS A WHOLE
Headache, asthenia/fatigue, and chest pain.
CARDIOVASCULAR
Bradycardia, arrhythmia, hypotension, hypertension, syncope, heart block, cerebral vascular accident, cerebral ischemia, cardiac failure, worsening of angina pectoris, palpitation, cardiac arrest, pulmonary edema, edema, claudication, Raynaud's phenomenon, and cold hands and feet.
DIGESTIVE
Nausea, diarrhea, dyspepsia, anorexia, and dry mouth.
IMMUNOLOGIC
Systemic lupus erythematosus.
NERVOUS SYSTEM/PSYCHIATRIC
Dizziness, increase in signs and symptoms of myasthenia gravis, paresthesia, somnolence, insomnia, nightmares, behavioral changes and psychic disturbances including depression, confusion, hallucinations, anxiety, disorientation, nervousness, and memory loss.
SKIN
Alopecia and psoriasiform rash or exacerbation of psoriasis.
HYPERSENSITIVITY
Signs and symptoms of systemic allergic reactions, including anaphylaxis, angioedema, urticaria, and localized and generalized rash.
RESPIRATORY
Bronchospasm (predominantly in patients with pre-existing bronchospastic disease), respiratory failure, dyspnea, nasal congestion, cough and upper respiratory infections.
ENDOCRINE
Masked symptoms of hypoglycemia in diabetic patients (see **WARNINGS**).
SPECIAL SENSES
Signs and symptoms of ocular irritation including conjunctivitis, blepharitis, keratitis, ocular pain, discharge (e.g., crusting), foreign body sensation, itching and tearing, and dry eyes; ptosis; decreased corneal sensitivity; cystoid macular edema; visual disturbances including refractive changes and diplopia; pseudopemphigoid; choroidal detachment following filtration surgery (see **PRECAUTIONS**, *General*); and tinnitus.
UROGENITAL
Retroperitoneal fibrosis, decreased libido, impotence, and Peyronie's disease.
The following additional adverse effects have been reported in clinical experience with ORAL timolol maleate or other ORAL beta-blocking agents and may be considered potential effects of ophthalmic timolol maleate: *Allergic:* Erythematous rash, fever combined with aching and sore throat, laryngospasm with respiratory distress; *Body as a Whole:* Extremity pain, decreased exercise tolerance, weight loss; *Cardiovascular:* Worsening of arterial insufficiency, vasodilatation; *Digestive:* Gastrointestinal pain, hepatomegaly, vomiting, mesenteric arterial thrombosis, ischemic colitis; *Hematologic:* Nonthrombocytopenic purpura; thrombocytopenic purpura, agranulocytosis; *Endocrine:* Hyperglycemia, hypoglycemia; *Skin:* Pruritus, skin irritation, increased pigmentation, sweating; *Musculoskeletal:* Arthralgia; *Nervous System/Psychiatric:* Vertigo, local weakness, diminished concentration, reversible mental depression progressing to catatonia, and acute reversible syndrome characterized by disorientation for time and place, emotional lability, slightly clouded sensorium, and decreased performance on neuropsychometrics; *Respiratory:* Rales, bronchial obstruction; *Urogenital:* Urination difficulties.
Overdosage
There have been reports of inadvertent overdosage with TIMOPTIC Ophthalmic Solution resulting in systemic effects similar to those seen with systemic beta-adrenergic blocking agents such as dizziness, headache, shortness of breath, bradycardia, bronchospasm, and cardiac arrest (see also ADVERSE REACTIONS).
Overdosage has been reported with Tablets BLOCADREN* (timolol maleate tablets). A 30 year old female ingested 650 mg of BLOCADREN (maximum recommended oral daily dose is 60 mg) and experienced second and third degree heart block. She recovered without treatment but approximately two months later developed irregular heartbeat, hypertension, dizziness, tinnitus, faintness, increased pulse rate, and borderline first degree heart block.
An *in vitro* hemodialysis study, using ^{14}C timolol added to human plasma or whole blood, showed that timolol was readily dialyzed from these fluids; however, a study of pa-

Continued on next page

Information on the Merck & Co., Inc., products listed on these pages is from the prescribing information in use August 31, 2004.

Timoptic—Cont.

tients with renal failure showed that timolol did not dialyze readily.

*Registered trademark of MERCK & CO., INC.

Dosage and Administration

TIMOPTIC Ophthalmic Solution is available in concentrations of 0.25 and 0.5 percent. The usual starting dose is one drop of 0.25 percent TIMOPTIC in the affected eye(s) twice a day. If the clinical response is not adequate, the dosage may be changed to one drop of 0.5 percent solution in the affected eye(s) twice a day.

Since in some patients the pressure-lowering response to TIMOPTIC may require a few weeks to stabilize, evaluation should include a determination of intraocular pressure after approximately 4 weeks of treatment with TIMOPTIC.

If the intraocular pressure is maintained at satisfactory levels, the dosage schedule may be changed to one drop a day in the affected eye(s). Because of diurnal variations in intraocular pressure, satisfactory response to the once-a-day dose is best determined by measuring the intraocular pressure at different times during the day.

Dosages above one drop of 0.5 percent TIMOPTIC twice a day generally have not been shown to produce further reduction in intraocular pressure. If the patient's intraocular pressure is still not at a satisfactory level on this regimen, concomitant therapy with other agent(s) for lowering intraocular pressure can be instituted. The concomitant use of two topical beta-adrenergic blocking agents is not recommended. (See PRECAUTIONS, *Drug Interactions, Beta-adrenergic blocking agents*.)

How Supplied

Sterile Ophthalmic Solution TIMOPTIC is a clear, colorless to light yellow solution.
No. 8895—TIMOPTIC Ophthalmic Solution, 0.25% timolol equivalent, is supplied in an OCUMETER®* PLUS container, a translucent, natural HDPE plastic ophthalmic dispenser with a white polystyrene cap with color coded label, and a controlled drop tip as follows:
NDC 0006-8895-35, 5 mL a 7.5 mL bottle
NDC 0006-8895-36, 10 mL in an 18 mL bottle.
No. 8896—TIMOPTIC Ophthalmic Solution, 0.5% timolol equivalent, is supplied in an OCUMETER®* PLUS container, a translucent, natural HDPE plastic ophthalmic dispenser with a white polystyrene cap with color coded label, and a controlled drop tip as follows:
NDC 0006-8896-35, 5 mL in a 7.5 mL bottle
NDC 0006-8896-36, 10 mL in an 18 mL bottle.

Storage

Store at room temperature, 15–30°C (59–86°F). Protect from freezing. Protect from light.

*Registered trademark of MERCK & CO., INC.

INSTRUCTIONS FOR USE

Please follow these instructions carefully when using TIMOPTIC*. Use TIMOPTIC as prescribed by your doctor.

1. If you use other topically applied ophthalmic medications, they should be administered at least 10 minutes before or after TIMOPTIC.
2. Wash hands before each use.
3. Before using the medication for the first time, be sure the Safety Strip on the front of the bottle is unbroken. A gap between the bottle and the cap is normal for an unopened bottle.

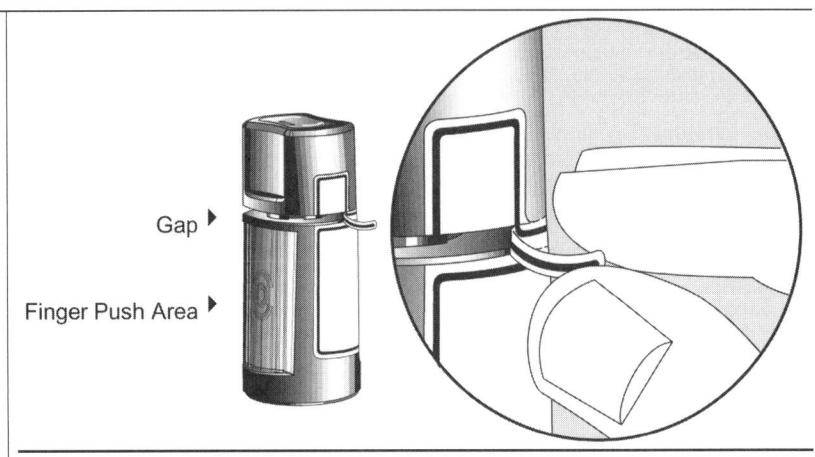

4. Tear off the Safety Strip to break the seal. [See first graphic above]
5. To open the bottle, unscrew the cap by turning as indicated by the arrows.

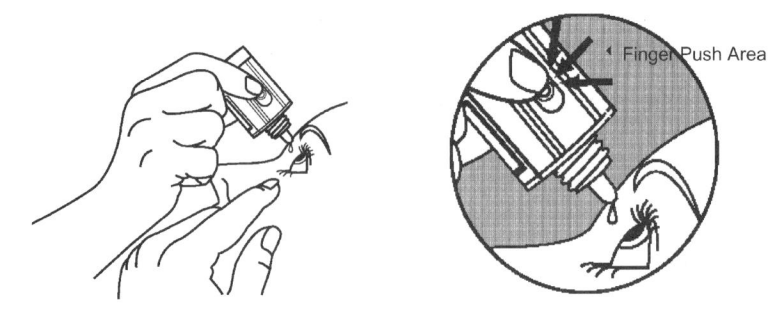

6. Tilt your head back and pull your lower eyelid down slightly to form a pocket between your eyelid and your eye. [See figure at top of next column]
7. Invert the bottle, and press lightly with the thumb or index finger over the "Finger Push Area" (as shown) until a single drop is dispensed into the eye as directed by your doctor. [See second graphic above]

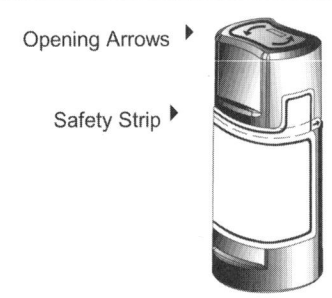

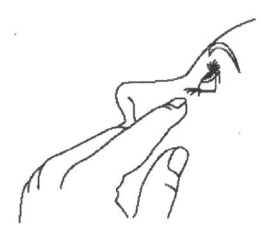

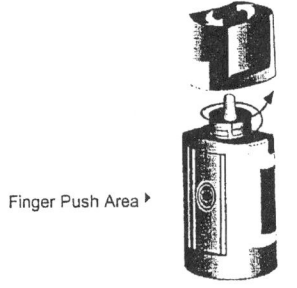

DO NOT TOUCH YOUR EYE OR EYELID WITH THE DROPPER TIP.
Ophthalmic medications, if handled improperly, can become contaminated by common bacteria known to cause eye infections. Serious damage to the eye and subsequent loss of vision may result from using contaminated ophthalmic medications. If you think your medication may be contaminated, or if you develop an eye infection, contact your doctor immediately concerning continued use of this bottle.

8. Repeat steps 6 & 7 with the other eye if instructed to do so by your doctor.
9. Replace the cap by turning until it is firmly touching the bottle. Do not overtighten the cap.
10. The dispenser tip is designed to provide a pre-measured drop; therefore, do NOT enlarge the hole of the dispenser tip.
11. After you have used all doses, there will be some TIMOPTIC left in the bottle. You should not be concerned since an extra amount of TIMOPTIC has been added and you will get the full amount of TIMOPTIC that your doctor prescribed. Do not attempt to remove excess medicine from the bottle.

WARNING: Keep out of reach of children.
If you have any questions about the use of TIMOPTIC, please consult your doctor.

*Registered trademark of MERCK & CO., Inc.

Manuf. for:
Merck & Co., Inc., Whitehouse Station, NJ 08889, USA
By: Laboratories Merck Sharp & Dohme-Chibret
63963 Clermont-Ferrand Cedex 9, France
9391003   Issued September 2002
COPYRIGHT © MERCK & CO., INC., 1985, 1995
All rights reserved

Shown in Product Identification Guide, page 105

TIMOPTIC® ℞
0.25% and 0.5%
(timolol maleate ophthalmic solution)
in OCUDOSE® (dispenser)
Preservative-Free Sterile Ophthalmic Solution in a Sterile Ophthalmic Unit Dose Dispenser

Description
Timolol maleate is a non-selective beta-adrenergic receptor blocking agent. Its chemical name is (-)-1-(*tert*-butylamino)-3-[(4-morpholino-1,2,5-thiadiazol-3-yl)oxy]-2-propanol maleate (1:1) (salt). Timolol maleate possesses an asymmetric carbon atom in its structure and is provided as the levo-isomer. The nominal optical rotation of timolol maleate is

$$[\alpha]_{405\,nm}^{25°} \text{ in } 1.0N \text{ HCl } (C = 5\%) = -12.2° \quad (-11.7° \text{ to } -12.5°).$$

Its molecular formula is $C_{13}H_{24}N_4O_3S \cdot C_4H_4O_4$ and its structural formula is:

Timolol maleate has a molecular weight of 432.50. It is a white, odorless, crystalline powder which is soluble in water, methanol, and alcohol. Timolol maleate is stable at room temperature.

Timolol maleate ophthalmic solution is supplied in two formulations: Ophthalmic Solution TIMOPTIC* (timolol maleate ophthalmic solution), which contains the preservative benzalkonium chloride; and Ophthalmic Solution TIMOPTIC* (timolol maleate ophthalmic solution), the preservative-free formulation.

Preservative-free Ophthalmic Solution The pH of the solution is approximately 7.0, and the osmolarity is 252–328 mOsm. TIMOPTIC is supplied in OCUDOSE*, a unit dose container, as a sterile, isotonic, buffered, aqueous solution of timolol maleate in two dosage strengths: Each mL of Preservative-free TIMOPTIC in OCUDOSE 0.25% contains 2.5 mg of timolol (3.4 mg of timolol maleate). Each mL of Preservative-free TIMOPTIC in OCUDOSE 0.5% contains 5 mg of timolol (6.8 mg of timolol maleate). Inactive ingredients: monobasic and dibasic sodium phosphate, sodium hydroxide to adjust pH, and water for injection.

*Registered trademark of MERCK & CO., INC.

Clinical Pharmacology
Mechanism of Action
Timolol maleate is a $beta_1$ and $beta_2$ (non-selective) adrenergic receptor blocking agent that does not have significant intrinsic sympathomimetic, direct myocardial depressant, or local anesthetic (membrane-stabilizing) activity.
Beta-adrenergic receptor blockade reduces cardiac output in both healthy subjects and patients with heart disease. In patients with severe impairment of myocardial function beta-adrenergic receptor blockade may inhibit the stimulatory effect of the sympathetic nervous system necessary to maintain adequate cardiac function.
Beta-adrenergic receptor blockade in the bronchi and bronchioles results in increased airway resistance from unopposed parasympathetic activity. Such an effect in patients with asthma or other bronchospastic conditions is potentially dangerous.
TIMOPTIC (timolol maleate ophthalmic solution), when applied topically on the eye, has the action of reducing elevated as well as normal intraocular pressure, whether or not accompanied by glaucoma. Elevated intraocular pressure is a major risk factor in the pathogenesis of glaucomatous visual field loss. The higher the level of intraocular pressure, the greater the likelihood of glaucomatous visual field loss and optic nerve damage.
The onset of reduction in intraocular pressure following administration of TIMOPTIC (timolol maleate ophthalmic solution) can usually be detected within one-half hour after a single dose. The maximum effect usually occurs in one to two hours and significant lowering of intraocular pressure can be maintained for periods as long as 24 hours with a single dose. Repeated observations over a period of one year indicate that the intraocular pressure-lowering effect of TIMOPTIC (timolol maleate ophthalmic solution) is well maintained.
The precise mechanism of the ocular hypotensive action of TIMOPTIC (timolol maleate ophthalmic solution) is not clearly established at this time. Tonography and fluorophotometry studies in man suggest that its predominant action may be related to reduced aqueous formation. However, in some studies a slight increase in outflow facility was also observed.

Pharmacokinetics
In a study of plasma drug concentration in six subjects, the systemic exposure to timolol was determined following twice daily administration of TIMOPTIC 0.5%. The mean peak plasma concentration following morning dosing was 0.46 ng/mL and following afternoon dosing was 0.35 ng/mL.

Clinical Studies
In controlled multiclinic studies in patients with untreated intraocular pressures of 22 mmHg or greater, TIMOPTIC (timolol maleate ophthalmic solution) 0.25 percent or 0.5 percent administered twice a day produced a greater reduction in intraocular pressure than 1,2,3, or 4 percent pilocarpine solution administered four times a day or 0.5, 1, or 2 percent epinephrine hydrochloride solution administered twice a day.
In these studies, TIMOPTIC (timolol maleate ophthalmic solution) was generally well tolerated and produced fewer and less severe side effects than either pilocarpine or epinephrine. A slight reduction of resting heart rate in some patients receiving TIMOPTIC (timolol maleate ophthalmic solution) (mean reduction 2.9 beats/minute standard deviation 10.2) was observed.

Indications and Usage
Preservative-free TIMOPTIC in OCUDOSE is indicated in the treatment of elevated intraocular pressure in patients with ocular hypertension or open-angle glaucoma.
Preservative-free TIMOPTIC in OCUDOSE may be used when a patient is sensitive to the preservative in TIMOPTIC (timolol maleate ophthalmic solution), benzalkonium chloride, or when use of a preservative-free topical medication is advisable.

Contraindications
Preservative-free TIMOPTIC in OCUDOSE is contraindicated in patients with (1) bronchial asthma; (2) a history of bronchial asthma; (3) severe chronic obstructive pulmonary disease (see **WARNINGS**); (4) sinus bradycardia; (5) second or third degree atrioventricular block; (6) overt cardiac failure (see **WARNINGS**); (7) cardiogenic shock; or (8) hypersensitivity to any component of this product.

Warnings
As with many topically applied ophthalmic drugs, this drug is absorbed systemically.
The same adverse reactions found with systemic administration of beta-adrenergic blocking agents may occur with topical administration. For example, severe respiratory reactions and cardiac reactions, including death due to bronchospasm in patients with asthma, and rarely death in association with cardiac failure, have been reported following systemic or ophthalmic administration of timolol maleate (see CONTRAINDICATIONS).

Cardiac Failure
Sympathetic stimulation may be essential for support of the circulation in individuals with diminished myocardial contractility, and its inhibition by beta-adrenergic receptor blockade may precipitate more severe failure.
In Patients Without a History of Cardiac Failure continued depression of the myocardium with beta-blocking agents over a period of time can, in some cases, lead to cardiac failure. At the first sign or symptom of cardiac failure Preservative-free TIMOPTIC in OCUDOSE should be discontinued.

Obstructive Pulmonary Disease
Patients with chronic obstructive pulmonary disease (e.g., chronic bronchitis, emphysema) of mild or moderate severity, bronchospastic disease, or a history of bronchospastic disease (other than bronchial asthma or a history of bronchial asthma, in which TIMOPTIC in OCUDOSE is contraindicated [see **CONTRAINDICATIONS**]) should, in general, not receive beta-blockers, including Preservative-free TIMOPTIC in OCUDOSE.

Major Surgery
The necessity or desirability of withdrawal of beta-adrenergic blocking agents prior to major surgery is controversial. Beta-adrenergic receptor blockade impairs the ability of the heart to respond to beta-adrenergically mediated reflex stimuli. This may augment the risk of general anesthesia in surgical procedures. Some patients receiving beta-adrenergic receptor blocking agents have experienced protracted severe hypotension during anesthesia. Difficulty in restarting and maintaining the heartbeat has also been reported. For these reasons, in patients undergoing elective surgery, some authorities recommend gradual withdrawal of beta-adrenergic receptor blocking agents.
If necessary during surgery, the effects of beta-adrenergic blocking agents may be reversed by sufficient doses of adrenergic agonists.

Diabetes Mellitus
Beta-adrenergic blocking agents should be administered with caution in patients subject to spontaneous hypoglycemia or to diabetic patients (especially those with labile diabetes) who are receiving insulin or oral hypoglycemic agents. Beta-adrenergic receptor blocking agents may mask the signs and symptoms of acute hypoglycemia.

Thyrotoxicosis
Beta-adrenergic blocking agents may mask certain clinical signs (e.g., tachycardia) of hyperthyroidism. Patients suspected of developing thyrotoxicosis should be managed carefully to avoid abrupt withdrawal of beta-adrenergic blocking agents that might precipitate a thyroid storm.

Continued on next page

Information on the Merck & Co., Inc., products listed on these pages is from the prescribing information in use August 31, 2004.

Timoptic in Ocudose—Cont.

Precautions
General
Because of potential effects of beta-adrenergic blocking agents on blood pressure and pulse, these agents should be used with caution in patients with cerebrovascular insufficiency. If signs or symptoms suggesting reduced cerebral blood flow develop following initiation of therapy with Preservative-free TIMOPTIC in OCUDOSE, alternative therapy should be considered.

Choroidal detachment after filtration procedures has been reported with the administration of aqueous suppressant therapy (e.g. timolol).

Angle-closure glaucoma: In patients with angle-closure glaucoma, the immediate objective of treatment is to reopen the angle. This requires constricting the pupil. Timolol maleate has little or no effect on the pupil. TIMOPTIC in OCUDOSE should not be used alone in the treatment of angle-closure glaucoma.

Anaphylaxis: While taking beta-blockers, patients with a history of atopy or a history of severe anaphylactic reactions to a variety of allergens may be more reactive to repeated accidental, diagnostic, or therapeutic challenge with such allergens. Such patients may be unresponsive to the usual doses of epinephrine used to treat anaphylactic reactions.

Muscle Weakness: Beta-adrenergic blockade has been reported to potentiate muscle weakness consistent with certain myasthenic symptoms (e.g., diplopia, ptosis, and generalized weakness). Timolol has been reported rarely to increase muscle weakness in some patients with myasthenia gravis or myasthenic symptoms.

Information for Patients
Patients should be instructed about the use of Preservative-free TIMOPTIC in OCUDOSE. Since sterility cannot be maintained after the individual unit is opened, patients should be instructed to use the product immediately after opening, and to discard the individual unit and any remaining contents immediately after use.

Patients with bronchial asthma, a history of bronchial asthma, severe chronic obstructive pulmonary disease, sinus bradycardia, second or third degree atrioventricular block, or cardiac failure should be advised not to take this product. (See **CONTRAINDICATIONS**.)

Drug Interactions
Although TIMOPTIC (timolol maleate ophthalmic solution) used alone has little or no effect on pupil size, mydriasis resulting from concomitant therapy with TIMOPTIC (timolol maleate ophthalmic solution) and epinephrine has been reported occasionally.

Beta-adrenergic blocking agents: Patients who are receiving a beta-adrenergic blocking agent orally and Preservative-free TIMOPTIC in OCUDOSE should be observed for potential additive effects of beta-blockade, both systemic and on intraocular pressure. The concomitant use of two topical beta-adrenergic blocking agents is not recommended.

Calcium antagonists: Caution should be used in the coadministration of beta-adrenergic blocking agents, such as Preservative-free TIMOPTIC in OCUDOSE, and oral or intravenous calcium antagonists, because of possible atrioventricular conduction disturbances, left ventricular failure, and hypotension. In patients with impaired cardiac function, coadministration should be avoided.

Catecholamine-depleting drugs: Close observation of the patient is recommended when a beta blocker is administered to patients receiving catecholamine-depleting drugs such as reserpine, because of possible additive effects and the production of hypotension and/or marked bradycardia, which may result in vertigo, syncope, or postural hypotension.

Digitalis and calcium antagonists: The concomitant use of beta-adrenergic blocking agents with digitalis and calcium antagonists may have additive effects in prolonging atrioventricular conduction time.

Quinidine: Potentiated systemic beta-blockade (e.g., decreased heart rate) has been reported during combined treatment with quinidine and timolol, possibly because quinidine inhibits the metabolism of timolol via the P-450 enzyme, CYP2D6.

Clonidine: Oral beta-adrenergic blocking agents may exacerbate the rebound hypertension which can follow the withdrawal of clonidine. There have been no reports of exacerbation of rebound hypertension with ophthalmic timolol maleate.

Injectable epinephrine: (See **PRECAUTIONS**, *General, Anaphylaxis*)

Carcinogenesis, Mutagenesis, Impairment of Fertility
In a two-year oral study of timolol maleate administered orally to rats, there was a statistically significant increase in the incidence of adrenal pheochromocytomas in male rats administered 300 mg/kg/day (approximately 42,000 times the systemic exposure following the maximum recommended human ophthalmic dose). Similar differences were not observed in rats administered oral doses equivalent to approximately 14,000 times the maximum recommended human ophthalmic dose.

In a lifetime oral study in mice, there were statistically significant increases in the incidence of benign and malignant pulmonary tumors, benign uterine polyps and mammary adenocarcinomas in female mice at 500 mg/kg/day (approximately 71,000 times the systemic exposure following the maximum recommended human ophthalmic dose), but not at 5 or 50 mg/kg/day (approximately 700 or 7,000 times, respectively, the systemic exposure following the maximum recommended human ophthalmic dose). In a subsequent study in female mice, in which post-mortem examinations were limited to the uterus and the lungs, a statistically significant increase in the incidence of pulmonary tumors was again observed at 500 mg/kg/day.

The increased occurrence of mammary adenocarcinomas was associated with elevations in serum prolactin which occurred in female mice administered oral timolol at 500 mg/kg/day, but not at doses of 5 or 50 mg/kg/day. An increased incidence of mammary adenocarcinomas in rodents has been associated with administration of several other therapeutic agents that elevate serum prolactin, but no correlation between serum prolactin levels and mammary tumors has been established in humans. Furthermore, in adult human female subjects who received oral dosages of up to 60 mg of timolol maleate (the maximum recommended human oral dosage), there were no clinically meaningful changes in serum prolactin.

Timolol maleate was devoid of mutagenic potential when tested *in vivo* (mouse) in the micronucleus test and cytogenetic assay (doses up to 800 mg/kg) and *in vitro* in a neoplastic cell transformation assay (up to 100 mcg/mL). In Ames tests the highest concentrations of timolol employed, 5000 or 10,000 mcg/plate, were associated with statistically significant elevations of revertants observed with tester strain TA 100 (in seven replicate assays), but not in the remaining three strains. In the assays with tester strain TA 100, no consistent dose response relationship was observed, and the ratio of test to control revertants did not reach 2. A ratio of 2 is usually considered the criterion for a positive Ames test.

Reproduction and fertility studies in rats demonstrated no adverse effect on male or female fertility at doses up to 21,000 times the systemic exposure following the maximum recommended human ophthalmic dose.

Pregnancy:
Teratogenic Effects—Pregnancy Category C. Teratogenicity studies with timolol in mice, rats and rabbits at oral doses up to 50 mg/kg/day (7,000 times the systemic exposure following the maximum recommended human ophthalmic dose) demonstrated no evidence of fetal malformations. Although delayed fetal ossification was observed at this dose in rats, there were no adverse effects on postnatal development of offspring. Doses of 1000 mg/kg/day (142,000 times the systemic exposure following the maximum recommended human ophthalmic dose) were maternotoxic in mice and resulted in an increased number of fetal resorptions. Increased fetal resorptions were also seen in rabbits at doses of 14,000 times the systemic exposure following the maximum recommended human ophthalmic dose, in this case without apparent maternotoxicity.

There are no adequate and well-controlled studies in pregnant women. Preservative-free TIMOPTIC in OCUDOSE should be used during pregnancy only if the potential benefit justifies the potential risk to the fetus.

Nursing Mothers
Timolol maleate has been detected in human milk following oral and ophthalmic drug administration. Because of the potential for serious adverse reactions from timolol in nursing infants, a decision should be made whether to discontinue nursing or to discontinue the drug, taking into account the importance of the drug to the mother.

Pediatric Use
Safety and effectiveness in pediatric patients have not been established.

Geriatric Use
No overall differences in safety or effectiveness have been observed between elderly and younger patients.

Adverse Reactions
The most frequently reported adverse experiences have been burning and stinging upon instillation (approximately one in eight patients).

The following additional adverse experiences have been reported less frequently with ocular administration of this or other timolol maleate formulations:

BODY AS A WHOLE
 Headache, asthenia/fatigue, chest pain.

CARDIOVASCULAR
 Bradycardia, arrhythmia, hypotension, hypertension, syncope, heart block, cerebral vascular accident, cerebral ischemia, cardiac failure, worsening of angina pectoris, palpitation, cardiac arrest, pulmonary edema, edema, claudication, Raynaud's phenomenon, and cold hands and feet.

DIGESTIVE
 Nausea, diarrhea. dyspepsia, anorexia, and dry mouth.

IMMUNOLOGIC
 Systemic lupus erythematosus.

NERVOUS SYSTEM/PSYCHIATRIC
 Dizziness, increase in signs and symptoms of myasthenia gravis, paresthesia, somnolence, insomnia, nightmares, behavioral changes and psychic disturbances including depression, confusion, hallucinations, anxiety, disorientation, nervousness, and memory loss.

SKIN
 Alopecia and psoriasiform rash or exacerbation of psoriasis.

HYPERSENSITIVITY
 Signs and symptoms of systemic allergic reactions, including anaphylaxis, angioedema, urticaria, and localized and generalized rash.

RESPIRATORY

Bronchospasm (predominantly in patients with pre-existing bronchospastic disease), respiratory failure, dyspnea, nasal congestion, cough and upper respiratory infections.

ENDOCRINE

Masked symptoms of hypoglycemia in diabetic patients (see **WARNINGS**).

SPECIAL SENSES

Signs and symptoms of ocular irritation including conjunctivitis, blepharitis, keratitis, ocular pain, discharge (e.g., crusting), foreign body sensation, itching and tearing, and dry eyes; ptosis; decreased corneal sensitivity; cystoid macular edema; visual disturbances including refractive changes and diplopia; pseudopemphigoid; choroidal detachment following filtration surgery (see **PRECAUTIONS**, *General*); and tinnitus.

UROGENITAL

Retroperitoneal fibrosis, decreased libido, impotence, and Peyronie's disease.

The following additional adverse effects have been reported in clinical experience with ORAL timolol maleate or other ORAL beta blocking agents, and may be considered potential effects of ophthalmic timolol maleate: *Allergic:* Erythematous rash, fever combined with aching and sore throat, laryngospasm with respiratory distress; *Body as a Whole:* Extremity pain, decreased exercise tolerance, weight loss; *Cardiovascular:* Worsening of arterial insufficiency, vasodilatation; *Digestive:* Gastrointestinal pain, hepatomegaly, vomiting, mesenteric arterial thrombosis, ischemic colitis; *Hematologic:* Nonthrombocytopenic purpura; thrombocytopenic purpura; agranulocytosis; *Endocrine:* Hyperglycemia, hypoglycemia; *Skin:* Pruritus, skin irritation, increased pigmentation, sweating; *Musculoskeletal:* Arthralgia; *Nervous System/Psychiatric:* Vertigo, local weakness, diminished concentration, reversible mental depression progressing to catatonia, an acute reversible syndrome characterized by disorientation for time and place, emotional lability, slightly clouded sensorium, and decreased performance on neuropsychometrics; *Respiratory:* Rales, bronchial obstruction; *Urogenital:* Urination difficulties.

Overdosage

There have been reports of inadvertent overdosage with Ophthalmic Solution TIMOPTIC (timolol maleate ophthalmic solution) resulting in systemic effects similar to those seen with systemic beta-adrenergic blocking agents such as dizziness, headache, shortness of breath, bradycardia, bronchospasm, and cardiac arrest (see also **ADVERSE REACTIONS**).

Overdosage has been reported with Tablets BLOCADREN* (timolol maleate tablets). A 30 year old female ingested 650 mg of BLOCADREN (maximum recommended oral daily dose is 60 mg) and experienced second and third degree heart block. She recovered without treatment but approximately two months later developed irregular heartbeat, hypertension, dizziness, tinnitus, faintness, increased pulse rate, and borderline first degree heart block.

An *in vitro* hemodialysis study, using ^{14}C timolol added to human plasma or whole blood, showed that timolol was readily dialyzed from these fluids; however, a study of patients with renal failure showed that timolol did not dialyze readily.

---

* Registered trademark of MERCK & CO., INC.

Dosage and Administration

Preservative-free TIMOPTIC in OCUDOSE is a sterile solution that does not contain a preservative. The solution from one individual unit is to be used immediately after opening for administration to one or both eyes. Since sterility cannot be guaranteed after the individual unit is opened, the remaining contents should be discarded immediately after administration.

Preservative-free TIMOPTIC in OCUDOSE is available in concentrations of 0.25 and 0.5 percent. The usual starting dose is one drop of 0.25 percent Preservative-free TIMOPTIC in OCUDOSE in the affected eye(s) administered twice a day. Apply enough gentle pressure on the individual container to obtain a single drop of solution. If the clinical response is not adequate, the dosage may be changed to one drop of 0.5 percent solution in the affected eye(s) administered twice a day.

Since in some patients the pressure-lowering response to Preservative-free TIMOPTIC in OCUDOSE may require a few weeks to stabilize, evaluation should include a determination of intraocular pressure after approximately 4 weeks of treatment with Preservative-free TIMOPTIC in OCUDOSE.

If the intraocular pressure is maintained at satisfactory levels, the dosage schedule may be changed to one drop once a day in the affected eye(s). Because of diurnal variations in intraocular pressure, satisfactory response to the once-a-day dose is best determined by measuring the intraocular pressure at different times during the day.

Dosages above one drop of 0.5 percent TIMOPTIC (timolol maleate ophthalmic solution) twice a day generally have not been shown to produce further reduction in intraocular pressure. If the patient's intraocular pressure is still not at a satisfactory level on this regimen, concomitant therapy with other agent(s) for lowering intraocular pressure can be instituted taking into consideration that the preparation(s) used concomitantly may contain one or more preservatives. The concomitant use of two topical beta-adrenergic blocking agents is not recommended. (See **PRECAUTIONS**, *Drug Interactions, Beta-adrenergic blocking agents.*)

How Supplied

Preservative-free Sterile Ophthalmic Solution TIMOPTIC in OCUDOSE is a clear, colorless to light yellow solution.

No. 9689—Preservative-free TIMOPTIC, 0.25% timolol equivalent, is supplied in OCUDOSE, a clear low density polyethylene unit dose container. Each individual unit contains 0.2 mL of solution, and is available in a foil laminate overwrapped pouch as follows:

NDC 0006-9689-60; 60 Individual Unit Doses
No. 9690—Preservative-free TIMOPTIC, 0.5% timolol equivalent, is supplied in OCUDOSE, a clear low density polyethylene unit dose container. Each individual unit contains 0.2 mL of solution, and is available in a foil laminate overwrapped pouch as follows:

NDC 0006-9690-60; 60 Individual Unit Doses

Storage

Store at room temperature, 15–30°C (59–86°F). Protect from freezing. Protect from light.

Because evaporation can occur through the unprotected polyethylene unit dose container and prolonged exposure to direct light can modify the product, the unit dose container should be kept in the protective foil overwrap and used within one month after the foil package has been opened.

Manuf. for:

Merck & Co., Inc., Whitehouse Station, NJ 08889, USA

By: Laboratoires Merck Sharp & Dohme-Chibret
    63963 Clermont-Ferrand Cedex 9, France
    9351204   Issued September 2002

COPYRIGHT © MERCK & CO., INC., 1986, 1995

All rights reserved

Shown in Product Identification Guide, page 105

TIMOPTIC-XE®   ℞
0.25% and 0.5%
(timolol maleate ophthalmic gel forming solution)
Sterile Ophthalmic Gel Forming Solution

Description

TIMOPTIC-XE* (timolol maleate ophthalmic gel forming solution) is a non-selective beta-adrenergic receptor blocking agent. Its chemical name is (-)-1-(*tert*-butyl-amino)-3-[(4-morpholino-1,2,5-thiadiazol-3-yl)oxy]-2-propanol maleate (1:1) (salt). Timolol maleate possesses an asymmetric carbon atom in its structure and is provided as the levo-isomer. The optical rotation of timolol maleate is:

$[\alpha]\ 25°$ in 1.0N HCl (C=5%) = $-12.2°$
                         ($-11.7°$ to $-12.5°$).
405 nm

Its molecular formula is $C_{13}H_{24}N_4O_3S \cdot C_4H_4O_4$ and its structural formula is:

Timolol maleate has a molecular weight of 432.50. It is a white, odorless, crystalline powder which is soluble in water, methanol, and alcohol.

TIMOPTIC-XE Sterile Ophthalmic Gel Forming Solution is supplied as a sterile, isotonic, buffered, aqueous solution of timolol maleate in two dosage strengths. The pH of the solution is approximately 7.0, and the osmolarity is 260–330 mOsm. Each mL of TIMOPTIC-XE 0.25% contains 2.5 mg of timolol (3.4 mg of timolol maleate). Each mL of TIMOPTIC-XE 0.5% contains 5 mg of timolol (6.8 mg of timolol maleate). Inactive ingredients: GELRITE* gellan gum, tromethamine, mannitol, and water for injection. Preservative: benzododecinium bromide 0.012%.

GELRITE is a purified anionic heteropolysaccharide derived from gellan gum. An aqueous solution of GELRITE, in the presence of a cation, has the ability to gel. Upon contact with the precorneal tear film, TIMOPTIC-XE forms a gel that is subsequently removed by the flow of tears.

---

* Registered trademark of MERCK & CO., INC.

Clinical Pharmacology

Mechanism of Action

Timolol maleate is a beta$_1$ and beta$_2$ (non-selective) adrenergic receptor blocking agent that does not have significant intrinsic sympathomimetic, direct myocardial depressant, or local anesthetic (membrane-stabilizing) activity.

TIMOPTIC-XE, when applied topically on the eye, has the action of reducing elevated, as well as normal intraocular pressure, whether or not accompanied by glaucoma. Elevated intraocular pressure is a major risk factor in the pathogenesis of glaucomatous visual field loss and optic nerve damage.

The precise mechanism of the ocular hypotensive action of TIMOPTIC-XE is not clearly established at this time. Tonography and fluoro-

Continued on next page

Information on the Merck & Co., Inc., products listed on these pages is from the prescribing information in use August 31, 2004.

Timoptic-XE—Cont.

photometry studies of TIMOPTIC* (timolol maleate ophthalmic solution) in man suggest that its predominant action may be related to reduced aqueous formation. However, in some studies, a slight increase in outflow facility was also observed.

Beta-adrenergic receptor blockade reduces cardiac output in both healthy subjects and patients with heart disease. In patients with severe impairment of myocardial function betaadrenergic receptor blockade may inhibit the stimulatory effect of the sympathetic nervous system necessary to maintain adequate cardiac function.

Beta-adrenergic receptor blockade in the bronchi and bronchioles results in increased airway resistance from unopposed parasympathetic activity. Such an effect in patients with asthma or other bronchospastic conditions is potentially dangerous.

Pharmacokinetics
In a study of plasma drug concentration in six subjects, the systemic exposure to timolol was determined following once daily administration of TIMOPTIC-XE 0.5% in the morning. The mean peak plasma concentration following this morning dose was 0.28 ng/mL.

Clinical Studies
In controlled, double-masked, multicenter clinical studies, comparing TIMOPTIC-XE 0.25% to TIMOPTIC 0.25% and TIMOPTIC-XE 0.5% to TIMOPTIC 0.5%, TIMOPTIC-XE administered once a day was shown to be equally effective in lowering intraocular pressure as the equivalent concentration of TIMOPTIC administered twice a day. The effect of timolol in lowering intraocular pressure was evident for 24 hours with a single dose of TIMOPTIC-XE. Repeated observations over a period of six months indicate that the intraocular pressure-lowering effect of TIMOPTIC-XE was consistent. The results from the largest U.S. and international clinical trials comparing TIMOPTIC-XE 0.5% to TIMOPTIC 0.5% are shown in Figure 1.

Figure 1

Mean IOP and Std Deviation (mm Hg) by Treatment Group

U.S. Study

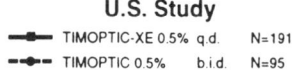

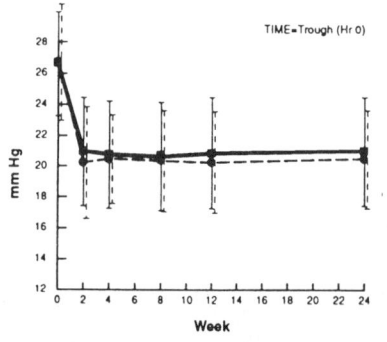

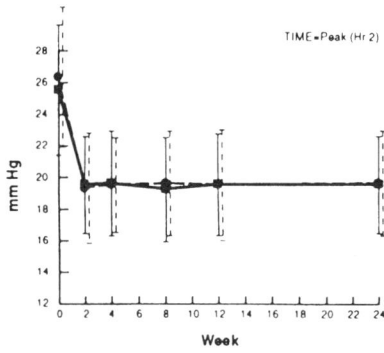

International Study

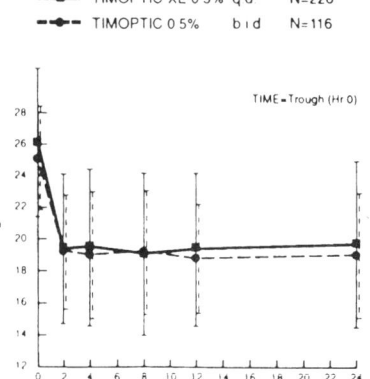

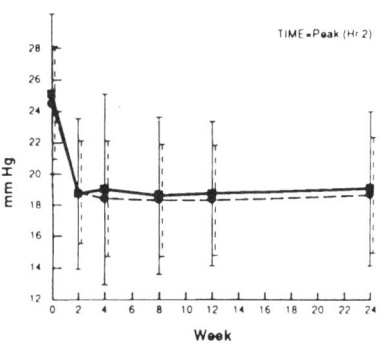

TIMOPTIC-XE administered once daily had a safety profile similar to that of an equivalent concentration of TIMOPTIC administered twice daily. Due to the physical characteristics of the formulation, there was a higher incidence of transient blurred vision in patients administered TIMOPTIC-XE. A slight reduction in resting heart rate was observed in some patients receiving TIMOPTIC-XE 0.5% (mean reduction 24 hours post-dose 0.8 beats/minute, mean reduction 2 hours post-dose 3.8 beats/minute). (See **ADVERSE REACTIONS**.)
TIMOPTIC-XE has not been studied in patients wearing contact lenses.

* Registered trademark of MERCK & CO., INC.

Indications and Usage
TIMOPTIC-XE Sterile Ophthalmic Gel Forming Solution is indicated in the treatment of elevated intraocular pressure in patients with ocular hypertension or open-angle glaucoma.

Contraindications
TIMOPTIC-XE is contraindicated in patients with (1) bronchial asthma; (2) a history of bronchial asthma; (3) severe chronic obstructive pulmonary disease (see **WARNINGS**); (4) sinus bradycardia; (5) second or third degree atrioventricular block; (6) overt cardiac failure (see **WARNINGS**); (7) cardiogenic shock; or (8) hypersensitivity to any component of this product.

Warnings
As with many topically applied ophthalmic drugs, this drug is absorbed systemically.
The same adverse reactions found with systemic administration of beta-adrenergic blocking agents may occur with topical ophthalmic administration. For example, severe respiratory reactions and cardiac reactions, including death due to bronchospasm in patients with asthma, and rarely death in association with cardiac failure, have been reported following systemic or ophthalmic administration of timolol maleate. (See CONTRAINDICATIONS.)

Cardiac Failure
Sympathetic stimulation may be essential for support of the circulation in individuals with diminished myocardial contractility, and its inhibition by beta-adrenergic receptor blockade may precipitate more severe failure.

In Patients Without a History of Cardiac Failure, continued depression of the myocardium with beta-blocking agents over a period of time can, in some cases, lead to cardiac failure. At the first sign or symptom of cardiac failure, TIMOPTIC-XE should be discontinued.

Obstructive Pulmonary Disease
Patients with chronic obstructive pulmonary disease (e.g., chronic bronchitis, emphysema) of mild or moderate severity, bronchospastic disease, or a history of bronchospastic disease (other than bronchial asthma or a history of bronchial asthma, in which TIMOPTIC-XE is contraindicated [see **CONTRAINDICATIONS**]) should, in general, not receive betablockers, including TIMOPTIC-XE.

Major Surgery
The necessity or desirability of withdrawal of beta-adrenergic blocking agents prior to major surgery is controversial. Beta-adrenergic receptor blockade impairs the ability of the heart to respond to beta-adrenergically mediated reflex stimuli. This may augment the risk of general anesthesia in surgical procedures. Some patients receiving beta-adrenergic receptor blocking agents have experienced protracted, severe hypotension during anesthesia. Difficulty in restarting and maintaining the heartbeat has also been reported. For these reasons, in patients undergoing elective surgery, some authorities recommend gradual withdrawal of beta-adrenergic receptor blocking agents.
If necessary during surgery, the effects of beta-adrenergic blocking agents may be reversed by sufficient doses of adrenergic agonists.

Diabetes Mellitus
Beta-adrenergic blocking agents should be administered with caution in patients subject to spontaneous hypoglycemia or to diabetic patients (especially those with labile diabetes) who are receiving insulin or oral hypoglycemic agents. Beta-adrenergic receptor blocking agents may mask the signs and symptoms of acute hypoglycemia.

Thyrotoxicosis
Beta-adrenergic blocking agents may mask certain clinical signs (e.g., tachycardia) of hyperthyroidism. Patients suspected of developing thyrotoxicosis should be managed carefully to avoid abrupt withdrawal of beta-adrenergic blocking agents that might precipitate a thyroid storm.

Precautions

General

Because of potential effects of beta-adrenergic blocking agents on blood pressure and pulse, these agents should be used with caution in patients with cerebrovascular insufficiency. If signs or symptoms suggesting reduced cerebral blood flow develop following initiation of therapy with TIMOPTIC-XE, alternative therapy should be considered.

There have been reports of bacterial keratitis associated with the use of multiple dose containers of topical ophthalmic products. These containers had been inadvertently contaminated by patients who, in most cases, had a concurrent corneal disease or a disruption of the ocular epithelial surface. (See **PRECAUTIONS,** *Information for Patients.*)

Choroidal detachment after filtration procedures has been reported with the administration of aqueous suppressant therapy (e.g. timolol).

Angle-closure glaucoma: In patients with angle-closure glaucoma, the immediate objective of treatment is to reopen the angle. This may require constricting the pupil. Timolol maleate has little or no effect on the pupil. TIMOPTIC-XE should not be used alone in the treatment of angle-closure glaucoma.

Anaphylaxis: While taking beta-blockers, patients with a history of atopy or a history of severe anaphylactic reactions to a variety of allergens may be more reactive to repeated accidental, diagnostic, or therapeutic challenge with such allergens. Such patients may be unresponsive to the usual doses of epinephrine used to treat anaphylactic reactions.

Muscle Weakness: Beta-adrenergic blockade has been reported to potentiate muscle weakness consistent with certain myasthenic symptoms (e.g., diplopia, ptosis, and generalized weakness). Timolol has been reported rarely to increase muscle weakness in some patients with myasthenia gravis or myasthenic symptoms.

Information for Patients

Patients should be instructed to avoid allowing the tip of the dispensing container to contact the eye or surrounding structures.

Patients should also be instructed that ocular solutions, if handled improperly or if the tip of the dispensing container contacts the eye or surrounding structures, can become contaminated by common bacteria known to cause ocular infections. Serious damage to the eye and subsequent loss of vision may result from using contaminated solutions. (See **PRECAUTIONS,** *General.*)

Patients should also be advised that if they have ocular surgery or develop an intercurrent ocular condition (e.g., trauma or infection), they should immediately seek their physician's advice concerning the continued use of the present multidose container.

Patients should be instructed to invert the closed container and shake once before each use. It is not necessary to shake the container more than once.

Patients requiring concomitant topical ophthalmic medications should be instructed to administer these at least 10 minutes before instilling TIMOPTIC-XE.

Patients with bronchial asthma, a history of bronchial asthma, severe chronic obstructive pulmonary disease, sinus bradycardia, second or third degree atrioventricular block, or cardiac failure should be advised not to take this product. (See **CONTRAINDICATIONS.**)

Transient blurred vision, generally lasting from 30 seconds to 5 minutes, following instillation, and potential visual disturbances may impair the ability to perform hazardous tasks such as operating machinery or driving a motor vehicle.

Drug Interactions

Beta-adrenergic blocking agents: Patients who are receiving a beta-adrenergic blocking agent orally and TIMOPTIC-XE should be observed for potential additive effects of beta-blockade, both systemic and on intraocular pressure. The concomitant use of two topical beta-adrenergic blocking agents is not recommended.

Calcium antagonists: Caution should be used in the coadministration of beta-adrenergic blocking agents, such as TIMOPTIC-XE, and oral or intravenous calcium antagonists because of possible atrioventricular conduction disturbances, left ventricular failure, or hypotension. In patients with impaired cardiac function, coadministration should be avoided.

Catecholamine-depleting drugs: Close observation of the patient is recommended when a beta blocker is administered to patients receiving catecholamine-depleting drugs such as reserpine, because of possible additive effects and the production of hypotension and/or marked bradycardia, which may result in vertigo, syncope, or postural hypotension.

Digitalis and calcium antagonists: The concomitant use of beta-adrenergic blocking agents with digitalis and calcium antagonists may have additive effects in prolonging atrioventricular conduction time.

Quinidine: Potentiated systemic beta-blockade (e.g., decreased heart rate) has been reported during combined treatment with quinidine and timolol, possibly because quinidine inhibits the metabolism of timolol via the P-450 enzyme, CYP2D6.

Clonidine: Oral beta-adrenergic blocking agents may exacerbate the rebound hypertension which can follow the withdrawal of clonidine. There have been no reports of exacerbation of rebound hypertension with ophthalmic timolol maleate.

Injectable epinephrine: (See **PRECAUTIONS,** *General, Anaphylaxis*)

Carcinogenesis, Mutagenesis, Impairment of Fertility

In a two-year study of timolol maleate administered orally to rats, there was a statistically significant increase in the incidence of adrenal pheochromocytomas in male rats administered 300 mg/kg/day (approximately 42,000 times the systemic exposure following the maximum recommended human ophthalmic dose). Similar differences were not observed in rats administered oral doses equivalent to approximately 14,000 times the maximum recommended human ophthalmic dose.

In a lifetime oral study in mice, there were statistically significant increases in the incidence of benign and malignant pulmonary tumors, benign uterine polyps, and mammary adenocarcinomas in female mice at 500 mg/kg/day (approximately 71,000 times the systemic exposure following the maximum recommended human ophthalmic dose), but not at 5 or 50 mg/kg/day (approximately 700 or 7,000, respectively, times the systemic exposure following the maximum recommended human ophthalmic dose). In a subsequent study in female mice, in which post-mortem examinations were limited to the uterus and the lungs, a statistically significant increase in the incidence of pulmonary tumors was again observed at 500 mg/kg/day.

The increased occurrence of mammary adenocarcinomas was associated with elevations in serum prolactin, which occurred in female mice administered oral timolol at 500 mg/kg/day, but not at oral doses of 5 or 50 mg/kg/day. An increased incidence of mammary adenocarcinomas in rodents has been associated with administration of several other therapeutic agents that elevate serum prolactin, but no correlation between serum prolactin levels and mammary tumors has been established in humans. Furthermore, in adult human female subjects who received oral dosages of up to 60 mg of timolol maleate (the maximum recommended human oral dosage), there were no clinically meaningful changes in serum prolactin.

Timolol maleate was devoid of mutagenic potential when tested *in vivo* (mouse) in the micronucleus test and cytogenetic assay (doses up to 800 mg) and *in vitro* in a neoplastic cell transformation assay (up to 100 mcg/mL). In Ames tests, the highest concentrations of timolol employed, 5,000 or 10,000 mcg/plate, were associated with statistically significant elevations of revertants observed with tester strain TA100 (in seven replicate assays), but not in the remaining three strains. In the assays with tester strain TA100, no consistent dose response relationship was observed, and the ratio of test to control revertants did not reach 2. A ratio of 2 is usually considered the criterion for a positive Ames test.

Reproduction and fertility studies in rats demonstrated no adverse effect on male or female fertility at doses up to 21,000 times the systemic exposure following the maximum recommended human ophthalmic dose.

Pregnancy:

Teratogenic Effects—Pregnancy Category C. Teratogenicity studies with timolol in mice and rabbits at oral doses up to 50 mg/kg/day (7,000 times the systemic exposure following the maximum recommended human ophthalmic dose) demonstrated no evidence of fetal malformations. Although delayed fetal ossification was observed at this dose in rats, there were no adverse effects on postnatal development of offspring. Doses of 1000 mg/kg/day (142,000 times the systemic exposure following the maximum recommended human ophthalmic dose) were maternotoxic in mice and resulted in an increased number of fetal resorptions. Increased fetal resorptions were also seen in rabbits at doses of 14,000 times the systemic exposure following the maximum recommended human ophthalmic dose, in this case without apparent maternotoxicity.

There are no adequate and well-controlled studies in pregnant women. TIMOPTIC-XE should be used during pregnancy only if the potential benefit justifies the potential risk to the fetus.

Nursing Mothers

Timolol maleate has been detected in human milk following oral and ophthalmic drug administration. Because of the potential for serious adverse reactions from TIMOPTIC-XE in nursing infants, a decision should be made whether to discontinue nursing or to discontinue the drug, taking into account the importance of the drug to the mother.

Pediatric Use

Safety and effectiveness in pediatric patients have not been established.

Geriatric Use

No overall differences in safety or effectiveness have been observed between elderly and younger patients.

Adverse Reactions

In clinical trials, transient blurred vision upon instillation of the drop was reported in approximately one in three patients (lasting from 30 seconds to 5 minutes). Less than 1% of patients discontinued from the studies due to blurred vision. The frequency of patients reporting burning and stinging upon instillation

Continued on next page

Information on the Merck & Co., Inc., products listed on these pages is from the prescribing information in use August 31, 2004.

Timoptic-XE—Cont.

was comparable between TIMOPTIC-XE and TIMOPTIC (approximately one in eight patients).

Adverse experiences reported in 1–5% of patients were:
Ocular: Pain, conjunctivitis, discharge (e.g. crusting), foreign body sensation, itching and tearing;
Systemic: Headache, dizziness, and upper respiratory infections.

The following additional adverse experiences have been reported with the ocular administration of this or other timolol maleate formulations:
BODY AS A WHOLE
Asthenia/fatigue, and chest pain.
CARDIOVASCULAR
Bradycardia, arrhythmia, hypotension, hypertension, syncope, heart block, cerebral vascular accident, cerebral ischemia, cardiac failure, worsening of angina pectoris, palpitation, cardiac arrest, pulmonary edema, edema, claudication, Raynaud's phenomenon, and cold hands and feet.
DIGESTIVE
Nausea, diarrhea, dyspepsia, anorexia, and dry mouth.
IMMUNOLOGIC
Systemic lupus erythematosus.
NERVOUS SYSTEM/PSYCHIATRIC
Increase in signs and symptoms of myasthenia gravis, paresthesia, somnolence, insomnia, nightmares, behavioral changes and psychic disturbances including depression, confusion, hallucinations, anxiety, disorientation, nervousness, and memory loss.
SKIN
Alopecia and psoriasiform rash or exacerbation of psoriasis.
HYPERSENSITIVITY
Signs and symptoms of systemic allergic reactions including anaphylaxis, angioedema, urticaria, localized and generalized rash.
RESPIRATORY
Bronchospasm (predominantly in patients with preexisting bronchospastic disease), respiratory failure, dyspnea, nasal congestion, and cough.
ENDOCRINE
Masked symptoms of hypoglycemia in diabetic patients (see **WARNINGS**).
SPECIAL SENSES
Signs and symptoms of ocular irritation including blepharitis, keratitis, and dry eyes; ptosis; decreased corneal sensitivity; cystoid macular edema; visual disturbances including refractive changes and diplopia; pseudopemphigoid; choroidal detachment following filtration surgery (see **PRECAUTIONS**, *General*); and tinnitus.
UROGENITAL
Retroperitoneal fibrosis, decreased libido, impotence, and Peyronie's disease.

The following additional adverse effects have been reported in clinical experience with ORAL timolol maleate or other ORAL beta-blocking agents and may be considered potential effects of ophthalmic timolol maleate: *Allergic:* Erythematous rash, fever combined with aching and sore throat, laryngospasm with respiratory distress; *Body as a Whole:* Extremity pain, decreased exercise tolerance, weight loss; *Cardiovascular:* Worsening of arterial insufficiency, vasodilatation; *Digestive:* Gastrointestinal pain, hepatomegaly, vomiting, mesenteric arterial thrombosis, ischemic colitis; *Hematologic:* Nonthrombocytopenic purpura, thrombocytopenic purpura, agranulocytosis; *Endocrine:* Hyperglycemia, hypoglycemia; *Skin:* Pruritus, skin irritation, increased pigmentation, sweating; *Musculoskeletal:* Arthralgia; *Nervous System/Psychiatric:* Vertigo, local weakness, diminished concentration, reversible mental depression progressing to catatonia; an acute reversible syndrome characterized by disorientation for time and place, emotional lability, slightly clouded sensorium, and decreased performance on neuropsychometrics; *Respiratory:* Rales, bronchial obstruction; *Urogenital:* Urination difficulties.

Overdosage
No data are available in regard to human overdosage with or accidental oral ingestion of TIMOPTIC-XE.
There have been reports of inadvertent overdosage with TIMOPTIC Ophthalmic Solution resulting in systemic effects similar to those seen with systemic beta-adrenergic blocking agents such as dizziness, headache, shortness of breath, bradycardia, bronchospasm, and cardiac arrest (see also **ADVERSE REACTIONS**).
Overdosage has been reported with Tablets BLOCADREN* (timolol maleate tablets). A 30 year old female ingested 650 mg of BLOCADREN (maximum recommended oral daily dose is 60 mg) and experienced second and third degree heart block. She recovered without treatment but approximately two months later developed irregular heartbeat, hypertension, dizziness, tinnitus, faintness, increased pulse rate, and borderline first degree heart block.
An *in vitro* hemodialysis study, using ^{14}C timolol added to human plasma or whole blood, showed that timolol was readily dialyzed from these fluids; however, a study of patients with renal failure showed that timolol did not dialyze readily.

---
*Registered trademark of MERCK & CO., Inc.

Dosage and Administration
Patients should be instructed to invert the closed container and shake once before each use. It is not necessary to shake the container more than once. Other topically applied ophthalmic medications should be administered at least 10 minutes before TIMOPTIC-XE. (See **PRECAUTIONS**, *Information for Patients* and accompanying INSTRUCTIONS FOR USE.)
TIMOPTIC-XE Sterile Ophthalmic Gel Forming Solution is available in concentrations of 0.25% and 0.5%. The dose is one drop of TIMOPTIC-XE (either 0.25% or 0.5%) in the affected eye(s) once a day.
Because in some patients the pressure-lowering response to TIMOPTIC-XE may require a few weeks to stabilize, evaluation should include a determination of intraocular pressure after approximately 4 weeks of treatment with TIMOPTIC-XE.
Dosages higher than one drop of 0.5% TIMOPTIC-XE once a day have not been studied. If the patient's intraocular pressure is still not at a satisfactory level on this regimen, concomitant therapy can be considered. The concomitant use of two topical beta-adrenergic blocking agents is not recommended. (See **PRECAUTIONS**, *Drug Interactions, Beta-adrenergic blocking agents*.)
When patients have been switched from therapy with TIMOPTIC administered twice daily to TIMOPTIC-XE administered once daily, the ocular hypotensive effect has remained consistent.

How Supplied
TIMOPTIC-XE Sterile Ophthalmic Gel Forming Solution is a colorless to nearly colorless, slightly opalescent, and slightly viscous solution.
No. 3557—TIMOPTIC-XE Sterile Ophthalmic Gel Forming Solution, 0.25% timolol equivalent, is supplied in OCUMETER*, a white, opaque, LDPE, plastic, ophthalmic dispenser with a controlled drop tip and color coded polypropylene cap as follows:
NDC 0006-3557-32, 2.5 mL in a 5 mL bottle.
NDC 0006-3557-03, 5 mL in a 7.5 mL bottle.
No. 3558—TIMOPTIC-XE Sterile Ophthalmic Gel Forming Solution, 0.5% timolol equivalent, is supplied in OCUMETER, a white, opaque, LDPE, plastic, ophthalmic dispenser with a controlled drop tip and color coded polypropylene cap as follows:
NDC 0006-3558-32, 2.5 mL in a 5 mL bottle.
NDC 0006-3558-03, 5 mL in a 7.5 mL bottle.
Storage
Store between 15° and 25°C (59° and 77°F).
AVOID FREEZING. Protect from light.

---
*Registered trademark of MERCK & CO., INC.
 9028714   Issued September 2002
COPYRIGHT© MERCK & CO., INC., 1993
All rights reserved

TIMOPTIC-XE®
0.25% AND 0.5%
(timolol maleate ophthalmic gel forming solution)

INSTRUCTIONS FOR USE
Please follow these instructions carefully when using TIMOPTIC-XE*. Use TIMOPTIC-XE as prescribed by your doctor.

1. If you use other topically applied ophthalmic medications, they should be administered at least 10 minutes before TIMOPTIC-XE.
2. Wash hands before each use.
3. Invert the closed bottle and shake ONCE before each use. (It is not necessary to shake the bottle more than once.)

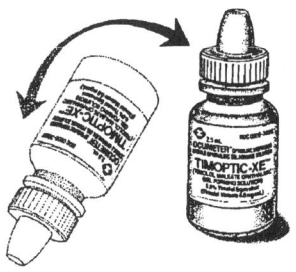

4. Remove the cap from the bottle carefully so that the dispenser tip does not touch anything. Place the cap in a clean, dry area.
5. Hold the bottle between the thumb and index finger. Use the index finger of the other hand to pull down the lower eyelid to form a pocket for the eye drop. Tilt your head back.

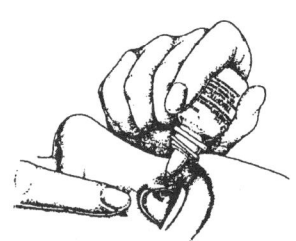

6. Place the dispenser tip close to your eye and gently squeeze the bottle to administer one drop. Remove pressure after a single drop has been released. If instructed, repeat steps 5 and 6 in the other eye.

DO NOT ALLOW THE DISPENSER TIP TO TOUCH THE EYE OR SURROUNDING AREAS.

Ophthalmic medications, if handled improperly, can become contaminated by common bacteria known to cause eye infections. Serious damage to the eye and subsequent loss of vision may result from using contaminated ophthalmic medications. If you think your medication may be contaminated, or you develop an eye infection, contact your doctor immediately concerning continued use of this bottle.

7. Replace the cap. Store the bottle at room temperature in an upright position in a clean area.
8. The dispenser tip is designed to provide a pre-measured drop; therefore, do NOT enlarge the hole of the dispenser.
9. Do NOT wash the tip of the dispenser with water, soap, or any other cleaner.

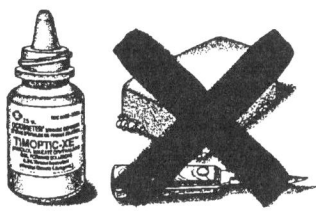

WARNING: Keep out of reach of children. If you have any questions about the use of TIMOPTIC-XE, please consult your doctor.

*Registered trademark of MERCK & CO., Inc.
COPYRIGHT © MERCK & CO., Inc., 1995
All rights reserved
Issued September 2002
MERCK & CO., Inc.
Whitehouse Station, NJ 08889, USA
Shown in Product Identification Guide, page 105

TRUSOPT® ℞
Sterile Ophthalmic Solution 2%
(dorzolamide hydrochloride ophthalmic solution)

Description
TRUSOPT* (dorzolamide hydrochloride ophthalmic solution) is a carbonic anhydrase inhibitor formulated for topical ophthalmic use. Dorzolamide hydrochloride is described chemically as: (4S-trans)-4-(ethylamino)-5,6-dihydro-6-methyl-4H-thieno [2,3-b]thiopyran-2-sulfonamide 7,7-dioxide monohydrochloride. Dorzolamide hydrochloride is optically active. The specific rotation is

$$\alpha_{405}^{25°} \ (C=1, \text{water}) = \sim -17°.$$

Its empirical formula is $C_{10}H_{16}N_2O_4S_3 \cdot HCl$ and its structural formula is:

Dorzolamide hydrochloride has a molecular weight of 360.9 and a melting point of about 264°C. It is a white to off-white, crystalline powder, which is soluble in water and slightly soluble in methanol and ethanol.
TRUSOPT Sterile Ophthalmic Solution is supplied as a sterile, isotonic, buffered, slightly viscous, aqueous solution of dorzolamide hydrochloride. The pH of the solution is approximately 5.6, and the osmolarity is 260–330 mOsM. Each mL of TRUSOPT 2% contains 20 mg dorzolamide (22.3 mg of dorzolamide hydrochloride). Inactive ingredients are hydroxyethyl cellulose, mannitol, sodium citrate dihydrate, sodium hydroxide (to adjust pH) and water for injection. Benzalkonium chloride 0.0075% is added as a preservative.

*Registered trademark of MERCK & CO., Inc.

Clinical Pharmacology
Mechanism of Action
Carbonic anhydrase (CA) is an enzyme found in many tissues of the body including the eye. It catalyzes the reversible reaction involving the hydration of carbon dioxide and the dehydration of carbonic acid. In humans, carbonic anhydrase exists as a number of isoenzymes, the most active being carbonic anhydrase II (CA-II), found primarily in red blood cells (RBCs), but also in other tissues. Inhibition of carbonic anhydrase in the ciliary processes of the eye decreases aqueous humor secretion, presumably by slowing the formation of bicarbonate ions with subsequent reduction in sodium and fluid transport. The result is a reduction in intraocular pressure (IOP).
TRUSOPT Ophthalmic Solution contains dorzolamide hydrochloride, an inhibitor of human carbonic anhydrase II. Following topical ocular administration, TRUSOPT reduces elevated intraocular pressure. Elevated intraocular pressure is a major risk factor in the pathogenesis of optic nerve damage and glaucomatous visual field loss.

Pharmacokinetics/Pharmacodynamics
When topically applied, dorzolamide reaches the systemic circulation. To assess the potential for systemic carbonic anhydrase inhibition following topical administration, drug and metabolite concentrations in RBCs and plasma and carbonic anhydrase inhibition in RBCs were measured. Dorzolamide accumulates in RBCs during chronic dosing as a result of binding to CA-II. The parent drug forms a single N-desethyl metabolite, which inhibits CA-II less potently than the parent drug but also inhibits CA-I. The metabolite also accumulates in RBCs where it binds primarily to CA-I. Plasma concentrations of dorzolamide and metabolite are generally below the assay limit of quantitation (15nM). Dorzolamide binds moderately to plasma proteins (approximately 33%). Dorzolamide is primarily excreted unchanged in the urine; the metabolite also is excreted in urine. After dosing is stopped, dorzolamide washes out of RBCs nonlinearly, resulting in a rapid decline of drug concentration initially, followed by a slower elimination phase with a half-life of about four months.
To simulate the systemic exposure after long-term topical ocular administration, dorzolamide was given orally to eight healthy subjects for up to 20 weeks. The oral dose of 2 mg b.i.d. closely approximates the amount of drug delivered by topical ocular administration of TRUSOPT 2% t.i.d. Steady state was reached within 8 weeks. The inhibition of CA-II and total carbonic anhydrase activities was below the degree of inhibition anticipated to be necessary for a pharmacological effect on renal function and respiration in healthy individuals.

Clinical Studies
The efficacy of TRUSOPT was demonstrated in clinical studies in the treatment of elevated intraocular pressure in patients with glaucoma or ocular hypertension (baseline IOP ≥23 mmHg). The IOP-lowering effect of TRUSOPT was approximately 3 to 5 mmHg throughout the day and this was consistent in clinical studies of up to one year duration. The efficacy of TRUSOPT when dosed less frequently than three times a day (alone or in combination with other products) has not been established.
In a one year clinical study, the effect of TRUSOPT 2% t.i.d. on the corneal endothelium was compared to that of betaxolol ophthalmic solution b.i.d. and timolol maleate ophthalmic solution 0.5% b.i.d. There were no statistically significant differences between groups in corneal endothelial cell counts or in corneal thickness measurements. There was a mean loss of approximately 4% in the endothelial cell counts for each group over the one year period.

Indications and Usage
TRUSOPT Ophthalmic Solution is indicated in the treatment of elevated intraocular pressure in patients with ocular hypertension or open-angle glaucoma.

Contraindications
TRUSOPT is contraindicated in patients who are hypersensitive to any component of this product.

Warnings
TRUSOPT is a sulfonamide and although administered topically is absorbed systemically. Therefore, the same types of adverse reactions that are attributable to sulfonamides may occur with topical administration with TRUSOPT. Fatalities have occurred, although rarely, due to severe reactions to sulfonamides including Stevens-Johnson syndrome, toxic epidermal necrolysis, fulminant hepatic necrosis, agranulocytosis, aplastic anemia, and other blood dyscrasias. Sensitization may recur when a sulfonamide is readministered irrespective of the route of administration. If signs of serious reactions or hypersensitivity occur, discontinue the use of this preparation.

Precautions
General
The management of patients with acute angle-closure glaucoma requires therapeutic interventions in addition to ocular hypotensive agents. TRUSOPT has not been studied in patients with acute angle-closure glaucoma.
TRUSOPT has not been studied in patients with severe renal impairment (CrCl < 30 mL/min). Because TRUSOPT and its metabolite are excreted predominantly by the kidney, TRUSOPT is not recommended in such patients.
TRUSOPT has not been studied in patients with hepatic impairment and should therefore be used with caution in such patients.
In clinical studies, local ocular adverse effects, primarily conjunctivitis and lid reactions, were reported with chronic administration of TRUSOPT. Many of these reactions had the clinical appearance and course of an allergic-type reaction that resolved upon discontinuation of drug therapy. If such reactions are observed, TRUSOPT should be discontinued and the patient evaluated before considering restarting the drug. (See **ADVERSE REACTIONS**.)
There is a potential for an additive effect on the known systemic effects of carbonic anhydrase inhibition in patients receiving an oral carbonic anhydrase inhibitor and TRUSOPT. The concomitant administration of TRUSOPT and oral carbonic anhydrase inhibitors is not recommended.
There have been reports of bacterial keratitis associated with the use of multiple dose containers of topical ophthalmic products. These containers had been inadvertently contami-

Continued on next page

Information on the Merck & Co., Inc., products listed on these pages is from the prescribing information in use August 31, 2004.

Trusopt—Cont.

nated by patients who, in most cases, had a concurrent corneal disease or a disruption of the ocular epithelial surface.

Choroidal detachment has been reported with administration of aqueous suppressant therapy (e.g., dorzolamide) after filtration procedures.

Information for Patients

TRUSOPT is a sulfonamide and although administered topically is absorbed systemically. Therefore the same types of adverse reactions that are attributable to sulfonamides may occur with topical administration. Patients should be advised that if serious or unusual reactions or signs of hypersensitivity occur, they should discontinue the use of the product (see **WARNINGS**).

Patients should be advised that if they develop any ocular reactions, particularly conjunctivitis and lid reactions, they should discontinue use and seek their physician's advice.

Patients should be instructed to avoid allowing the tip of the dispensing container to contact the eye or surrounding structures.

Patients should also be instructed that ocular solutions, if handled improperly or if the tip of the dispensing container contacts the eye or surrounding structures, can become contaminated by common bacteria known to cause ocular infections. Serious damage to the eye and subsequent loss of vision may result from using contaminated solutions.

Patients also should be advised that if they have ocular surgery or develop an intercurrent ocular condition (e.g., trauma or infection), they should immediately seek their physician's advice concerning the continued use of the present multidose container.

If more than one topical ophthalmic drug is being used, the drugs should be administered at least ten minutes apart.

Patients should be advised that TRUSOPT contains benzalkonium chloride which may be absorbed by soft contact lenses. Contact lenses should be removed prior to administration of the solution. Lenses may be reinserted 15 minutes following TRUSOPT administration.

Drug Interactions

Although acid-base and electrolyte disturbances were not reported in the clinical trials with TRUSOPT, these disturbances have been reported with oral carbonic anhydrase inhibitors and have, in some instances, resulted in drug interactions (e.g., toxicity associated with high-dose salicylate therapy). Therefore, the potential for such drug interactions should be considered in patients receiving TRUSOPT.

Carcinogenesis, Mutagenesis, Impairment of Fertility

In a two-year study of dorzolamide hydrochloride administered orally to male and female Sprague-Dawley rats, urinary bladder papillomas were seen in male rats in the highest dosage group of 20 mg/kg/day (250 times the recommended human ophthalmic dose). Papillomas were not seen in rats given oral doses equivalent to approximately 12 times the recommended human ophthalmic dose. No treatment-related tumors were seen in a 21-month study in female and male mice given oral doses up to 75 mg/kg/day (900 times the recommended human ophthalmic dose).

The increased incidence of urinary bladder papillomas seen in the high-dose male rats is a class-effect of carbonic anhydrase inhibitors in rats. Rats are particularly prone to developing papillomas in response to foreign bodies, compounds causing crystalluria, and diverse sodium salts.

No changes in bladder urothelium were seen in dogs given oral dorzolamide hydrochloride for one year at 2 mg/kg/day (25 times the recommended human ophthalmic dose) or monkeys dosed topically to the eye at 0.4 mg/kg/day (5 times the recommended human ophthalmic dose) for one year.

The following tests for mutagenic potential were negative: (1) *in vivo* (mouse) cytogenetic assay; (2) *in vitro* chromosomal aberration assay; (3) alkaline elution assay; (4) V-79 assay; and (5) Ames test.

In reproduction studies of dorzolamide hydrochloride in rats, there were no adverse effects on the reproductive capacity of males or females at doses up to 188 or 94 times, respectively, the recommended human ophthalmic dose.

Pregnancy

Teratogenic Effects. Pregnancy Category C. Developmental toxicity studies with dorzolamide hydrochloride in rabbits at oral doses of ≥2.5 mg/kg/day (31 times the recommended human ophthalmic dose) revealed malformations of the vertebral bodies. These malformations occurred at doses that caused metabolic acidosis with decreased body weight gain in dams and decreased fetal weights. No treatment-related malformations were seen at 1.0 mg/kg/day (13 times the recommended human ophthalmic dose). There are no adequate and well-controlled studies in pregnant women. TRUSOPT should be used during pregnancy only if the potential benefit justifies the potential risk to the fetus.

Nursing Mothers

In a study of dorzolamide hydrochloride in lactating rats, decreases in body weight gain of 5 to 7% in offspring at an oral dose of 7.5 mg/kg/day (94 times the recommended human ophthalmic dose) were seen during lactation. A slight delay in postnatal development (incisor eruption, vaginal canalization and eye openings), secondary to lower fetal body weight, was noted.

It is not known whether this drug is excreted in human milk. Because many drugs are excreted in human milk and because of the potential for serious adverse reactions in nursing infants from TRUSOPT, a decision should be made whether to discontinue nursing or to discontinue the drug, taking into account the importance of the drug to the mother.

Pediatric Use

Safety and effectiveness in pediatric patients have not been established.

Geriatric Use

No overall differences in safety and effectiveness have been observed between elderly and younger patients.

Adverse Reactions

Controlled clinical trials: The most frequent adverse events associated with TRUSOPT were ocular burning, stinging, or discomfort immediately following ocular administration (approximately one-third of patients). Approximately one-quarter of patients noted a bitter taste following administration. Superficial punctate keratitis occurred in 10–15% of patients and signs and symptoms of ocular allergic reaction in approximately 10%. Events occurring in approximately 1–5% of patients were conjunctivitis and lid reactions (see PRECAUTIONS, *General*), blurred vision, eye redness, tearing, dryness, and photophobia. Other ocular events and systemic events were reported infrequently, including headache, nausea, asthenia/fatigue; and, rarely, skin rashes, urolithiasis, and iridocyclitis.

Clinical practice: The following adverse events have occurred either at low incidence (<1%) during clinical trials or have been reported during the use of TRUSOPT in clinical practice where these events were reported voluntarily from a population of unknown size and frequency of occurrence cannot be determined precisely. They have been chosen for inclusion based on factors such as seriousness, frequency of reporting, possible causal connection to TRUSOPT, or a combination of these factors: signs and symptoms of systemic allergic reactions including angioedema, bronchospasm, pruritus, and urticaria; dizziness, paresthesia; ocular pain, transient myopia, choroidal detachment following filtration surgery, eyelid crusting; dyspnea; contact dermatitis, epistaxis, dry mouth and throat irritation.

Overdosage

Electrolyte imbalance, development of an acidotic state, and possible central nervous system effects may occur. Serum electrolyte levels (particularly potassium) and blood pH levels should be monitored.

Dosage and Administration

The dose is one drop of TRUSOPT Ophthalmic Solution in the affected eyes(s) three times daily.

TRUSOPT may be used concomitantly with other topical ophthalmic drug products to lower intraocular pressure. If more than one topical ophthalmic drug is being used, the drugs should be administered at least ten minutes apart.

How Supplied

TRUSOPT Ophthalmic Solution is a slightly opalescent, nearly colorless, slightly viscous solution.

No. 3519—TRUSOPT Ophthalmic Solution 2% is supplied in OCUMETER®* PLUS container, a white, opaque, plastic ophthalmic dispenser with a controlled drop tip as follows:

NDC 0006-3519-35, 5 mL
NDC 0006-3519-36, 10 mL.

Storage

Store TRUSOPT Ophthalmic Solution at 15–30°C (59–86°F). Protect from light.

---

*Registered trademark of MERCK & CO., Inc.

INSTRUCTIONS FOR USE

Please follow these instructions carefully when using TRUSOPT*. Use TRUSOPT as prescribed by your doctor.

1. If you use other topically applied ophthalmic medications, they should be administered at least 10 minutes before or after TRUSOPT.
2. Wash hands before each use.
3. Before using the medication for the first time, be sure the Safety Strip on the front of the bottle is unbroken. A gap between the bottle and the cap is normal for an unopened bottle.

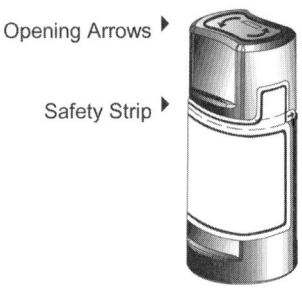

4. Tear off the Safety Strip to break the seal. [See first graphic at top of next page]
5. To open the bottle, unscrew the cap by turning as indicated by the arrows. [See first figure at top of next column]
6. Tilt your head back and pull your lower eyelid down slightly to form a pocket between your eyelid and your eye. [See second figure at top of next column]
7. Invert the bottle, and press lightly with the thumb or index finger over the "Finger Push Area" (as shown) until a single drop is dispensed into the eye as directed by your doctor.

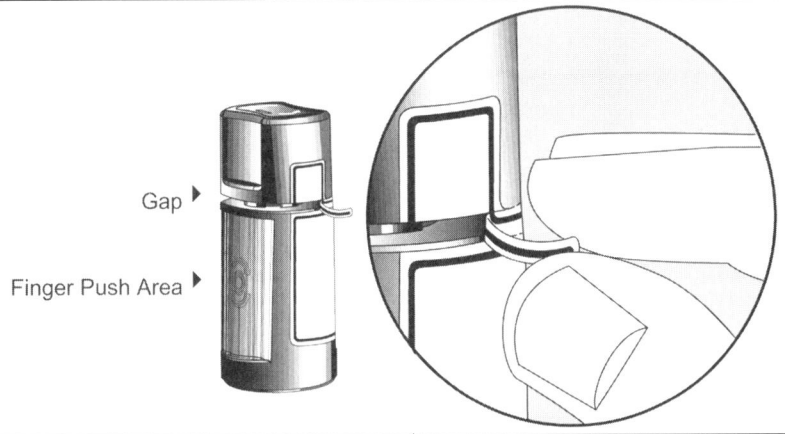

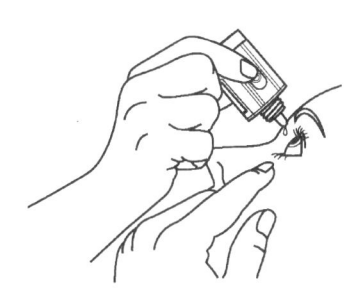

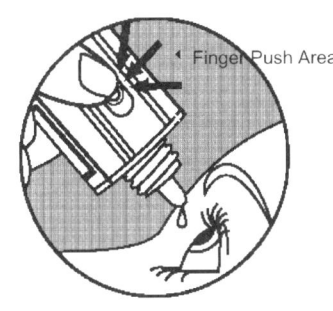

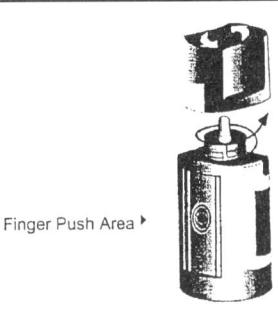

Finger Push Area ▶

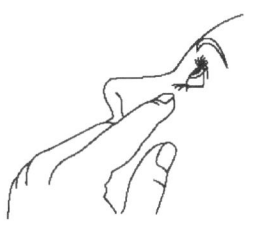

[See second graphic above]
DO NOT TOUCH YOUR EYE OR EYELID WITH THE DROPPER TIP.
Ophthalmic medications, if handled improperly, can become contaminated by common bacteria known to cause eye infections. Serious damage to the eye and subsequent loss of vision may result from using contaminated ophthalmic medications. If you think your medication may be contaminated, or if you develop an eye infection, contact your doctor immediately concerning continued use of this bottle.

8. Repeat steps 6 & 7 with the other eye if instructed to do so by your doctor.
9. Replace the cap by turning until it is firmly touching the bottle. Do not overtighten the cap.
10. The dispenser tip is designed to provide a pre-measured drop; therefore, do NOT enlarge the hole of the dispenser tip.
11. After you have used all doses, there will be some TRUSOPT left in the bottle. You should not be concerned since an extra amount of TRUSOPT has been added and you will get the full amount of TRUSOPT that your doctor prescribed. Do not attempt to remove excess medicine from the bottle.

WARNING: Keep out of reach of children.
If you have any questions about the use of TRUSOPT, please consult your doctor.

*Registered trademark of MERCK & CO., Inc.
Manuf. for:
Merck & Co., Inc., Whitehouse Station, NJ 08889, USA
By: Laboratories Merck Sharp & Dohme-Chibret
    63963 Clermont-Ferrand Cedex 9, France
    9368203   Issued October 2001
COPYRIGHT© MERCK & CO., Inc., 2000
All rights reserved
Shown in Product Identification Guide, page 105

Refer to Section 8 for information on Intraocular Products.

Monarch Pharmaceuticals

Please see King Pharmaceuticals, Inc.

Novartis Pharmaceuticals Corporation
ONE HEALTH PLAZA
EAST HANOVER, NJ 07936

Direct Inquiries to:
Customer Service 888-669-6682
www.novartisophthalmics.com

GENTEAL® MILD   OTC
Lubricant Eye Drops
How Supplied: 15mL, 25mL

GENTEAL®   OTC
Lubricant Eye Drops
How Supplied: 15mL, 25mL

GENTEAL® GEL   OTC
Lubricant Eye Gel
How Supplied: 3.5mL, 10mL

GENTEAL® PF   OTC
Lubricant Eye Drops (Preservative Free)
How Supplied: 36 Single - (0.015 fl. oz. ea.) Use Containers

HYPOTEARS®   OTC
Sterile Lubricant Eye Drops
How Supplied: 15mL, 30mL

HYPOTEARS® PF   OTC
Lubricant Eye Drops (Preservative Free)
How Supplied: 30 Single-Use Containers (0.015 fl. oz. each)

LIVOSTIN® 0.05% (levocabastine HCl ophthalmic suspension)   ℞
How Supplied: 5mL, 10mL

MIOCHOL®-E (acetylcholine chloride intraocular solution) 1:100 with electrolyte diluent   ℞
How Supplied: Miochol®-E System Pak: One Miochol®-E 2mL sterile univial, One pack Novartis Ophthalmics Steri-Tags™ sterile labels, One B-D 3mL sterile syringe, One Dyna Gard™ 0.2 micron sterile filter

VASOCON®-A   OTC
Itching/Redness Reliever Eye Drops
(antazoline phosphate 0.5%, naphazoline hydrochloride 0.05%)
How Supplied: 15mL

VISUDYNE® (verteporfin for injection)   ℞
How Supplied: 15mg, and
Patient Treatment Kit:
3 ea. 12 cc Syringes
1 ea. 30 cc Syringe
1 ea. PCA Extension Set (38.5″)
1 ea. Sterile Acrodisc 1.2 micron filter
1 ea. B-D Intima IV Catheter System with Y adapter (22 ga.)
1 ea. 50mL Dextrose 5% Sterile Solution (D5W)
5 ea. 19 Gauge Needles
6 ea. Alcohol Wipes
1 ea. 20mL Sterile Water for Injection
1 ea. Glasses, Amber Solar Shields
1 ea. Patient Wrist Band
1 ea. Booklet, "A Patient Guide to Visudyne Therapy"
1 ea. Insert, Infusion Line Set-up

VOLTAREN OPHTHALMIC®   ℞
(diclofenac sodium ophthalmic solution) 0.1%
How Supplied: 2.5mL, 5mL

Continued on next page

ZADITOR™ Ketotifen Fumarate ℞
Ophthalmic Solution, 0.025%
How Supplied: 5mL

GENTEAL® Mild	OTC
GENTEAL®	OTC
GENTEAL® Gel	OTC
GENTEAL® PF	OTC

A product for every level of Dry Eye.

GenTeal® Mild, GenTeal®, and GenTeal® Gel contain GenAqua™, a disappearing preservative that turns into pure water and oxygen upon contact with your eye, thereby minimizing the irritation that may be caused by traditional preservatives while still providing the convenience and economy of the multidose form. All you feel is the soothing relief of the moisturizing ingredients, with the added assurance that each drop is as pure as the first.
GenTeal® Mild and GenTeal® are available in 15 and 25mL bottles. Made in Canada for Novartis Pharmaceuticals Corporation, East Hanover, NJ 07936
GenTeal® Gel is a clear lubricant eye gel that liquifies upon contact with your eye, forming a non-blurring, protective film. GenTeal® Gel is available in 3.5 mL and 10 mL tubes. Made in Puerto Rico for Novartis Pharmaceuticals Corporation, East Hanover, NJ07936
GenTeal® PF is a hypotonic and preservative-free solution, specially formulated to be a soothing lubricant. GenTeal® PF is available in a pack of 36 single-use containers 0.105 fl. oz. in each container. Made in Canada for Novartis Pharmaceuticals Corporation, East Hanover NJ 07936

GenTeal® Mild
Active ingredient:
Hypromellose
0.2% .... Lubricant
Inactive Ingredients:
Boric acid, calcium chloride dihydrate, GenAqua™ (sodium perborate), phosphonic acid, potassium chloride, purified water, and sodium chloride
Mild dry eye sufferers may experience gritty sensation, tearing, mild redness, burning, mild itching. These symptoms may be signs of other eye conditions. Consult your eye doctor.
NDC 58768-791-15   NDC 58768-791-25

GenTeal®
Active Ingredient:
Hypromellose
0.3% .... Lubricant
Inactive Ingredients:
Boric acid, GenAqua™ (sodium perborate), phosphonic acid, potassium chloride, purified water, and sodium chloride
Moderate dry eye sufferers may experience irritation, redness, itching, significant burning, and mucous discharge. These symptoms may be signs of other eye conditions. Consult your eye doctor.
NDC 58768-788-15   NDC 58768-788-25

GenTeal® Lubricant Eye Gel
Active Ingredients:
Hypromellose
0.3% .... Lubricant
Inactive Ingredients:
Carbopol 980, GenAqua™ (sodium perborate), phosphonic acid, purified water, sodium hydroxide, and sorbitol
Severe dry eye sufferers may experience pain, persistent redness, blurred vision, severe itching, and frequent mucous discharge. These symptoms may be signs of other eye conditions. Consult your eye doctor.
NDC 58768-790-36   58768-790-35

GenTeal® PF
Active Ingredients:
Hypromellose
0.3% .... Lubricant

Inactive Ingredients:
Boric acid, calcium chloride, magnesium chloride, potassium chloride, purified water, sodium borate, sodium chloride, and zinc sulfate
Convenient single-use containers for mild to moderate dry eye relief.
NDC 58768-789-15

Uses for GenTeal® products:
- Relieves dryness of the eye.
- Temporarily relieves discomfort due to minor irritations of the eye from exposure to wind, sun, or other irritants.
- As a protectant against further irritation.

Warnings:
Do not use if solution or gel changes color or becomes cloudy.
When using GenTeal® Mild, GenTeal®, and GenTeal® Gel do not touch tip of container to any surface. Replace cap after using.
When using GenTeal® PF do not touch tip of container to any surface.
Stop use and ask a doctor if you experience any of the following: eye pain, changes in vision, continued redness or irritation, or if the conditions worsen or persist for more than 72 hours.
Directions for GenTeal® Mild, GenTeal®, and GenTeal® Gel:
Instill 1 or 2 drops in the affected eye(s) as needed.
Directions for GenTeal® PF:
To open, twist the top of the container. Apply 1 to 2 drops as needed in the affected eye(s). Discard container after use.
Other Information:
- Store between 15°–30°C (59°–86°F)
- Keep out of reach of children

Questions? Call 1-866-393-6336
Shown in Product Identification Guide, page 105

VISUDYNE® ℞
(verteporfin for injection)

Description: VISUDYNE® (verteporfin for injection) is a light activated drug used in photodynamic therapy. The finished drug product is a lyophilized dark green cake. Verteporfin is a 1:1 mixture of two regioisomers (I and II), represented by the following structures:

The chemical names for the verteporfin regioisomers are: 9-methyl (I) and 13-methyl (II) trans-(±)-18-ethenyl-4,4a-dihydro-3,4-bis(methoxycarbonyl)-4a,8,14,19-tetramethyl-23H, 25H-benzo[b]porphine-9,13-dipropanoate
The molecular formula is $C_{41}H_{42}N_4O_8$ with a molecular weight of approximately 718.8.
Each mL of reconstituted VISUDYNE contains:
ACTIVE: Verteporfin, 2 mg
INACTIVES: Lactose, egg phosphatidylglycerol, dimyristoyl phosphatidylcholine, ascorbyl palmitate and butylated hydroxytoluene

Clinical Pharmacology:
Mechanism of Action
VISUDYNE therapy is a two-stage process requiring administration of both verteporfin for injection and nonthermal red light.
Verteporfin is transported in the plasma primarily by lipoproteins. Once verteporfin is activated by light in the presence of oxygen, highly reactive, short-lived singlet oxygen and reactive oxygen radicals are generated. Light activation of verteporfin results in local damage to neovascular endothelium, resulting in vessel occlusion. Damaged endothelium is known to release procoagulant and vasoactive factors through the lipo-oxygenase (leukotriene) and cyclo-oxygenase (eicosanoids such as thromboxane) pathways, resulting in platelet aggregation, fibrin clot formation and vasoconstriction. Verteporfin appears to somewhat preferentially accumulate in neovasculature, including choroidal neovasculature. However, animal models indicate that the drug is also present in the retina. Therefore, there may be collateral damage to retinal structures following photoactivation including the retinal pigmented epithelium and outer nuclear layer of the retina. The temporary occlusion of choroidal neovascularization (CNV) following VISUDYNE therapy has been confirmed in humans by fluorescein angiography.

Pharmacokinetics
Following intravenous infusion, verteporfin exhibits a bi-exponential elimination with a terminal elimination half-life of approximately 5–6 hours. The extent of exposure and the maximal plasma concentration are proportional to the dose between 6 and 20 mg/m². At the intended dose, pharmacokinetic parameters are not significantly affected by gender. Verteporfin is metabolized to a small extent to its diacid metabolite by liver and plasma esterases. NADPH-dependent liver enzyme systems (including the cytochrome P450 isozymes) do not appear to play a role in the metabolism of verteporfin. Elimination is by the fecal route, with less than 0.01% of the dose recovered in urine.
In a study of patients with mild hepatic insufficiency (defined as having two abnormal hepatic function tests at enrollment), AUC and C_{max} were not significantly different from the control group, half-life however was significantly increased by approximately 20%.

Clinical Studies
Age-Related Macular Degeneration (AMD)
Two adequate and well-controlled, double-masked, placebo-controlled, randomized studies were conducted in patients with classic-containing subfoveal CNV secondary to age-related macular degeneration. A total of 609 patients (VISUDYNE 402, placebo 207) were enrolled in these two studies. During these studies, retreatment was allowed every 3 months if fluorescein angiograms showed any recurrence or persistence of leakage. The placebo control (sham treatment) consisted of intravenous administration of Dextrose 5% in Water, followed by light application identical to that used for VISUDYNE therapy.
The difference between treatment groups statistically favored VISUDYNE at the 1-year and 2 year analyses for visual acuity endpoints.
The subgroup of patients with predominantly classic CNV lesions was more likely to exhibit a treatment benefit (N=242; VISUDYNE 159, placebo 83). Predominantly classic CNV lesions were defined as those in which the classic component comprised 50% or more of the area of the entire lesion. For the primary efficacy endpoint (percentage of patients who lost less than 3 lines of visual acuity), these patients showed a difference of approximately 25% between treatment groups at both Months 12 and 24 (67% for VISUDYNE patients compared to 40% for placebo patients, at month 12; and 59% for VISUDYNE patients compared to 31% for placebo patients, at Month 24). Severe vision loss (≥6 lines of visual acuity from baseline) was experienced by 12% of VISUDYNE-treated patients compared to 34% of placebo-treated patients at Month 12, and by 15% of VISUDYNE-treated patients compared to 36% of placebo-treated patients at Month 24.
Patients with predominantly classic CNV lesions that did not contain occult CNV exhib-

ited the greatest benefit (N=134; VISUDYNE 90, placebo 44). At 1 year, these patients demonstrated a 49% difference between treatment groups when assessed by the <3 lines-lost definition (77% vs. 27%). Older patients (≥75 years), patients with dark irides, patients with occult lesions or patients with less than 50% classic CNV were less likely to benefit from VISUDYNE therapy.
The safety and efficacy of VISUDYNE beyond 2 years have not been demonstrated.

Pathologic Myopia
One adequate and well-controlled, double-masked, placebo-controlled, randomized study was conducted in patients with subfoveal CNV secondary to pathologic myopia. A total of 120 patients (VISUDYNE 81, placebo 39) were enrolled in the study. The treatment dosing and retreatments were the same as in the AMD studies. The difference between treatment groups statistically favored VISUDYNE at the 1-year analysis but not at the 2-year analysis for visual acuity endpoints. For the primary efficacy endpoint (percentage of patients who lost less than 3 lines of visual acuity), patients at the 1-year time point showed a difference of approximately 19% between treatment groups (86% for VISUDYNE patients compared to 67% for placebo patients). However, by the 2-year timepoint, the effect was no longer statistically significant (79% for VISUDYNE patients compared to 72% for placebo patients).

Presumed Ocular Histoplasmosis
One open-label study was conducted in patients with subfoveal CNV secondary to presumed ocular histoplasmosis. A total of 26 patients were treated with VISUDYNE in the study. The treatment dosing and retreatments for VISUDYNE were the same as in the AMD studies. VISUDYNE-treated patients compare favorably with historical control data demonstrating a reduction in the number of episodes of severe visual acuity loss (>6 lines of loss).

Indications and Usage: VISUDYNE therapy is indicated for the treatment of patients with predominantly classic subfoveal choroidal neovascularization due to age-related macular degeneration, pathologic myopia or presumed ocular histoplasmosis.
There is insufficient evidence to indicate VISUDYNE for the treatment of predominantly occult subfoveal choroidal neovascularization.

Contraindications: VISUDYNE is contraindicated for patients with porphyria or a known hypersensitivity to any component of this preparation.

Warnings: Following injection with VISUDYNE, care should be taken to avoid exposure of skin or eyes to direct sunlight or bright indoor light for 5 days. In the event of extravasation during infusion, the extravasation area must be thoroughly protected from direct light until the swelling and discoloration have faded in order to prevent the occurrence of a local burn which could be severe. If emergency surgery is necessary within 48 hours after treatment, as much of the internal tissue as possible should be protected from intense light.
Patients who experience severe decrease of vision of 4 lines or more within 1 week after treatment should not be retreated, at least until their vision completely recovers to pretreatment levels and the potential benefits and risks of subsequent treatment are carefully considered by the treating physician.
Use of incompatible lasers that do not provide the required characteristics of light for the photoactivation of VISUDYNE could result in incomplete treatment due to partial photoactivation of VISUDYNE, overtreatment due to overactivation of VISUDYNE, or damage to surrounding normal tissue.

Precautions:
General
Standard precautions should be taken during infusion of VISUDYNE to avoid extravasation. Examples of standard precautions include, but are not limited to:
- A free-flowing intravenous (IV) line should be established before starting VISUDYNE infusion and the line should be carefully monitored.
- Due to the possible fragility of vein walls of some elderly patients, it is strongly recommended that the largest arm vein possible, preferably antecubital, be used for injection.
- Small veins in the back of the hand should be avoided.

If extravasation does occur, the infusion should be stopped immediately and cold compresses applied (see Warnings).
VISUDYNE therapy should be considered carefully in patients with moderate to severe hepatic impairment or biliary obstruction since there is no clinical experience with verteporfin in such patients.
There is no clinical data related to the use of VISUDYNE in anesthetized patients. At a >10-fold higher dose given by bolus injection to sedated or anesthetized pigs, verteporfin caused severe hemodynamic effects, including death, probably as a result of complement activation. These effects were diminished or abolished by pretreatment with antihistamine and they were not seen in conscious non-sedated pigs. VISUDYNE resulted in a concentration-dependent increase in complement activation in human blood in vitro. At 10 µg/mL (approximately 5 times the expected plasma concentration in human patients), there was mild to moderate complement activation. At ≥100 µg/mL, there was significant complement activation. Signs [chest pain, syncope, dyspnea, and flushing] consistent with complement activation have been observed in <1% of patients administered VISUDYNE. Patients should be supervised during VISUDYNE infusion.

Information for Patients
Patients who receive VISUDYNE will become temporarily photosensitive after the infusion. Patients should wear a wrist band to remind them to avoid direct sunlight for 5 days. During that period, patients should avoid exposure of unprotected skin, eyes or other body organs to direct sunlight or bright indoor light. Sources of bright light include, but are not limited to, tanning salons, bright halogen lighting and high power lighting used in surgical operating rooms or dental offices. Prolonged exposure to light from light-emitting medical devices such as pulse oximeters should also be avoided for 5 days following VISUDYNE administration.
If treated patients must go outdoors in daylight during the first 5 days after treatment, they should protect all parts of their skin and their eyes by wearing protective clothing and dark sunglasses. UV sunscreens are not effective in protecting against photosensitivity reactions because photoactivation of the residual drug in the skin can be caused by visible light. Patients should not stay in the dark and should be encouraged to expose their skin to ambient indoor light, as it will help inactivate the drug in the skin through a process called photobleaching.

Drug Interactions
Drug interaction studies in humans have not been conducted with VISUDYNE.
Verteporfin is rapidly eliminated by the liver, mainly as unchanged drug. Metabolism is limited and occurs by liver and plasma esterases. Microsomal cytochrome P450 does not appear to play a role in verteporfin metabolism.

Based on the mechanism of action of verteporfin, many drugs used concomitantly could influence the effect of VISUDYNE therapy. Possible examples include the following:
Calcium channel blockers, polymyxin B or radiation therapy could enhance the rate of VISUDYNE uptake by the vascular endothelium. Other photosensitizing agents (e.g., tetracyclines, sulfonamides, phenothiazines, sulfonyl urea hypoglycemic agents, thiazide diuretics and griseofulvin) could increase the potential for skin photosensitivity reactions. Compounds that quench active oxygen species or scavenge radicals, such as dimethyl sulfoxide, β-carotene, ethanol, formate and mannitol, would be expected to decrease VISUDYNE activity. Drugs that decrease clotting, vasoconstriction or platelet aggregation, e.g., thromboxane A_2 inhibitors, could also decrease the efficacy of VISUDYNE therapy.

Carcinogenesis, Mutagenesis, Impairment of Fertility
No studies have been conducted to evaluate the carcinogenic potential of verteporfin.
Photodynamic therapy (PDT) as a class has been reported to result in DNA damage including DNA strand breaks, alkali-labile sites, DNA degradation, and DNA-protein cross links which may result in chromosomal aberrations, sister chromatid exchanges (SCE), and mutations. In addition, other photodynamic therapeutic agents have been shown to increase the incidence of SCE in Chinese hamster ovary (CHO) cells irradiated with visible light and in Chinese hamster lung fibroblasts irradiated with near UV light, increase mutations and DNA-protein cross-linking in mouse L5178 cells, and increase DNA-strand breaks in malignant human cervical carcinoma cells, but not in normal cells. Verteporfin was not evaluated in these latter systems. It is not known how the potential for DNA damage with PDT agents translates into human risk.
No effect on male or female fertility has been observed in rats following intravenous administration of verteporfin for injection up to 10 mg/kg/day (approximately 60- and 40-fold human exposure at 6 mg/m² based on AUC_{inf} in male and female rats, respectively).

Pregnancy
Teratogenic Effects: Pregnancy Category C.
Rat fetuses of dams administered verteporfin for injection intravenously at ≥10 mg/kg/day during organogenesis (approximately 40-fold human exposure at 6 mg/m² based on AUC_{inf} in female rats) exhibited an increase in the incidence of anophthalmia/microphthalmia. Rat fetuses of dams administered 25 mg/kg/day (approximately 125 fold the human exposure at 6 mg/m² based on AUC_{inf} in female rats) had an increased incidence of wavy ribs and anophthalmia/microphthalmia.
In pregnant rabbits, a decrease in body weight gain and food consumption was observed in animals that received verteporfin for injection intravenously at ≥ 10 mg/kg/day during organogenesis. The no observed adverse effect level (NOAEL) for maternal toxicity was 3 mg/kg/day (approximately 7-fold human exposure at 6 mg/m² based on body surface area). There were no teratogenic effects observed in rabbits at doses up to 10 mg/kg/day.
There are no adequate and well-controlled studies in pregnant women. VISUDYNE should be used during pregnancy only if the benefit justifies the potential risk to the fetus.

Nursing Mothers
It is not known whether verteporfin for injection is excreted in human milk. Because many drugs are excreted in human milk, caution should be exercised when VISUDYNE is administered to a woman who is nursing.

Continued on next page

Visudyne—Cont.

Pediatric Use
Safety and effectiveness in pediatric patients have not been established.

Geriatric Use
Approximately 90% of the patients treated with VISUDYNE in the clinical efficacy trials were over the age of 65. A reduced treatment effect was seen with increasing age.

Adverse Reactions: The most frequently reported adverse events to VISUDYNE are injection site reactions (including extravasation and rashes) and visual disturbances (including blurred vision, decreased visual acuity and visual field defects). These events occurred in approximately 10–30% of patients. The following events, listed by Body System, were reported more frequently with VISUDYNE therapy than with placebo therapy and occurred in 1–10% of patients:

Ocular Treatment Site: Blepharitis, cataracts, conjunctivitis/conjunctival injection, dry eyes, ocular itching, severe vision loss with or without subretinal or vitreous hemorrhage

Body as a Whole: Asthenia, back pain (primarily during infusion), fever, flu syndrome, photosensitivity reactions

Cardiovascular: Atrial fibrillation, hypertension, peripheral vascular disorder, varicose veins

Dermatologic: Eczema

Digestive: Constipation, gastrointestinal cancers, nausea

Hemic and Lymphatic: Anemia, white blood cell count decreased, white blood cell count increased

Hepatic: Elevated liver function tests

Metabolic/Nutritional: Albuminuria, creatinine increased

Musculoskeletal: Arthralgia, arthrosis, myasthenia

Nervous System: Hypesthesia, sleep disorder, vertigo

Respiratory: Cough, pharyngitis, pneumonia

Special Senses: Cataracts, decreased hearing, diplopia, lacrimation disorder

Urogenital: Prostatic disorder

Severe vision decrease, equivalent of 4 lines or more, within 7 days after treatment has been reported in 1–5% of patients. Partial recovery of vision was observed in some patients. Photosensitivity reactions usually occurred in the form of skin sunburn following exposure to sunlight. The higher incidence of back pain in the VISUDYNE group occurred primarily during infusion.

The following adverse events have occurred either at low incidence (<1%) during clinical trials or have been reported during the use of VISUDYNE in clinical practice where these events were reported voluntarily from a population of unknown size and frequency of occurrence cannot be determined precisely. They have been chosen for inclusion based on factors such as seriousness, frequency of reporting, possible causal connection to VISUDYNE, or a combination of these factors:

Ocular Treatment Site: Retinal detachment (nonrhegmatogenous), retinal or choroidal vessel nonperfusion

Non-ocular Events: Chest pain and other musculoskeletal pain during infusion, hypersensitivity reactions (which can be severe), syncope, severe allergic reactions with dyspnea and flushing, and vaso-vagal reactions.

Overdosage: Overdose of drug and/or light in the treated eye may result in nonperfusion of normal retinal vessels with the possibility of severe decrease in vision that could be permanent. An overdose of drug will also result in the prolongation of the period during which the patient remains photosensitive to bright light. In such cases, it is recommended to extend the photosensitivity precautions for a time proportional to the overdose.

Dosage and Administration: A course of VISUDYNE therapy is a two-step process requiring administration of both drug and light. The first step is the intravenous infusion of VISUDYNE. The second step is the activation of VISUDYNE with light from a nonthermal diode laser.

The physician should re-evaluate the patient every 3 months and if choroidal neovascular leakage is detected on fluorescein angiography, therapy should be repeated.

Lesion Size Determination
The greatest linear dimension (GLD) of the lesion is estimated by fluorescein angiography and color fundus photography. All classic and occult CNV, blood and/or blocked fluorescence, and any serous detachments of the retinal pigment epithelium should be included for this measurement. Fundus cameras with magnification within the range of 2.4–2.6X are recommended. The GLD of the lesion on the fluorescein angiogram must be corrected for the magnification of the fundus camera to obtain the GLD of the lesion of the retina.

Spot Size Determination
The treatment spot size should be 1000 microns larger than the GLD of the lesion on the retina to allow a 500 micron border, ensuring full coverage of the lesion. The maximum spot size used in the clinical trials was 6400 microns.

The nasal edge of the treatment spot must be positioned at least 200 microns from the temporal edge of the optic disc, even if this will result in lack of photoactivation of CNV within 200 microns of the optic nerve.

VISUDYNE Administration
Reconstitute each vial of VISUDYNE with 7 mL of sterile Water for Injection to provide 7.5 mL containing 2 mg/mL. Reconstituted VISUDYNE should be protected from light and used within 4 hours. It is recommended that reconstituted VISUDYNE be inspected visually for particulate matter and discoloration prior to administration. Reconstituted VISUDYNE is an opaque dark green solution. The volume of reconstituted VISUDYNE required to achieve the desired dose of 6 mg/m^2 body surface area is withdrawn from the vial and diluted with 5% Dextrose for Injection to a total infusion volume of 30 mL. The full infusion volume is administered intravenously over 10 minutes at a rate of 3 mL/minute, using an appropriate syringe pump and in-line filter. The clinical studies were conducted using a standard infusion line filter of 1.2 microns. Precautions should be taken to prevent extravasation at the injection site. If extravasation occurs, protect the site from light (See Precautions).

Light Administration
Initiate 689 nm wavelength laser light delivery to the patient 15 minutes after the start of the 10-minute infusion with VISUDYNE.

Photoactivation of VISUDYNE is controlled by the total light dose delivered. In the treatment of choroidal neovascularization, the recommended light dose is 50 J/cm^2 of neovascular lesion administered at an intensity of 600 mW/cm^2. This dose is administered over 83 seconds.

Light dose, light intensity, ophthalmic lens magnification factor and zoom lens setting are important parameters for the appropriate delivery of light to the predetermined treatment spot. Follow the laser system manuals for procedure set up and operation.

The laser system must deliver a stable power output at a wavelength of 689±3 nm. Light is delivered to the retina as a single circular spot via a fiber optic and a slit lamp, using a suitable ophthalmic magnification lens.

The following laser systems have been tested for compatibility with VISUDYNE and are approved for delivery of a stable power output at a wavelength of 689±3 nm:

Coherent Opal Photoactivator laser console and modified Coherent LaserLink adapter, Manufactured by Lumenis, Inc., Santa Clara, CA

Zeiss VISULAS 690s laser and VISULINK PDT/U adapter, Manufactured by Carl Zeiss Inc., Thornwood, NY

Concurrent Bilateral Treatment
The controlled trials only allowed treatment of one eye per patient. In patients who present with eligible lesions in both eyes, physicians should evaluate the potential benefits and risks of treating both eyes concurrently. If the patient has already received previous VISUDYNE therapy in one eye with an acceptable safety profile, both eyes can be treated concurrently after a single administration of VISUDYNE. The more aggressive lesion should be treated first, at 15 minutes after the start of infusion. Immediately at the end of light application to the first eye, the laser settings should be adjusted to introduce the treatment parameters for the second eye, with the same light dose and intensity as for the first eye, starting no later than 20 minutes from the start of infusion.

In patients who present for the first time with eligible lesions in both eyes without prior VISUDYNE therapy, it is prudent to treat only one eye (the most aggressive lesion) at the first course. One week after the first course, if no significant safety issues are identified, the second eye can be treated using the same treatment regimen after a second VISUDYNE infusion. Approximately 3 months later, both eyes can be evaluated and concurrent treatment following a new VISUDYNE infusion can be started if both lesions still show evidence of leakage.

How Supplied: VISUDYNE is supplied in a single use glass vial with a gray bromobutyl stopper and aluminum flip-off cap. It contains a lyophilized cake with 15 mg verteporfin. The product is intended for intravenous injection only.

A Patient Treatment Kit contains three 12 cc Syringes, one 30 cc Syringe, one PCA Extension Set (38.5″), one Sterile Acrodisc 1.2 micron filter, one B-D Intima IV Catheter System with Y adapter (22 ga.), one 50 mL Dextrose 5% Sterile Solution (D5W), five 19 Gauge Needles, six Alcohol Wipes, one 20 mL Sterile Water for Injection, one Glasses, Amber Solar Shields, one Patient Wrist Band, one Booklet, "A Patient Guide to Visudyne Therapy", one Insert, Infusion Line Set-up.

Spills and Disposal
Spills of VISUDYNE should be wiped up with a damp cloth. Skin and eye contact should be avoided due to the potential for photosensitivity reactions upon exposure to light. Use of rubber gloves and eye protection is recommended. All materials should be disposed of properly.

Accidental Exposure
Because of the potential to induce photosensitivity reactions, it is important to avoid contact with the eyes and skin during preparation and administration of VISUDYNE. Any exposed person must be protected from bright light (See Warnings).

NDC 58768-150-15

Store VISUDYNE between 20°C and 25°C (68°F–77°F).

℞ Only

Manufactured by: Parkedale Pharmaceuticals, Inc., Rochester, MI 48307

or Cardinal Health
Albuquerque, NM 87107

For: QLT PhotoTherapeutics Inc., Seattle, WA 98101

Co-developed and Distributed by:
Novartis Pharmaceuticals Corporation, East Hanover NJ 07936
Effective: April, 2003
I6154E

Shown in Product Identification Guide, page 105

VOLTAREN OPHTHALMIC® ℞
(diclofenac sodium ophthalmic solution) 0.1%
Sterile Ophthalmic Solution

Prescribing Information:

Description: Voltaren Ophthalmic (diclofenac sodium ophthalmic solution) 0.1% solution is a sterile, topical, nonsteroidal, anti-inflammatory product for ophthalmic use. Diclofenac sodium is designated chemically as 2-[(2,6-dichlorophenyl)amino] benzeneacetic acid, monosodium salt, with an empirical formula of $C_{14}H_{10}Cl_2NO_2Na$. The structural formula of diclofenac sodium is:

Voltaren Ophthalmic is available as a sterile solution which contains diclofenac sodium 0.1% (1 mg/mL).

Inactive Ingredients: polyoxyl 35 castor oil, Boric acid, tromethamine, sorbic acid (2 mg/mL), edetate disodium (1 mg/mL), and purified water.

Diclofenac sodium is a faintly yellow-white to light-beige, slightly hygroscopic crystalline powder. It is freely soluble in methanol, sparingly soluble in water, very slightly soluble in acetonitrile, and insoluble in chloroform and in 0.1N hydrochloric acid. Its molecular weight is 318.14. Voltaren Ophthalmic 0.1% is an iso-osmotic solution with an osmolality of about 300 mOsmol/1000 g, buffered at approximately pH 7.2. Voltaren Ophthalmic solution has a faint characteristic odor of castor oil.

Clinical Pharmacology:
Pharmacodynamics
Diclofenac sodium is one of a series of phenylacetic acids that has demonstrated anti-inflammatory and analgesic properties in pharmacological studies. It is thought to inhibit the enzyme cyclooxygenase, which is essential in the biosynthesis of prostaglandins.

Animal Studies
Prostaglandins have been shown in many animal models to be mediators of certain kinds of intraocular inflammation. In studies performed in animal eyes, prostaglandins have been shown to produce disruption of the blood-aqueous humor barrier, vasodilation, increased vascular permeability, leukocytosis, and increased intraocular pressure.

Pharmacokinetics
Results from a bioavailability study established that plasma levels of diclofenac following ocular instillation of two drops of Voltaren Ophthalmic to each eye were below the limit of quantification (10 ng/mL) over a 4-hour period. This study suggests that limited, if any, systemic absorption occurs with Voltaren Ophthalmic.

Clinical Trials:
Postoperative Anti-Inflammatory Effects:
In two double-masked, controlled, efficacy studies of postoperative inflammation, a total of 206 cataract patients were treated with Voltaren Ophthalmic and 103 patients were treated with vehicle placebo. Voltaren Ophthalmic was favored over vehicle placebo over a 2-week period for the clinical assessments of inflammation as measured by anterior chamber cells and flare.

In double-masked, controlled studies of corneal refractive surgery (radial keratotomy (RK) and laser photorefractive keratectomy (PRK)) patients were treated with Voltaren Ophthalmic and/or vehicle placebo. The efficacy of Voltaren Ophthalmic given before and shortly after surgery was favored over vehicle placebo during the 6-hour period following surgery for the clinical assessments of pain and photophobia. Patients were permitted to use a hydrogel soft contact lens with Voltaren Ophthalmic for up to three days after PRK.

Indications and Usage: Voltaren Ophthalmic is indicated for the treatment of postoperative inflammation in patients who have undergone cataract extraction and for the temporary relief of pain and photophobia in patients undergoing corneal refractive surgery.

Contraindications: Voltaren Ophthalmic is contraindicated in patients who are hypersensitive to any component of the medication.

Warnings: The refractive stability of patients undergoing corneal refractive procedures and treated with Voltaren has not been established. Patients should be monitored for a year following use in this setting.

With some nonsteroidal anti-inflammatory drugs, there exists the potential for increased bleeding time due to interference with thrombocyte aggregation. There have been reports that ocularly applied nonsteroidal anti-inflammatory drugs can cause increased bleeding of ocular tissues (including hyphemas) in conjunction with ocular surgery.

There is the potential for cross-sensitivity to acetylsalicylic acid, phenylacetic acid derivatives, and other nonsteroidal anti-inflammatory agents. Therefore, caution should be used when treating individuals who have previously exhibited sensitivities to these drugs.

Precautions:
General
All topical nonsteroidal anti-inflammatory drugs (NSAIDs) may slow or delay healing. Topical corticosteroids are also known to slow or delay healing. Concomitant use of topical NSAIDs and topical steroids may increase the potential for healing problems.

Use of topical NSAIDs may result in keratitis. In some susceptible patients continued use of topical NSAIDs may result in epithelial breakdown, corneal thinning, corneal infiltrates, corneal erosion, corneal ulceration, and corneal perforation. These events may be sight threatening. Patients with evidence of corneal epithelial breakdown should immediately discontinue use of topical NSAIDs and should be closely monitored for corneal health.

Postmarketing experience with topical NSAIDs suggests that patients experiencing complicated ocular surgeries, corneal denervation, corneal epithelial defects, diabetes mellitus, ocular surface disease (e.g., dry eye syndrome), rheumatoid arthritis, or repeat ocular surgeries within a short period-of-time may be at increased risk for corneal adverse events, which may become sight threatening. Topical NSAIDs should be used with caution in these patients.

Postmarketing experience with topical NSAIDs also suggests that use more than 24 hours prior to surgery or use beyond 14 days post surgery may increase patient risk for occurrence and severity of corneal adverse events.

It is recommended that Voltaren Ophthalmic, like other NSAIDs, be used with caution in patients with known bleeding tendencies or who are receiving other medications which may prolong bleeding time.

Results from clinical studies indicate that Voltaren Ophthalmic has no significant effect upon ocular pressure. However, elevations in intraocular pressure may occur following cataract surgery.

Information for Patients
Except for the use of a bandage hydrogel soft contact lens during the first 3 days following refractive surgery, Voltaren Ophthalmic should not be used by patients currently wearing soft contact lenses due to adverse events that have occurred in other circumstances.

Carcinogenesis, Mutagenesis, Impairment of Fertility
Long-term carcinogenicity studies in rats given Voltaren in oral doses up to 2 mg/kg/day (approximately 500 times the human oral dose) revealed no significant increases in tumor incidence. A 2-year carcinogenicity study conducted in mice employing oral Voltaren up to 2 mg/kg/day did not reveal any oncogenic potential. Voltaren did not show mutagenic potential in various mutagenicity studies including the Ames test. Voltaren administered to male and female rats at 4 mg/kg/day (approximately 1000 times the human ophthalmic dose) did not affect fertility.

Geriatric Use:
No overall differences in safety or effectiveness have been observed between elderly and younger adult patients.

PREGNANCY:
Teratogenic Effects
Pregnancy Category C. Reproduction studies performed in mice at oral doses up to 5,000 times (20 mg/kg/day) and in rats and rabbits at oral doses up to 2,500 times (10 mg/kg/day) the human topical dose have revealed no evidence of teratogenicity due to Voltaren despite the induction of maternal toxicity and fetal toxicity. In rats, maternally toxic doses were associated with dystocia, prolonged gestation, reduced fetal weights and growth, and reduced fetal survival. Voltaren has been shown to cross the placental barrier in mice and rats.

There are, however, no adequate and well-controlled studies in pregnant women. Because animal reproduction studies are not always predictive of human response, this drug should be used during pregnancy only if clearly needed.

Non-teratogenic Effects
Because of the known effects of prostaglandin biosynthesis-inhibiting drugs on the fetal cardiovascular system (closure of ductus arteriosus), the use of Voltaren Ophthalmic during late pregnancy should be avoided.

Pediatric Use
Safety and effectiveness in pediatric patients have not been established.

Adverse Reactions:
Clinical Practice: The following events have been identified during postmarketing use of topical diclofenac sodium ophthalmic solution, 0.1% in clinical practice. Because they are reported voluntarily from a population of unknown size, estimates of frequency cannot be made. The events, which have been chosen for inclusion due to their seriousness, frequency of reporting, possible causal connection to topical diclofenac sodium ophthalmic solution, 0.1%, or a combination of these factors, include corneal erosion, corneal infiltrates, corneal perforation, corneal thinning, corneal ulceration, epithelial breakdown, and superficial punctate keratitis, (see **Precautions, General**)

Ocular: Transient burning and stinging were reported in approximately 15% of patients across studies with the use of Voltaren Ophthalmic. In cataract surgery studies, keratitis was reported in up to 28% of patients receiving Voltaren Ophthalmic, although in many of these cases keratitis was initially noted prior to the initiation of treatment. Elevated intraocular pressure following cataract surgery was reported in approximately 15% of patients undergoing cataract surgery. Lacrimation complaints were reported in approxi-

Continued on next page

Voltaren—Cont.

mately 30% of case studies undergoing incisional refractive surgery.
The following adverse reactions were reported in approximately 5% or less of the patients: abnormal vision, acute elevated IOP, blurred vision, conjunctivitis, corneal deposits, corneal edema, corneal opacity, corneal lesions, discharge, eyelid swelling, injection, iritis, irritation, itching, lacrimation disorder and ocular allergy.

Systemic: The following adverse reactions were reported in 3% or less of the patients: abdominal pain, asthenia, chills, dizziness, facial edema, fever, headache, insomnia, nausea, pain, rhinitis, viral infection, and vomiting.

Overdosage: Overdosage will not ordinarily cause acute problems. If Voltaren Ophthalmic is accidentally ingested, fluids should be taken to dilute the medication.

Dosage and Administration:
Cataract Surgery: One drop of Voltaren Ophthalmic should be applied to the affected eye, 4 times daily beginning 24 hours after cataract surgery and continuing throughout the first 2 weeks of the post operative period.

Corneal Refractive Surgery: One or two drops of Voltaren Ophthalmic should be applied to the operative eye within the hour prior to corneal refractive surgery. Within 15 minutes after surgery, one or two drops should be applied to the operative eye and continued 4 times daily for up to 3 days.

How Supplied: Voltaren Ophthalmic 0.1% (1 mg/mL) Sterile Solution is supplied in a low density polyethylene (LDPE) white bottle with a LDPE Dropper Tip and Polypropylene grey closure. The 2.5 mL fill is supplied in a 7.5 mL size bottle. The 5.0 mL fill is supplied in a 10.0 mL size bottle.

Bottles of 2.5 mL   NDC 58768-100-02
Bottles of 5 mL   NDC 58768-100-05
Store at 15° to 25°C (59° to 77°F). Protect from light.
Dispense in original, unopened container only.
R Only
Printed in Canada
Made in Canada. Manufactured for:
Novartis Ophthalmics, Duluth, Georgia 30097
NOVARTIS   CS 665635G
September 2003

ZADITOR™   R
Ketotifen Fumarate
Ophthalmic Solution, 0.025%

Description: ZADITOR™ is a sterile ophthalmic solution containing ketotifen for topical administration to the eyes. Ketotifen fumarate is a finely crystalline powder with an empirical formula of $C_{23}H_{23}NO_5S$ and a molecular weight of 425.50.

Established Name: ketotifen fumarate ophthalmic solution
Chemical Name:
4-(1-Methyl-4-piperidylidene)-4H-benzo[4,5] cyclohepta[1,2-b] thiophen-10(9H)-one hydrogen fumarate
Each mL of ZADITOR™ contains:
Active: 0.345 mg ketotifen fumarate equivalent to 0.25 mg ketotifen.

Inactives: glycerol, sodium hydroxide/hydrochloric acid (to adjust pH) and purified water.
Preservative: benzalkonium chloride 0.01%. It has a pH of 4.4 to 5.8 and an osmolality of 210–300 mOsm/kg.

Clinical Pharmacology: Ketotifen is a relatively selective, non-competitive histamine antagonist (H1-receptor) and mast cell stabilizer. Ketotifen inhibits the release of mediators from cells involved in hypersensitivity reactions. Decreased chemotaxis and activation of eosinophils has also been demonstrated.
Ketotifen has been shown to have little systemic exposure following topical ocular administration. A study conducted with 15 healthy volunteers dosed bilaterally with ketotifen fumarate ophthalmic solution twice daily for 14 days demonstrated plasma concentrations generally below the quantitation limit of assay (< 20 pg/mL).
In human conjunctival allergen challenge studies, ZADITOR™ was significantly more effective than placebo in preventing ocular itching associated with allergic conjunctivitis. The action of ketotifen occurs rapidly with an effect seen within minutes after administration.

Indications and Usage: ZADITOR™ (ketotifen fumarate ophthalmic solution) is indicated for the temporary prevention of itching of the eye due to allergic conjunctivitis.

Contraindications: ZADITOR™ is contraindicated in persons with a known hypersensitivity to any component of this product.

Warnings: For topical ophthalmic use only. Not for injection or oral use.

Precautions: Information for Patients: To prevent contaminating the dropper tip and solution, care should be taken not to touch the eyelids or surrounding areas with the dropper tip of the bottle. Keep the bottle tightly closed when not in use. Patients should be advised not to wear a contact lens if their eye is red. ZADITOR™ should not be used to treat contact lens related irritation. The preservative in ZADITOR™, benzalkonium chloride, may be absorbed by soft contact lenses. Patients who wear soft contact lenses and whose eyes are not red, should be instructed to wait at least ten minutes after instilling ZADITOR™ before they insert their contact lenses.

Carcinogenesis, Mutagenesis, Impairment of Fertility: Ketotifen fumarate was determined to be non-mutagenic in a battery of *in vitro* and *in vivo* mutagenicity assays including: Ames test, *in vitro* chromosomal aberration test with V79 Chinese hamster cells, *in vivo* micronucleus assay in mouse, and mouse dominant lethal test.

Treatment of male rats with oral doses of ketotifen ≥ 10 mg/kg/day orally [6,667 times the maximum recommended human ocular dose of 0.0015 mg/kg/day on a mg/kg basis (MRHOD)] for 70 days prior to mating resulted in mortality and a decrease in fertility. Treatment with ketotifen did not impair fertility in female rats receiving up to 50 mg/kg/day of ketotifen orally (33,333 times the MRHOD) for 15 days prior to mating.

Pregnancy: Pregnancy Category C
Oral treatment of pregnant rabbits during organogenesis with 45 mg/kg/day of ketotifen (30,000 times the MRHOD) resulted in an increased incidence of retarded ossification of the sternebrae. However, no effects were observed in rabbits treated with up to 15 mg/kg/day (10,000 times the MRHOD). Similar treatment of rats during organogenesis with 100 mg/kg/day of ketotifen (66,667 times the MRHOD) did not reveal any biologically relevant effects.
Oral treatment of pregnant rats (up to 100 mg/kg/day or 66,667 times the MRHOD) and rabbits (up to 45 mg/kg/day or 30,000 times the MRHOD) during organogenesis did not result in any biologically relevant embryofetal toxicity. In the offspring of the rats that received ketotifen orally from day 15 of pregnancy to day 21 post partum at 50 mg/kg/day (33,333 times the MRHOD), a maternally toxic treatment protocol, the incidence of postnatal mortality was slightly increased, and body weight gain during the first four days post partum was slightly decreased.

Nursing Mothers: Ketotifen fumarate has been identified in breast milk in rats following oral administration. It is not known whether topical ocular administration could result in sufficient systemic absorption to produce detectable quantities in breast milk. Nevertheless, caution should be exercised when ketotifen fumarate is administered to a nursing mother.

Pediatric Use: Safety and effectiveness in pediatric patients below the age of 3 years have not been established.

Adverse Reactions: In controlled clinical studies, conjunctival injection, headaches, and rhinitis were reported at an incidence of 10 to 25%. The occurrence of these side effects was generally mild. Some of these events were similar to the underlying ocular disease being studied.
The following ocular and non-ocular adverse reactions were reported at an incidence of less than 5%:

Ocular: Allergic reactions, burning or stinging, conjunctivitis, discharge, dry eyes, eye pain, eyelid disorder, itching, keratitis, lacrimation disorder, mydriasis, photophobia, and rash.

Non-Ocular: Flu syndrome, pharyngitis.

Overdosage: Oral ingestion of the contents of a 5 mL bottle would be equivalent to 1.725 mg of ketotifen fumarate. Clinical results have shown no serious signs or symptoms after the ingestion of up to 20 mg of ketotifen fumarate.

Dosage and Administration: The recommended dose is one drop in the affected eye(s) twice daily, every 8 to 12 hours.

How Supplied: NDC 58768-102-05
ZADITOR™ 5 mL is supplied in a white Polypropylene (PP) 7.5 cc container with a PP dropper tip and closure.

Storage: Store at 4°–25°C (39°–77°F).
R Only   October, 2002
Made in Canada by CIBA Vision Sterile Mfg. for
Novartis Pharmaceuticals Corporation
East Hanover, NJ 07936
I6137-E

Shown in Product Identification Guide, page 106

Pfizer Consumer Healthcare

Pfizer Inc
182 TABOR ROAD
MORRIS PLAINS, NJ 07950
ATTN: CONSUMER AFFAIRS

Direct Inquiries to:
Consumer Affairs
1-800-223-0182

VISINE® ADVANCED RELIEF   OTC
Lubricant/Redness Reliever Eye Drops
Redness & Irritation Relief

Description: Visine Advanced Relief is a unique eye drop formulation that combines the proven redness-relieving power of Visine with the additional benefit of three moisturizing ingredients that cool, soothe and refresh irritated eyes fast.
Visine Advanced Relief combines the redness reliever, tetrahydrozoline hydrochloride with the demulcents, polyethylene glycol 400, povidone, and dextran 70. The redness reliever

provides symptomatic relief of conjunctival hyperemia secondary to minor irritations, while the demulcents provide effective lubrication and protection against further irritation.

Active Ingredients: **Purpose:**
Dextran 70 0.1% .... Lubricant
Polyethylene glycol 400 1% .... Lubricant
Povidone 1% .... Lubricant
Tetrahydrozoline
  HCl 0.05% .... Redness reliever

Uses:
- for the relief of redness of the eye due to minor eye irritations
- for use as a protectant against further irritation or to relieve dryness of the eye

Warnings:
Ask a doctor before use if you have narrow angle glaucoma
When using this product
- pupils may become enlarged temporarily
- overuse may cause more eye redness
- remove contact lenses before using
- do not use if this solution changes color or becomes cloudy
- do not touch tip of container to any surface to avoid contamination
- replace cap after each use

Stop use and ask a doctor if
- you feel eye pain
- changes in vision occur
- redness or irritation of the eye lasts
- condition worsens or lasts more than 72 hours

If pregnant or breast-feeding, ask a health professional before use.
Keep out of reach of children. If swallowed, get medical help or contact a Poison Control Center right away.
Directions:
- put 1 or 2 drops in the affected eye(s) up to 4 times daily
- children under 6 years of age: ask a doctor

Other Information:
- store at 15° to 25°C (59° to 77°F)

Inactive Ingredients: benzalkonium chloride, boric acid, edetate disodium, purified water, sodium borate, and sodium chloride

Shown in Product Identification Guide, page 105

VISINE-A® OTC
Antihistamine & Redness Reliever Eye Drops
Eye Allergy Relief

Description: Visine-A® is an antihistamine/redness reliever eye drop, formerly available by prescription only, that provides temporary relief of itchy, red eyes due to pollen, ragweed, grass, animal hair and dander.

Active Ingredients: **Purpose:**
Naphazoline
  hydrochloride 0.025% .... Redness reliever
Pheniramine maleate 0.3% ..... Antihistamine
Uses: temporarily relieves itchy, red eyes due to:
- pollen • ragweed • grass • animal hair and dander

Warnings:
Do not use
- if you are sensitive to any ingredient in this product

Ask a doctor before use if you have
- heart disease
- high blood pressure
- narrow angle glaucoma
- trouble urinating due to an enlarged prostate gland

When using this product
- pupils may become enlarged temporarily
- do not touch tip of container to any surface to avoid contamination
- replace cap after each use
- remove contact lenses before using
- do not use if this solution changes color or becomes cloudy
- overuse may cause more eye redness

Stop use and ask a doctor if
- you feel eye pain
- changes in vision occur
- redness or irritation of the eye lasts
- condition worsens or lasts more than 72 hours

Keep out of reach of children. If swallowed, get medical help or contact a Poison Control Center right away. Accidental swallowing by infants and children may lead to coma and marked reduction in body temperature.

Directions:
- adults and children 6 years of age and over: put 1 or 2 drops in the affected eye(s) up to 4 times a day
- children under 6 years of age: consult a doctor

Other Information:
- some users may experience a brief tingling sensation
- store between 15° and 25°C (59° and 77°F)

Inactive Ingredients: boric acid and sodium borate buffer system preserved with benzalkonium chloride (0.01%) and edetate disodium (0.1%), sodium hydroxide and/or hydrochloric acid (to adjust pH), and purified water.

Shown in Product Identification Guide, page 106

VISINE A.C.® OTC
Astringent/Redness Reliever Eye Drops
Seasonal Itching & Redness Relief

Description: Visine A.C. is a sterile, isotonic, buffered ophthalmic solution containing tetrahydrozoline hydrochloride and zinc sulfate. Visine A.C. is a fast-acting, dual-action ophthalmic solution combining the redness reliever, tetrahydrozoline hydrochloride, with the astringent, zinc sulfate. The redness reliever provides temporary relief of conjunctival hyperemia while the astringent helps to relieve itching, burning, watery eyes due to pollen, dust and ragweed.

Active Ingredients: **Purpose:**
Tetrahydrozoline HCl 0.05% . Redness reliever
Zinc sulfate 0.25% .... Astringent
Use:
- for temporary relief of discomfort and redness of the eye due to minor eye irritations

Warnings:
Ask a doctor before use if you have narrow angle glaucoma
When using this product
- pupils may become enlarged temporarily
- overuse may cause more eye redness
- remove contact lenses before using
- do not use if this solution changes color or becomes cloudy
- do not touch tip of container to any surface to avoid contamination
- replace cap after each use

Stop use and ask a doctor if
- you feel eye pain
- changes in vision occur
- redness or irritation of the eye lasts
- condition worsens or lasts more than 72 hours

If pregnant or breast feeding, ask a health professional before use.
Keep out of reach of children. If swallowed, get medical help or contact a Poison Control Center right away.
Directions:
- put 1 or 2 drops in the affected eye(s) up to 4 times daily
- children under 6 years of age: ask a doctor

Other Information:
- some users may experience a brief tingling sensation
- store at 15° to 25°C (59° to 77°F)

Inactive Ingredients: benzalkonium chloride, boric acid, edetate disodium, purified water; sodium chloride, and sodium citrate

Shown in Product Identification Guide, page 105

VISINE FOR CONTACTS® OTC
Lubricating & Rewetting Drops
Contact Lens Relief

Description: Visine For Contacts Lubricating & Rewetting Drops is for use while wearing daily and extended wear soft (hydrophilic) contact lenses. It refreshes eyes, moistens your lenses and helps remove particulate matter that can cause irritation and discomfort.
Contains: Visine For Contacts Lubricating & Rewetting Drops is a sterile, isotonic solution with a borate buffer system, hypromellose and glycerin, with potassium sorbate and edetate disodium as the preservatives.
Indications (Uses): Visine For Contacts Lubricating & Rewetting Drops may be used with daily and extended wear soft (hydrophilic) contact lenses for the following:
- Moistening of daily wear soft lenses while on the eyes during the day
- Moistening of extended wear soft lenses upon awakening and as needed during the day
- Moistening of extended wear soft lenses prior to retiring at night

Contraindications (Reasons Not To Use): Patients allergic to any ingredient in Visine For Contacts Lubricating & Rewetting Drops should not use this product.
Warnings:
- PROBLEMS WITH CONTACT LENSES AND LENS CARE PRODUCTS COULD RESULT IN SERIOUS INJURY TO THE EYE. It is essential that you follow your eye care professional's direction and all labeling instructions for proper use of your lenses and lens care products. EYE PROBLEMS, INCLUDING CORNEAL ULCERS, CAN DEVELOP RAPIDLY AND LEAD TO LOSS OF VISION; THEREFORE, IF YOU EXPERIENCE EYE DISCOMFORT, EXCESSIVE TEARING, VISION CHANGES, REDNESS OF THE EYE, IMMEDIATELY REMOVE YOUR LENSES AND PROMPTLY CONTACT YOUR EYE CARE PROFESSIONAL.
- All contact lens wearers must see their eye care professionals as directed. If your lenses are for extended wear, your eye care professional may prescribe more frequent visits.
- Never touch the dropper tip of the container to any surface, since this may contaminate the solution. If drops turn yellow, do not use and discard immediately. Replace cap after every use.

Directions: Visine For Contacts Lubricating & Rewetting Drops may be used as needed throughout the day. If minor irritation, discomfort or blurring occurs while wearing lenses, place 1 or 2 drops on the eye and blink 2 or 3 times. If discomfort continues, immediately remove lenses and immediately see your eye care professional.
Precautions:
- Always wash and rinse your hands before handling your lenses
- Store at room temperature
- Keep container tightly closed when not in use
- Use before the expiration date marked on the container and carton
- Keep this and all medications out of the reach of children

Adverse Reactions (Problems and What To Do): The following problems may occur while wearing contact lenses:

Continued on next page

Visine for Contacts—Cont.

- Eyes stinging, burning or itching (irritation)
- Excessive watering (tearing) of the eyes
- Unusual eye secretions
- Redness of the eyes
- Reduced sharpness of vision (visual acuity)
- Blurred vision
- Sensitivity to light (photophobia)
- Dry eyes

If you notice any of the above problems, immediately remove and examine your lenses. If the problem stops and the lenses appear to be undamaged, thoroughly clean, rinse and disinfect the lenses and reinsert them. If the problem continues or a lens appears to be damaged, IMMEDIATELY remove your lenses and IMMEDIATELY consult your eye care professional. **Do not reinsert a damaged lens.**

If any of the above symptoms occur, a serious condition such as infection, corneal ulcer, neovascularization or iritis may be present. Seek immediate professional identification of the problem and treatment to avoid serious eye damage.

Storage: Store between 15° and 25°C (59° and 77°F)

How Supplied: Visine For Contacts Lubricating & Rewetting Drops is produced through a process that ensures sterility and supplied in a 0.5 fl. oz. and 1 fl. oz. plastic bottles. The container and carton are marked with a lot number and expiration date.

Shown in Product Identification Guide, page 106

VISINE L.R.® OTC
Redness Reliever Eye Drops
Long Lasting Redness Relief

Description: Visine L.R. is a sterile, isotonic, buffered ophthalmic solution containing the redness reliever oxymetazoline hydrochloride. Visine L.R. is specifically formulated to relieve redness of the eye in minutes with effective relief that lasts up to 6 hours.

Active Ingredient: **Purpose:**
Oxymetazoline
HCl 0.025% .... Redness reliever

Use:
- for the relief of redness of the eye due to minor eye irritations

Warnings:
Ask a doctor before use if you have narrow angle glaucoma

When using this product
- overuse may cause more eye redness
- remove contact lenses before using
- do not use if this solution changes color or becomes cloudy
- do not touch tip of container to any surface to avoid contamination
- replace cap after each use

Stop use and ask a doctor if
- you feel eye pain
- changes in vision occur
- redness or irritation of the eye lasts
- condition worsens or lasts more than 72 hours

If pregnant or breast-feeding, ask a health professional before use.

Keep out of reach of children. If swallowed, get medical help or contact a Poison Control Center right away.

Directions:
- adults and children 6 years of age and over: put 1 or 2 drops in the affected eye(s)
- this may be repeated as needed every 6 hours or as directed by a doctor
- children under 6 years of age: ask a doctor

Other Information:
- store at 15° to 25°C (59° to 77°F)

Inactive Ingredients: benzalkonium chloride, boric acid, edetate disodium, purified water, sodium borate, and sodium chloride

Shown in Product Identification Guide, page 105

VISINE® ORIGINAL OTC
Redness Reliever Eye Drops
Redness Relief

Description: Visine Original is a redness reliever eye drop that gives fast relief of redness of the eye due to minor eye irritation caused by smoke, dust, other airborne pollutants and swimming.

Visine Original is a sterile, isotonic, buffered ophthalmic solution containing tetrahydrozoline hydrochloride. The effectiveness of Visine in relieving conjunctival hyperemia has been demonstrated by numerous clinicals, including several double-blind studies, involving more than 2,000 subjects suffering from acute or chronic hyperemia induced by a variety of conditions. Visine was found to be efficacious in providing relief from conjunctival hyperemia.

Active Ingredient: **Purpose:**
Tetrahydrozoline
HCl 0.05% .... Redness reliever

Use:
- for the relief of redness of the eye due to minor eye irritations

Warnings:
Ask a doctor before use if you have narrow angle glaucoma

When using this product
- pupils may become enlarged temporarily
- overuse may cause more eye redness
- remove contact lenses before using
- do not use if this solution changes color or becomes cloudy
- do not touch tip of container to any surface to avoid contamination
- replace cap after each use

Stop use and ask a doctor if
- you feel eye pain
- changes in vision occur
- redness or irritation of the eye lasts
- condition worsens or lasts more than 72 hours

If pregnant or breast-feeding, ask a health professional before use.

Keep out of reach of children. If swallowed, get medical help or contact a Poison Control Center right away.

Directions:
- put 1 to 2 drops in the affected eye(s) up to 4 times daily
- children under 6 years of age: ask a doctor

Other Information:
- store at 15° to 25°C (59° to 77°F)

Inactive Ingredients: benzalkonium chloride, boric acid, edetate disodium, purified water, sodium borate, and sodium chloride

Shown in Product Identification Guide, page 105

VISINE TEARS® OTC
Lubricant Eye Drops
Dry Eye Relief

Description: Visine Tears® Lubricant Eye Drops cools and comforts your dry, scratchy, irritated eyes, and helps them feel their best. It relieves the dryness caused by computer use, reading, wind, heat and air conditioning, while it protects your eyes from further irritation. Visine Tears is safe to use as often as needed.

Active Ingredients: **Purpose:**
Glycerin 0.2% .... Lubricant
Hypromellose 0.2% .... Lubricant
Polyethylene glycol 400 1% .... Lubricant

Uses:
- for the temporary relief of burning and irritation due to dryness of the eye
- for protection against further irritation

Warnings:
When using this product
- remove contact lenses before using
- do not use if this solution changes color or becomes cloudy
- do not touch tip of container to any surface to avoid contamination
- replace cap after each use

Stop use and ask a doctor if
- you feel eye pain
- changes in vision occur
- redness or irritation of the eye lasts
- condition worsens or lasts more than 72 hours

If pregnant or breast-feeding, ask a health professional before use.

Keep out of reach of children. If swallowed, get medical help or contact a Poison Control Center right away.

Directions:
- put 1 or 2 drops in the affected eye(s) as needed
- children under 6 years of age: ask a doctor

Other Information:
- store at 15° to 25°C (59° to 77°F)

Inactive Ingredients: ascorbic acid, benzalkonium chloride, boric acid, dextrose, disodium phosphate, glycine, magnesium chloride, potassium chloride, purified water, sodium borate, sodium chloride, sodium citrate, and sodium lactate

Shown in Product Identification Guide, page 106

VISINE TEARS® OTC
Preservative Free, Single-Use Containers
Lubricant Eye Drops
Dry Eye Relief

Description: Visine Tears® Preservative Free Lubricant Eye Drops cools and comforts your dry, scratchy irritated eyes, and helps them feel their best. It relieves the dryness caused by computer use, reading, wind, heat and air conditioning, while it protects your eyes from further irritation. Specially formulated for people whose eyes are sensitive to preservatives, Visine Tears Preservative Free is sealed in convenient single-use containers and is safe to use as often as needed.

Active Ingredients: **Purpose:**
Glycerin 0.2% .... Lubricant
Hypromellose 0.2% .... Lubricant
Polyethylene glycol 400 1% .... Lubricant

Uses:
- for the temporary relief of burning and irritation due to dryness of the eye
- for protection against further irritation

Warnings:
When using this product
- remove contact lenses before using
- do not use if this solution changes color or becomes cloudy
- do not touch tip of container to any surface to avoid contamination
- do not reuse; once opened, discard

Stop use and ask a doctor if
- you feel eye pain
- changes in vision occur
- redness or irritation of the eye lasts
- condition worsens or lasts more than 72 hours

If pregnant or breast-feeding, ask a health professional before use.

Keep out of reach of children. If swallowed, get medical help or contact a Poison Control Center right away.

Directions:
- put 1 or 2 drops in the affected eye(s) as needed

- children under 6 years of age: ask a doctor

Other Information:
- store at 15° to 25°C (59° to 77°F)

Inactive Ingredients: ascorbic acid, dextrose, disodium phosphate, glycine, magnesium chloride, potassium chloride, purified water, sodium chloride, sodium citrate, sodium lactate, and sodium phosphate

Shown in Product Identification Guide, page 106

Pharmacia & Upjohn
A Pfizer Company
235 EAST 42ND ST
NEW YORK, NY 10017

For Medical Information contact:
24 hours a day, 7 days a week:
(800) 438-1985

XALATAN® ℞
[ză-lă-tăn]
(latanoprost ophthalmic solution)
0.005% (50 μg/mL)

Description: Latanoprost is a prostaglandin $F_{2\alpha}$ analogue. Its chemical name is isopropyl - (Z)- 7 [(1R,2R,3R,5S) 3,5-dihydroxy-2-[(3R)-3-hydroxy-5-phenylpentyl] cyclopentyl] -5-heptenoate. Its molecular formula is $C_{26}H_{40}O_5$ and its chemical structure is:

M.W. 432.58

Latanoprost is a colorless to slightly yellow oil that is very soluble in acetonitrile and freely soluble in acetone, ethanol, ethyl acetate, isopropanol, methanol and octanol. It is practically insoluble in water.

XALATAN Sterile Ophthalmic Solution (latanoprost ophthalmic solution) is supplied as a sterile, isotonic, buffered aqueous solution of latanoprost with a pH of approximately 6.7 and an osmolality of approximately 267 mOsmol/kg. Each mL of XALATAN contains 50 micrograms of latanoprost. Benzalkonium chloride, 0.02% is added as a preservative. The inactive ingredients are: sodium chloride, sodium dihydrogen phosphate monohydrate, disodium hydrogen phosphate anhydrous and water for injection. One drop contains approximately 1.5 μg of latanoprost.

Clinical Pharmacology:
Mechanism of Action
Latanoprost is a prostanoid selective FP receptor agonist that is believed to reduce the intraocular pressure (IOP) by increasing the outflow of aqueous humor. Studies in animals and man suggest that the main mechanism of action is increased uveoscleral outflow. Elevated IOP represents a major risk factor for glaucomatous field loss. The higher the level of IOP, the greater the likelihood of optic nerve damage and visual field loss.

Pharmacokinetics/Pharmacodynamics
Absorption: Latanoprost is absorbed through the cornea where the isopropyl ester prodrug is hydrolyzed to the acid form to become biologically active. Studies in man indicate that the peak concentration in the aqueous humor is reached about two hours after topical administration.

Distribution: The distribution volume in humans is 0.16 ± 0.02 L/kg. The acid of latanoprost can be measured in aqueous humor during the first 4 hours, and in plasma only during the first hour after local administration.

Metabolism: Latanoprost, an isopropyl ester prodrug, is hydrolyzed by esterases in the cornea to the biologically active acid. The active acid of latanoprost reaching the systemic circulation is primarily metabolized by the liver to the 1,2-dinor and 1,2,3,4-tetranor metabolites via fatty acid β-oxidation.

Excretion: The elimination of the acid of latanoprost from human plasma is rapid ($t_{1/2}$ =17 min) after both intravenous and topical administration. Systemic clearance is approximately 7 mL/min/kg. Following hepatic β-oxidation, the metabolites are mainly eliminated via the kidneys. Approximately 88% and 98% of the administered dose is recovered in the urine after topical and intravenous dosing, respectively.

Animal Studies
In monkeys, latanoprost has been shown to induce increased pigmentation of the iris. The mechanism of increased pigmentation seems to be stimulation of melanin production in melanocytes of the iris, with no proliferative changes observed. The change in iris color may be permanent.

Ocular administration of latanoprost at a dose of 6 μg/eye/day (4 times the daily human dose) to cynomolgus monkeys has also been shown to induce increased palpebral fissure. This effect was reversible upon discontinuation of the drug.

Indications And Usage: XALATAN Sterile Ophthalmic Solution is indicated for the reduction of elevated intraocular pressure in patients with open-angle glaucoma or ocular hypertension.

Clinical Studies: Patients with mean baseline intraocular pressure of 24 – 25 mmHg who were treated for 6 months in multi-center, randomized, controlled trials demonstrated 6 – 8 mmHg reductions in intraocular pressure. This IOP reduction with XALATAN Sterile Ophthalmic Solution 0.005% dosed once daily was equivalent to the effect of timolol 0.5% dosed twice daily.

A 3-year open-label, prospective safety study with a 2-year extension phase was conducted to evaluate the progression of increased iris pigmentation with continuous use of XALATAN once-daily as adjunctive therapy in 519 patients with open-angle glaucoma. The analysis was based on observed-cases population of the 380 patients who continued in the extension phase.

Results showed that the onset of noticeable increased iris pigmentation occurred within the first year of treatment for the majority of the patients who developed noticeable increased iris pigmentation. Patients continued to show signs of increasing iris pigmentation throughout the five years of the study. Observation of increased iris pigmentation did not affect the incidence, nature or severity of adverse events (other than increased iris pigmentation) recorded in the study. IOP reduction was similar regardless of the development of increased iris pigmentation during the study.

Contraindications: Known hypersensitivity to latanoprost, benzalkonium chloride or any other ingredients in this product.

Warnings: XALATAN Sterile Ophthalmic Solution has been reported to cause changes to pigmented tissues. The most frequently reported changes have been increased pigmentation of the iris, periorbital tissue (eyelid) and eyelashes, and growth of eyelashes. Pigmentation is expected to increase as long as XALATAN is administered. After discontinuation of XALATAN, pigmentation of the iris is likely to be permanent while pigmentation of the periorbital tissue and eyelash changes have been reported to be reversible in some patients. Patients who receive treatment should be informed of the possibility of increased pigmentation. The effects of increased pigmentation beyond 5 years are not known.

Precautions:
General: XALATAN Sterile Ophthalmic Solution may gradually increase the pigmentation of the iris. The eye color change is due to increased melanin content in the stromal melanocytes of the iris rather than to an increase in the number of melanocytes. This change may not be noticeable for several months to years (see **Warnings**). Typically, the brown pigmentation around the pupil spreads concentrically towards the periphery of the iris and the entire iris or parts of the iris become more brownish. Neither nevi nor freckles of the iris appear to be affected by treatment. While treatment with XALATAN can be continued in patients who develop noticeably increased iris pigmentation, these patients should be examined regularly.

During clinical trials, the increase in brown iris pigment has not been shown to progress further upon discontinuation of treatment, but the resultant color change may be permanent. Eyelid skin darkening, which may be reversible, has been reported in association with the use of XALATAN (see **Warnings**).

XALATAN may gradually change eyelashes and vellus hair in the treated eye; these changes include increased length, thickness, pigmentation, the number of lashes or hairs, and misdirected growth of eyelashes. Eyelash changes are usually reversible upon discontinuation of treatment.

XALATAN should be used with caution in patients with a history of intraocular inflammation (iritis/uveitis) and should generally not be used in patients with active intraocular inflammation.

Macular edema, including cystoid macular edema, has been reported during treatment with XALATAN. These reports have mainly occurred in aphakic patients, in pseudophakic patients with a torn posterior lens capsule, or in patients with known risk factors for macular edema. XALATAN should be used with caution in patients who do not have an intact posterior capsule or who have known risk factors for macular edema.

There is limited experience with XALATAN in the treatment of angle closure, inflammatory or neovascular glaucoma.

There have been reports of bacterial keratitis associated with the use of multiple-dose containers of topical ophthalmic products. These containers had been inadvertently contaminated by patients who, in most cases, had a concurrent corneal disease or a disruption of the ocular epithelial surface (see **Precautions**, *Information for Patients*).

Contact lenses should be removed prior to the administration of XALATAN, and may be reinserted 15 minutes after administration (see **Precautions**, *Information for Patients*).

Information for Patients (see **Warnings** and **Precautions**): Patients should be advised about the potential for increased brown pigmentation of the iris, which may be permanent. Patients should also be informed about the possibility of eyelid skin darkening, which may be reversible after discontinuation of XALATAN.

Patients should also be informed of the possibility of eyelash and vellus hair changes in the treated eye during treatment with XALATAN. These changes may result in a disparity between eyes in length, thickness, pigmentation, number of eyelashes or vellus hairs, and/or direction of eyelash growth. Eyelash changes are usually reversible upon discontinuation of treatment.

Patients should be instructed to avoid allowing the tip of the dispensing container to contact the eye or surrounding structures because this could cause the tip to become contaminated by common bacteria known to cause ocular infec-

Continued on next page

Xalatan—Cont.

tions. Serious damage to the eye and subsequent loss of vision may result from using contaminated solutions.

Patients also should be advised that if they develop an intercurrent ocular condition (e.g., trauma, or infection) or have ocular surgery, they should immediately seek their physician's advice concerning the continued use of the multiple-dose container.

Patients should be advised that if they develop any ocular reactions, particularly conjunctivitis and lid reactions, they should immediately seek their physician's advice.

Patients should also be advised that XALATAN contains benzalkonium chloride, which may be absorbed by contact lenses. Contact lenses should be removed prior to administration of the solution. Lenses may be reinserted 15 minutes following administration of XALATAN.

If more than one topical ophthalmic drug is being used, the drugs should be administered at least five (5) minutes apart.

Drug Interactions: In vitro studies have shown that precipitation occurs when eye drops containing thimerosal are mixed with XALATAN. If such drugs are used they should be administered at least five (5) minutes apart.

Carcinogenesis, Mutagenesis, Impairment of Fertility: Latanoprost was not mutagenic in bacteria, in mouse lymphoma or in mouse micronucleus tests.

Chromosome aberrations were observed *in vitro* with human lymphocytes.

Latanoprost was not carcinogenic in either mice or rats when administered by oral gavage at doses of up to 170 µg/kg/day (approximately 2,800 times the recommended maximum human dose) for up to 20 and 24 months, respectively.

Additional *in vitro* and *in vivo* studies on unscheduled DNA synthesis in rats were negative. Latanoprost has not been found to have any effect on male or female fertility in animal studies.

Pregnancy: Teratogenic Effects: Pregnancy Category C.

Reproduction studies have been performed in rats and rabbits. In rabbits an incidence of 4 of 16 dams had no viable fetuses at a dose that was approximately 80 times the maximum human dose, and the highest nonembryocidal dose in rabbits was approximately 15 times the maximum human dose. There are no adequate and well-controlled studies in pregnant women. XALATAN should be used during pregnancy only if the potential benefit justifies the potential risk to the fetus.

Nursing Mothers: It is not known whether this drug or its metabolites are excreted in human milk. Because many drugs are excreted in human milk, caution should be exercised when XALATAN is administered to a nursing woman.

Pediatric Use: Safety and effectiveness in pediatric patients have not been established.

Geriatric Use: No overall differences in safety or effectiveness have been observed between elderly and younger patients.

Adverse Reactions:

Adverse events referred to in other sections of this insert:

Eyelash changes (increased length, thickness, pigmentation, and number of lashes); eyelid skin darkening; intraocular inflammation (iritis/uveitis); iris pigmentation changes; and macular edema, including cystoid macular edema (see **Warnings** and **Precautions**).

Controlled Clinical Trials:

The ocular adverse events and ocular signs and symptoms reported in 5 to 15% of the patients on XALATAN Sterile Ophthalmic Solution in the three 6-month, multi-center, double-masked, active-controlled trials were blurred vision, burning and stinging, conjunctival hyperemia, foreign body sensation, itching, increased pigmentation of the iris, and punctate epithelial keratopathy.

Local conjunctival hyperemia was observed; however, less than 1% of the patients treated with XALATAN required discontinuation of therapy because of intolerance to conjunctival hyperemia.

In addition to the above listed ocular events/signs and symptoms, the following were reported in 1 to 4% of the patients: dry eye, excessive tearing, eye pain, lid crusting, lid discomfort/pain, lid edema, lid erythema, and photophobia.

The following events were reported in less than 1% of the patients: conjunctivitis, diplopia and discharge from the eye.

During clinical studies, there were extremely rare reports of the following: retinal artery embolus, retinal detachment, and vitreous hemorrhage from diabetic retinopathy.

The most common systemic adverse events seen with XALATAN were upper respiratory tract infection/cold/flu, which occurred at a rate of approximately 4%. Chest pain/angina pectoris, muscle/joint/back pain, and rash/allergic skin reaction each occurred at a rate of 1 to 2%.

Clinical Practice:

The following events have been identified during postmarketing use of XALATAN in clinical practice. Because they are reported voluntarily from a population of unknown size, estimates of frequency cannot be made. The events, which have been chosen for inclusion due to either their seriousness, frequency of reporting, possible causal connection to XALATAN, or a combination of these factors, include: asthma and exacerbation of asthma; corneal edema and erosions; dyspnea; eyelash and vellus hair changes (increased length, thickness, pigmentation, and number); eyelid skin darkening; herpes keratitis; intraocular inflammation (iritis/uveitis); keratitis; macular edema, including cystoid macular edema; misdirected eyelashes sometimes resulting in eye irritation; and toxic epidermal necrolysis.

Overdosage: Apart from ocular irritation and conjunctival or episcleral hyperemia, the ocular effects of latanoprost administered at high doses are not known. Intravenous administration of large doses of latanoprost in monkeys has been associated with transient bronchoconstriction; however, in 11 patients with bronchial asthma treated with latanoprost, bronchoconstriction was not induced. Intravenous infusion of up to 3 µg/kg in healthy volunteers produced mean plasma concentrations 200 times higher than during clinical treatment and no adverse reactions were observed. Intravenous dosages of 5.5 to 10 µg/kg caused abdominal pain, dizziness, fatigue, hot flushes, nausea and sweating.

If overdosage with XALATAN Sterile Ophthalmic Solution occurs, treatment should be symptomatic.

Dosage And Administration: The recommended dosage is one drop (1.5 µg) in the affected eye(s) once daily in the evening.

The dosage of XALATAN Sterile Ophthalmic Solution should not exceed once daily since it has been shown that more frequent administration may decrease the intraocular pressure lowering effect.

Reduction of the intraocular pressure starts approximately 3 to 4 hours after administration and the maximum effect is reached after 8 to 12 hours.

XALATAN may be used concomitantly with other topical ophthalmic drug products to lower intraocular pressure. If more than one topical ophthalmic drug is being used, the drugs should be administered at least five (5) minutes apart.

How Supplied: XALATAN Sterile Ophthalmic Solution is a clear, isotonic, buffered, preserved colorless solution of latanoprost 0.005% (50 µg/mL). It is supplied as a 2.5 mL solution in a 5 mL clear low density polyethylene bottle with a clear low density polyethylene dropper tip, a turquoise high density polyethylene screw cap, and a tamper-evident clear low density polyethylene overcap.

2.5 mL fill, 0.005% (50 µg/mL)
Package of 1 bottle   NDC 0013-8303-04
Storage: Protect from light. Store unopened bottle(s) under refrigeration at 2° to 8°C (36° to 46°F). During shipment to the patient, the bottle may be maintained at temperatures up to 40°C (104°F) for a period not exceeding 8 days. Once a bottle is opened for use, it may be stored at room temperature up to 25°C (77°F) for 6 weeks.

℞ only
U.S. Patent Nos. 4,599,353; 5,296,504 and 5,422,368.
Manufactured for:
Pharmacia & Upjohn Company
A subsidiary of Pharmacia Corporation
Kalamazoo, MI 49001, USA
By:
Cardinal Health
Woodstock, IL 60098, USA
Revised September 2003   818 057 207
                                                 691211

Shown in Product Identification Guide, page 106

Santen Inc.

for further product information see VISTAKON® Pharmaceuticals, LLC

VISTAKON Pharmaceuticals LLC
7500 CENTURION PARKWAY
JACKSONVILLE, FL 32256

Direct Inquiries to:
Phone (866) 427-6815

ALAMAST®   ℞
[ăĺă-măst]
(pemirolast potassium ophthalmic solution) 0.1%

Description: ALAMAST® (pemirolast potassium ophthalmic solution) is a sterile, aqueous ophthalmic solution with a pH of approximately 8.0 containing 0.1% of the mast cell stabilizer, pemirolast potassium, for topical administration to the eyes.

Pemirolast potassium is a slightly yellow, water-soluble powder with a molecular weight of 266.3.

The chemical structure is presented below:

$C_{10}H_7KN_6O$

Chemical name:
9-methyl-3-(1H-tetrazol-5-yl)-4H-pyrido[1,2-α]pyrimidin-4-one potassium

Each mL contains: ACTIVE: pemirolast potassium 1 mg (0.1%); PRESERVATIVE: lauralkonium chloride 0.005%; INACTIVES: glycerin, dibasic sodium phosphate, monobasic sodium phosphate, phosphoric acid and/or sodium hydroxide to adjust pH, and purified water. The osmolality of ALAMAST® ophthalmic solution is approximately 240 mOsmol/kg.

Clinical Pharmacology:

Mechanism of Action: Pemirolast potassium is a mast cell stabilizer that inhibits the *in vivo* Type I immediate hypersensitivity reaction.

In vitro and *in vivo* studies have demonstrated that pemirolast potassium inhibits the antigen-induced release of inflammatory mediators (e.g., histamine, leukotriene C_4, D_4, E_4) from human mast cells.

In addition, pemirolast potassium inhibits the chemotaxis of eosinophils into ocular tissue and blocks the release of mediators from human eosinophils.

Although the precise mechanism of action is unknown, the drug has been reported to prevent calcium influx into mast cells upon antigen stimulation.

Pharmacokinetics: Topical ocular administration of one to two drops of ALAMAST® ophthalmic solution in each eye four times daily in 16 healthy volunteers for two weeks resulted in detectable concentrations in the plasma. The mean ($\pm$SE) peak plasma level of 4.7 $\pm$ 0.8 ng/mL occurred at 0.42 $\pm$ 0.05 hours and the mean $t_{1/2}$ was 4.5 $\pm$ 0.2 hours. When a single 10 mg pemirolast potassium dose was taken orally, a peak plasma concentration of 0.723 µg/mL was reached.

Following topical administration, about 10-15% of the dose was excreted unchanged in the urine.

Clinical Studies: In clinical environmental studies, ALAMAST® was significantly more effective than placebo after 28 days in preventing ocular itching associated with allergic conjunctivitis.

Indications and Usage:
ALAMAST® ophthalmic solution is indicated for the prevention of itching of the eye due to allergic conjunctivitis. Symptomatic response to therapy (decreased itching) may be evident within a few days, but frequently requires longer treatment (up to four weeks).

Contraindications:
ALAMAST® ophthalmic solution is contraindicated in patients with previously demonstrated hypersensitivity to any of the ingredients of this product.

Warnings:
For topical ophthalmic use only. Not for injection or oral use.

Precautions:
Information for patients: To prevent contaminating the dropper tip and solution, do not touch the eyelids or surrounding areas with the dropper tip. Keep the bottle tightly closed when not in use.

Patients should be advised not to wear contact lenses if their eyes are red. ALAMAST® should not be used to treat contact lens related irritation. The preservative in ALAMAST®, lauralkonium chloride, may be absorbed by soft contact lenses. Patients who wear soft contact lenses and whose eyes are not red should be instructed to wait at least ten minutes after instilling ALAMAST® before they insert their contact lenses.

Carcinogenesis, mutagenesis, impairment of fertility: Pemirolast potassium was not mutagenic or clastogenic when tested in a series of bacterial and mammalian tests for gene mutation and chromosomal injury *in vitro* nor was it clastogenic when tested *in vivo* in rats.

Pemirolast potassium had no effect on mating and fertility in rats at oral doses up to 250 mg/kg (approximately 20,000 fold the human dose at 2 drops/eye, 40 µL/drop, QID for a 50 kg adult). A reduced fertility and pregnancy index occurred in the F_1 generation when F_0 dams were treated with 400 mg/kg pemirolast potassium during late pregnancy and lactation period (approximately 30,000 fold the human dose).

Pregnancy:
Teratogenic effects: **Pregnancy Category C.** Pemirolast potassium caused an increased incidence of thymic remnant in the neck, interventricular septal defect, fetuses with wavy rib, splitting of thoracic vertebral body, and reduced numbers of ossified sternebrae, sacral and caudal vertebrae, and metatarsi when rats were given oral doses $\geq$250 mg/kg (approximately 20,000 fold the human dose at 2 drops/eye, 40 µL/drop, QID for a 50 kg adult) during organogenesis. Increased incidence of dilation of renal pelvis/ureter in the fetuses and neonates was also noted when rats were given an oral dose of 400 mg/kg pemirolast potassium (approximately 30,000 fold the human dose). Pemirolast potassium was not teratogenic in rabbits given oral doses up to 150 mg/kg (approximately 12,000 fold the human dose) during the same time period. There are no adequate and well-controlled studies in pregnant women. Because animal reproductive studies are not always predictive of human response, ALAMAST® ophthalmic solution should be used during pregnancy only if the benefit outweighs the risk.

Non-teratogenic effects: Pemirolast potassium produced increased pre- and post-implantation losses, reduced embryo/fetal and neonatal survival, decreased neonatal body weight, and delayed neonatal development in rats receiving an oral dose at 400 mg/kg (approximately 30,000 fold the human dose). Pemirolast potassium also caused a reduction in the number of corpus lutea, the number of implantations, and number of live fetuses in the F_1 generation in rats when F_0 dams were given oral dosages $\geq$250 mg/kg (approximately 20,000 fold the human dose) during late gestation and the lactation period.

Nursing Mothers: Pemirolast potassium is excreted in the milk of lactating rats at concentrations higher than those in plasma. It is not known whether pemirolast potassium is excreted in human milk. Because many drugs are excreted in human milk, caution should be exercised when ALAMAST® ophthalmic solution is administered to a nursing woman.

Pediatric Use: Safety and effectiveness in pediatric patients below the age of 3 years have not been established.

Adverse Reactions:
In clinical studies lasting up to 17 weeks with ALAMAST® ophthalmic solution, headache, rhinitis, and cold/flu symptoms were reported at an incidence of 10–25%. The occurrence of these side effects was generally mild. Some of these events were similar to the underlying ocular disease being studied.

The following ocular and non-ocular adverse reactions were reported at an incidence of less than 5%:

Ocular: burning, dry eye, foreign body sensation, and ocular discomfort.

Non-Ocular: allergy, back pain, bronchitis, cough, dysmenorrhea, fever, sinusitis, and sneezing/nasal congestion.

Overdosage:
No accounts of ALAMAST® ophthalmic solution overdose were reported following topical ocular application.

Oral ingestion of the contents of a 10 mL bottle would be equivalent to 10 mg of pemirolast potassium.

Dosage and Administration:
The recommended dose is one to two drops in each affected eye four times daily.

Symptomatic response to therapy (decreased itching) may be evident within a few days, but frequently requires longer treatment (up to four weeks).

How Supplied:
ALAMAST® (pemirolast potassium ophthalmic solution) 0.1% is supplied as follows:
10 mL in a white, low density polyethylene bottle with a controlled dropper tip, and a white polyethylene screw cap.
NDC 68669-711-10 10 mL fill in 10 cc container

Storage: Store at 15°–25°C (59°–77°F).
Rx only
Manufactured by:
Parkedale Pharmaceuticals, Inc., Rochester, MI 48307, USA
2.5 mL Physician Sample Manufactured by:
Santen Oy, PO Box 33
FIN-33721 Tampere, Finland
Santen®
Marketed by:
VISTAKON® Pharmaceuticals, LLC
Jacksonville, FL 32256
Licensed from Mitsubishi Pharma Corporation
Tokyo, Japan
March 2004 Version
U.S. Patent No. 5,034,230
VISTAKON® Pharmaceuticals, LLC
III-03

Shown in Product Identification Guide, page 106

BETIMOL® ℞
[*bāt'-ĭ-mŏl"*]
(timolol ophthalmic solution) 0.25%, 0.5%

Description: Betimol® (timolol ophthalmic solution), 0.25% and 0.5%, is a non-selective beta-adrenergic antagonist for ophthalmic use. The chemical name of the active ingredient is (S)-1-[(1,1-dimethylethyl)amino]-3-[[4-(4-morpholinyl)-1,2,5-thiadiazol-3-yl]oxy]-2-propanol. Timolol hemihydrate is the levo isomer. Specific rotation is $[\alpha]^{25}_{405nm} = -16°$ (C=10% as the hemihydrate form in 1N HCl).

The molecular formula of timolol is Formula $C_{13}H_{24}N_4O_3S$ and its structural formula is:

Timolol (as the hemihydrate) is a white, odorless, crystalline powder which is slightly soluble in water and freely soluble in ethanol. Timolol hemihydrate is stable at room temperature.

Betimol® is a clear, colorless, isotonic, sterile, microbiologically preserved phosphate buffered aqueous solution.

It is supplied in two dosage strengths, 0.25% and 0.5%.

Each mL of Betimol® 0.25% contains 2.56 mg of timolol hemihydrate equivalent to 2.5 mg timolol.

Each mL of Betimol® 05% contains 5.12 mg of timolol hemihydrate equivalent to 5.0 mg timolol.

Inactive ingredients: monosodium and disodium phosphate dihydrate to adjust pH (6.5 – 7.5) and water for injection, benzalkonium chloride 0.01% added as preservative.

The osmolality of Betimol® is 260 to 320 mOsmol/kg.

Clinical Pharmacology: Timolol is a non-selective beta-adrenergic antagonist.

It blocks both beta$_1$- and beta$_2$-adrenergic receptors. Timolol does not have significant intrinsic sympathomimetic activity, local anesthetic (membrane-stabilizing) or direct myocardial depressant activity.

Timolol, when applied topically in the eye, reduces normal and elevated intraocular pressure (IOP) whether or not accompanied by glaucoma. Elevated intraocular pressure is a

Continued on next page

Betimol—Cont.

major risk factor in the pathogenesis of glaucomatous visual field loss. The higher the level of IOP, the greater the likelihood of glaucomatous visual field loss and optic nerve damage. The predominant mechanism of ocular hypotensive action of topical beta-adrenergic blocking agents is likely due to a reduction in aqueous humor production.

In general, beta-adrenergic blocking agents reduce cardiac output both in healthy subjects and patients with heart diseases. In patients with severe impairment of myocardial function, beta-adrenergic receptor blocking agents may inhibit sympathetic stimulatory effect necessary to maintain adequate cardiac function. In the bronchi and bronchioles, beta-adrenergic receptor blockade may also increase airway resistance because of unopposed parasympathetic activity.

Pharmacokinetics
When given orally, timolol is well absorbed and undergoes considerable first pass metabolism. Timolol and its metabolites are primarily excreted in the urine. The half-life of timolol in plasma is approximately 4 hours.

Clinical Studies
In two controlled multicenter studies in the U.S., Betimol® 0.25% and 0.5% were compared with respective timolol maleate eyedrops. In these studies, the efficacy and safety profile of Betimol® was similar to that of timolol maleate.

Indications and Usage: Betimol® is indicated in the treatment of elevated intraocular pressure in patients with ocular hypertension or open-angle glaucoma.

Contraindications: Betimol® is contraindicated in patients with overt heart failure, cardiogenic shock, sinus bradycardia, second- or third-degree atrioventricular block, bronchial asthma or history of bronchial asthma, or severe chronic obstructive pulmonary disease, or hypersensitivity to any component of this product.

Warnings: As with other topically applied ophthalmic drugs, Betimol® is absorbed systemically. The same adverse reactions found with systemic administration of beta-adrenergic blocking agents may occur with topical administration. For example, severe respiratory and cardiac reactions, including death due to bronchospasm in patients with asthma, and rarely, death in association with cardiac failure have been reported following systemic or topical administration of beta-adrenergic blocking agents.

Cardiac Failure: Sympathetic stimulation may be essential for support of the circulation in individuals with diminished myocardial contractility, and its inhibition by beta-adrenergic receptor blockade may precipitate more severe cardiac failure.

In patients without a history of cardiac failure, continued depression of the myocardium with beta-blocking agents over a period of time can, in some cases, lead to cardiac failure. Betimol® should be discontinued at the first sign or symptom of cardiac failure.

Obstructive Pulmonary Disease: Patients with chronic obstructive pulmonary disease (e.g. chronic bronchitis, emphysema) of mild or moderate severity, bronchospastic disease, or a history of bronchospastic disease (other than bronchial asthma or a history of bronchial asthma which are contraindications) should in general not receive beta-blocking agents.

Major Surgery: The necessity or desirability of withdrawal of beta-adrenergic blocking agents prior to a major surgery is controversial. Beta-adrenergic receptor blockade impairs the ability of the heart to respond to beta-adrenergically mediated reflex stimuli. This may augment the risk of general anesthesia in surgical procedures. Some patients receiving beta-adrenergic receptor blocking agents have been subject to protracted severe hypotension during anesthesia. Difficulty in restarting and maintaining the heartbeat has also been reported. For these reasons, in patients undergoing elective surgery, gradual withdrawal of beta-adrenergic receptor blocking agents is recommended. If necessary during surgery, the effects of beta-adrenergic blocking agents may be reversed by sufficient doses of beta-adrenergic agonists.

Diabetes Mellitus: Beta-adrenergic blocking agents should be administered with caution in patients subject to spontaneous hypoglycemia or to diabetic patients (especially those with labile diabetes) who are receiving insulin or oral hypoglycemic agents. Beta-adrenergic receptor blocking agents may mask the signs and symptoms of acute hypoglycemia.

Thyrotoxicosis: Beta-adrenergic blocking agents may mask certain clinical signs (e.g. tachycardia) of hyperthyroidism. Patients suspected of developing thyrotoxicosis should be managed carefully to avoid abrupt withdrawal of beta-adrenergic blocking agents which might precipitate a thyroid storm.

Precautions:
General
Because of the potential effects of beta-adrenergic blocking agents relative to blood pressure and pulse, these agents should be used with caution in patients with cerebrovascular insufficiency. If signs or symptoms suggesting reduced cerebral blood flow develop following initiation of therapy with Betimol®, alternative therapy should be considered.

There have been reports of bacterial keratitis associated with the use of multiple dose containers of topical ophthalmic products. These containers had been inadvertently contaminated by patients who, in most cases, had a concurrent corneal disease or a disruption of the ocular epithelial suface. (See PRECAUTIONS, Information for Patients.)

Muscle Weakness: Beta-adrenergic blockade has been reported to potentiate muscle weakness consistent with certain myasthenic symptoms (e.g. diplopia, ptosis, and generalized weakness). Beta-adrenergic blocking agents have been reported rarely to increase muscle weakness in some patients with myasthenia gravis or myasthenic symptoms.

In angle-closure glaucoma, the goal of the treatment is to reopen the angle. This requires constricting the pupil. Betimol® has no effect on the pupil. Therefore, if timolol is used in angle-closure glaucoma, it should always be combined with a miotic and not used alone.

Anaphylaxis: While taking beta-blockers, patients with a history of atopy or a history of severe anaphylactic reactions to a variety of allergens may be more reactive to repeated accidental, diagnostic, or therapeutic challenge with such allergens. Such patients may be unresponsive to the usual doses of epinephrine used to treat anaphylactic reactions.

The preservative benzalkonium chloride may be absorbed by soft contact lenses. Patients who wear soft contact lenses should wait 5 minutes after instilling Betimol® before they insert their lenses.

Information for Patients
Patients should be instructed to avoid allowing the tip of the dispensing container to contact the eye or surrounding structures.

Patients should also be instructed that ocular solutions can become contaminated by common bacteria known to cause ocular infections. Serious damage to the eye and subsequent loss of vision may result from using contaminated solutions. (See PRECAUTIONS, General.)

Patients requiring concomitant topical ophthalmic medications should be instructed to administer these at least 5 minutes apart.

Patients with bronchial asthma, a history of bronchial asthma, severe chronic obstructive pulmonary disease, sinus bradycardia, second- or third-degree atrioventricular block, or cardiac failure should be advised not to take this product (See CONTRAINDICATIONS.)

Drug Interactions
Beta-adrenergic blocking agents: Patients who are receiving a beta-adrenergic blocking agent orally and Betimol® should be observed for a potential additive effect either on the intraocular pressure or on the known systemic effects of beta-blockade.

Patients should not usually receive two topical ophthalmic beta-adrenergic blocking agents concurrently.

Catecholamine-depleting drugs: Close observation of the patient is recommended when a beta-blocker is administered to patients receiving catecholamine-depleting drugs such as reserpine, because of possible additive effects and the production of hypotension and/or marked bradycardia, which may produce vertigo, syncope, or postural hypotension.

Calcium antagonists: Caution should be used in the co-administration of beta-adrenergic blocking agents and oral or intravenous calcium antagonists, because of possible atrioventricular conduction disturbances, left ventricular failure, and hypotension. In patients with impaired cardiac function, co-administration should be avoided.

Digitalis and calcium antagonists The concomitant use of beta-adrenergic blocking agents with digitalis and calcium antagonists may have additive effects in prolonging atrioventricular conduction time.

Injectable Epinephrine: (See PRECAUTIONS, General, Anaphylaxis.)

Carcinogenesis, Mutagenesis, Impairment of Fertility
Carcinogenicity of timolol (as the maleate) has been studied in mice and rats. In a two-year study orally administered timolol maleate (300mg/kg/day) (approximately 42,000 times the systemic exposure following the maximum recommended human ophthalmic dose) in male rats caused a significant increase in the incidence of adrenal pheochromocytomas; the lower doses, 25 mg or 100 mg/kg daily did not cause any changes.

In a life span study in mice the overall incidence of neoplasms was significantly increased in female mice at 500 mg/kg/day (approximately 71,000 times the systemic exposure following the maximum recommended human ophthalmic dose). Furthermore, significant increases were observed in the incidences of benign and malignant pulmonary tumors, benign uterine polyps, as well as mammary adenocarcinomas. These changes were not seen at the daily dose level of 5 or 50 mg/kg (approximately 700 or 7,000, respectively, times the systemic exposure following the maximum recommended human ophthalmic dose). For comparison, the maximum recommended human oral dose of timolol maleate is 1 mg/kg/day.

Mutagenic potential of timolol was evaluated *in vivo* in the micronucleus test and cytogenetic assay and *in vitro* in the neoplastic cell transformation assay and Ames test, In the bacterial mutagenicity test (Ames test) high concentrations of timolol maleate (5000 and 10,000 g/plate) statistically significantly increased the number of revertants in *Salmonella typhimurium* TA100, but not in the other three strains tested. However, no consistent dose-response was observed nor did the number of revertants reach the double of the control value, which is regarded as one of the criteria for a positive result in the Ames test. *In vivo* genotoxicity tests (the mouse micronucleus test and cytogenetic assay) and *in vitro* the neoplastic cell transformation assay were negative up to dose levels of 800 mg/kg and 100 g/mL, respectively.

No adverse effects on male and female fertility were reported in rats at timolol oral doses of up to 150 mg/kg/day (21,000 times the systemic exposure following the maximum recommended human ophthalmic dose).

Pregnancy Teratogenic effects:
Category C: Teratogenicity of timolol (as the maleate) after oral administration was studied in mice and rabbits. No fetal malformations were reported in mice or rabbits at a daily oral dose of 50 mg/kg (7,000 times the systemic exposure following the maximum recommended human ophthalmic dose). Although delayed fetal ossification was observed at this dose in rats, there were no adverse effects on postnatal development of offspring. Doses of 1000 mg/kg/day (142,000 times the systemic exposure following the maximum recommended human ophthalmic dose) were maternotoxic in mice and resulted in an increased number of fetal resorptions. Increased fetal resorptions were also seen in rabbits at doses of 14,000 times the systemic exposure following the maximum recommended human ophthalmic dose in this case without apparent maternotoxicity.

There are no adequate and well-controlled studies in pregnant women. Betimol® should be used during pregnancy only it the potential benefit justifies the potential risk to the fetus.

Nursing mothers:
Because of the potential for serious adverse reactions in nursing infants from timolol, a decision should be made whether to discontinue nursing or to discontinue the drug, taking into account the importance of the drug to the mother.

Pediatric use:
Safety and efficacy in pediatric patients have not been established.

Adverse Reactions: The most frequently reported ocular event in clinical trials was burning/stinging on instillation and was comparable between Betimol® and timolol maleate (approximately one in eight patients).

The following adverse events were associated with use of Betimol® in frequencies of more than 5% in two controlled, double-masked clinical studies in which 184 patients received 0.25% or 0.5% Betimol®:

OCULAR:
Dry eyes, itching, foreign body sensation, discomfort in the eye, eyelid erythema, conjunctival injection, and headache.

BODY AS A WHOLE:
Headache.

The following side effects were reported in frequencies of 1 to 5%:

OCULAR:
Eye pain, epiphora, photophobia, blurred or abnormal vision, corneal fluorescein staining, keratitis, blepharitis and cataract.

BODY AS A WHOLE:
Allergic reaction, asthenia, common cold and pain in extremities.

CARDIOVASCULAR:
Hypertension.

DIGESTIVE:
Nausea.

METABOLIC/NUTRITIONAL:
Peripheral edema.

NERVOUS SYSTEM/PSYCHIATRY:
Dizziness and dry mouth.

RESPIRATORY:
Respiratory infection and sinusitis.

In addition, the following adverse reactions have been reported with ophthalmic use of beta blockers:

OCULAR:
Conjunctivitis, blepharoptosis, decreased corneal sensitivity, visual disturbances including refractive changes, diplopia and retinal vascular disorder.

BODY AS A WHOLE:
Chest pain.

CARDIOVASCULAR:
Arrhythmia, palpitation, bradycardia, hypotension, syncope, heart block, cerebral vascular accident, cerebral ischemia, cardiac failure and cardiac arrest.

DIGESTIVE:
Diarrhea.

ENDOCRINE:
Masked symptoms of hypoglycemia in insulin dependent diabetics (See WARNINGS).

NERVOUS SYSTEM/PSYCHIATRY:
Depression, impotence, increase in signs and symptoms of myasthenia gravis and paresthesia.

RESPIRATORY:
Dyspnea, bronchospasm, respiratory failure and nasal congestion.

SKIN:
Alopecia, hypersensitivity including localized and generalized rash, urticaria.

Overdosage: No information is available on overdosage with Betimol®. Symptoms that might be expected with an overdose of a beta-adrenergic receptor blocking agent are bronchospasm, hypotension, bradycardia, and acute cardiac failure.

Dosage and Administration: Betimol® Ophthalmic Solution is available in concentrations of 0.25 and 0.5 percent. The usual starting dose is one drop of 0.25 percent Betimol® in the affected eye(s) twice a day. If the clinical response is not adequate, the dosage may be changed to one drop of 0.5 percent solution in the affected eye(s) twice a day.

If the intraocular pressure is maintained at satisfactory levels, the dosage schedule may be changed to one drop once a day in the affected eye(s). Because of diurnal variations in intraocular pressure, satisfactory response to the once-a-day dose is best determined by measuring the intraocular pressure at different times during the day.

Since in some patients the pressure-lowering response to Betimol® may require a few weeks to stabilize, evaluation should include a determination of intraocular pressure after approximately 4 weeks of treatment with Betimol®. Dosages above one drop of 0.5 percent Betimol® twice a day generally have not been shown to produce further reduction in intraocular pressure, If the patient's intraocular pressure is still not at a satisfactory level on this regimen, concomitant therapy with pilocarpine and other miotics, and/or epinephrine, and/or systemically administered carbonic anhydrase inhibitors, such as acetazolamide can be instituted.

How Supplied: Betimol® (timolol ophthalmic solution) is a clear, colorless solution.

Betimol® 0.25% is supplied in a white, opaque, plastic, ophthalmic dispenser bottle with a controlled drop tip as follows:
NDC 68669-522-05 5.0mL fill in 5 cc container
NDC 68669-522-10 10mL fill in 11 cc container
NDC 68669-522-15 15mL fill in 15 cc container

Betimol® 0.5% is supplied in a white, opaque, plastic, ophthalmic dispenser bottle with a controlled drop tip as follows:
NDC 68669-525-05 5.0mL fill in 5 cc container
NDC 68669-525-10 10mL fill in 11 cc container
NDC 68669-525-15 15mL fill in 15 cc container

Rx Only

STORAGE
Store between 15-30°C (59-86°F). Do not freeze. Protect from light.

MARKETED BY:
VISTAKON® Pharmaceuticals, LLC
Jacksonville, FL 32256 USA

MANUFACTURED BY:
Santen Oy, P.O. Box 33
FIN-33721 Tampere, Finland
Santen®
March 2004 Version

VISTAKON® Pharmaceuticals, LLC
Shown in Product Identification Guide, page 106

QUIXIN® ℞
[quik-sin]
(levofloxacin ophthalmic solution) 0.5%

Description: QUIXIN® (levofloxacin ophthalmic solution) 0.5% is a sterile topical ophthalmic solution. Levofloxacin is a fluoroquinolone antibacterial active against a broad spectrum of Gram-positive and Gram-negative ocular pathogens. Levofloxacin is the pure (-)-(S)-enantiomer of the racemic drug substance, ofloxacin. It is more soluble in water at neutral pH than ofloxacin.

Structural formula

levofloxacin hemihydrate

$C_{18}H_{20}FN_3O_4 \cdot 1/2\ H_2O$ Mol Wt 370.38

Chemical Name: (-)-(S)-9-fluoro-2,3-dihydro-3-methyl-10-(4-methyl-1-piperazinyl)-7-oxo-7H-pyrido[1,2,3-de]-1,4 benzoxazine-6-carboxylic acid hemihydrate.

Levofloxacin (hemihydrate) is a yellowish-white crystalline powder.

Each mL of QUIXIN® contains 5.12 mg of levofloxacin hemihydrate equivalent to 5 mg levofloxacin.

Contains:
Active: Levofloxacin 0.5% (5 mg/mL); **Preservative:** benzalkonium chloride 0.005%; **Inactives:** sodium chloride and water. May also contain hydrochloric acid and/or sodium hydroxide to adjust pH.

QUIXIN® solution is isotonic and formulated at pH 6.5 with an osmolality of approximately 300 mOsm/kg. Levofloxacin is a fluorinated 4-quinolone containing a six-member (pyridobenzoxazine) ring from positions 1 to 8 of the basic ring structure.

Clinical Pharmacology:
Pharmacokinetics:
Levofloxacin concentration in plasma was measured in 15 healthy adult volunteers at various time points during a 15-day course of treatment with QUIXIN® solution. The mean levofloxacin concentration in plasma 1 hour postdose, ranged from 0.86 ng/mL on Day 1 to 2.05 ng/mL on Day 15. The highest maximum mean levofloxacin concentration of 2.25 ng/mL was measured on Day 4 following 2 days of dosing every 2 hours for a total of 8 doses per day. Maximum mean levofloxacin concentrations increased from 0.94 ng/mL on Day 1 to 2.15 ng/mL on Day 15, which is more than 1,000 times lower than those reported after standard oral doses of levofloxacin.

Levofloxacin concentration in tears was measured in 30 healthy adult volunteers at various time points following instillation of a single drop of QUIXIN® solution. Mean levofloxacin concentrations in tears ranged from 34.9 to 221.1 μg/mL during the 60-minute period following the single dose. The mean tear concentrations measured 4 and 6 hours postdose were 17.0 and 6.6 μg/mL. The clinical significance of these concentrations is unknown.

Microbiology:
Levofloxacin is the L-isomer of the racemate, ofloxacin, a quinolone antimicrobial agent. The antibacterial activity of ofloxacin resides primarily in the L-isomer. The mechanism of ac-

Continued on next page

Quixin—Cont.

tion of levofloxacin and other fluoroquinolone antimicrobials involves the inhibition of bacterial topoisomerase IV and DNA gyrase (both of which are type II topoisomerases), enzymes required for DNA replication, transcription, repair, and recombination.

Levofloxacin has *in vitro* activity against a wide range of Gram-negative and Gram-positive microorganisms and is often bactericidal at concentrations equal to or slightly greater than inhibitory concentrations.

Fluoroquinolones, including levofloxacin, differ in chemical structure and mode of action from β-lactam antibiotics and aminoglycosides, and therefore may be active against bacteria resistant to β-lactam antibiotics and aminoglycosides. Additionally, β-lactam antibiotics and aminoglycosides may be active against bacteria resistant to levofloxacin.

Resistance to levofloxacin due to spontaneous mutation *in vitro* is a rare occurrence (range: 10^{-9} to 10^{-10}).

Levofloxacin has been shown to be active against most strains of the following microorganisms, both *in vitro* and in clinical infections as described in the INDICATIONS AND USAGE section:

AEROBIC GRAM-POSITIVE MICROORGANISMS
Corynebacterium species*
Staphylococcus aureus
Staphylococcus epidermidis
Streptococcus pneumoniae
Streptococcus (Groups C/F)
Streptococcus (Group G)
Viridans group streptococci

AEROBIC GRAM-NEGATIVE MICROORGANISMS
Acinetobacter lwoffii
Haemophilus influenzae
Serratia marcescens

*Efficacy for this organism was studied in fewer than 10 infections.

The following *in vitro* data are also available, but their clinical significance in ophthalmic infections is unknown. The safety and effectiveness of levofloxacin in treating ophthalmological infections due to these microorganisms have not been established in adequate and well-controlled trials.

These organisms are considered susceptible when evaluated using systemic breakpoints. However, a correlation between the *in vitro* systemic breakpoint and ophthalmological efficacy has not been established. The list of organisms is provided as guidance only in assessing the potential treatment of conjunctival infections. Levofloxacin exhibits *in vitro* minimal inhibitory concentrations (MICs) of 2 µg/mL or less (systemic susceptible breakpoint) against most (≥90%) strains of the following ocular pathogens.

AEROBIC GRAM-POSITIVE MICROORGANISMS
Enterococcus faecalis
Staphylococcus saprophyticus
Streptococcus agalactiae
Streptococcus pyogenes

AEROBIC GRAM-NEGATIVE MICROORGANISMS
Acinetobacter anitratus
Acinetobacter baumannii
Citrobacter diversus
Citrobacter freundii
Enterobacter aerogenes
Enterobacter agglomerans
Enterobacter cloacae
Escherichia coli
Haemophilus parainfluenzae
Klebsiella oxytoca
Klebsiella pneumoniae
Legionella pneumophila
Moraxella catarrhalis
Morganella morganii
Neisseria gonorrhoeae
Proteus mirabilis
Proteus vulgaris
Providencia rettgeri
Providencia stuartii
Pseudomonas aeruginosa
Pseudomonas fluorescens

Clinical Studies: In randomized, double-masked, multicenter controlled clinical trials where patients were dosed for 5 days, QUIXIN® demonstrated clinical cures in 79% of patients treated for bacterial conjunctivitis on the final study visit day (day 6-10). Microbial outcomes for the same clinical trials demonstrated an eradication rate for presumed pathogens of 90%.

Indications And Usage: QUIXIN® solution is indicated for the treatment of bacterial conjunctivitis caused by susceptible strains of the following organisms:

AEROBIC GRAM-POSITIVE MICROORGANISMS
Corynebacterium species*
Staphylococcus aureus
Staphylococcus epidermidis
Streptococcus pneumoniae
Streptococcus (Groups C/F)
Streptococcus (Group G)
Viridans group streptococci

AEROBIC GRAM-NEGATIVE MICROORGANISMS
Acinetobacter lwoffii
Haemophilus influenzae
Serratia marcescens

*Efficacy for this organism was studied in fewer than 10 infections.

Contraindications: QUIXIN® solution is contraindicated in patients with a history of hypersensitivity to levofloxacin, to other quinolones, or to any of the components in this medication.

Warnings: NOT FOR INJECTION.
QUIXIN® solution should not be injected subconjunctivally, nor should it be introduced directly into the anterior chamber of the eye.
In patients receiving systemic quinolones, serious and occasionally fatal hypersensitivity (anaphylactic) reactions have been reported, some following the first dose. Some reactions were accompanied by cardiovascular collapse, loss of consciousness, angioedema (including laryngeal, pharyngeal or facial edema), airway obstruction, dyspnea, urticaria, and itching. If an allergic reaction to levofloxacin occurs, discontinue the drug. Serious acute hypersensitivity reactions may require immediate emergency treatment. Oxygen and airway management should be administered as clinically indicated.

Precautions:

General:
As with other anti-infectives, prolonged use may result in overgrowth of non-susceptible organisms, including fungi. If superinfection occurs, discontinue use and institute alternative therapy. Whenever clinical judgment dictates, the patient should be examined with the aid of magnification, such as slit-lamp biomicroscopy, and, where appropriate, fluorescein staining.
Patients should be advised not to wear contact lenses if they have signs and symptoms of bacterial conjunctivitis.

Information for Patients:
Avoid contaminating the applicator tip with material from the eye, fingers or other source. Systemic quinolones have been associated with hypersensitivity reactions, even following a single dose. Discontinue use immediately and contact your physician at the first sign of a rash or allergic reaction.

Drug Interactions:
Specific drug interaction studies have not been conducted with QUIXIN®. However, the systemic administration of some quinolones has been shown to elevate plasma concentrations of theophylline, interfere with the metabolism of caffeine, and enhance the effects of the oral anticoagulant warfarin and its derivatives, and has been associated with transient elevations in serum creatinine in patients receiving systemic cyclosporine concomitantly.

Carcinogenesis, Mutagenesis, Impairment of Fertility:
In a long term carcinogenicity study in rats, levofloxacin exhibited no carcinogenic or tumorigenic potential following daily dietary administration for 2 years; the highest dose (100 mg/kg/day) was 875 times the highest recommended human ophthalmic dose.
Levofloxacin was not mutagenic in the following assays: Ames bacterial mutation assay (*S. typhimurium* and *E. coli*), CHO/HGPRT forward mutation assay, mouse micronucleus test, mouse dominant lethal test, rat unscheduled DNA synthesis assay, and the *in vivo* mouse sister chromatid exchange assay. It was positive in the *in vitro* chromosomal aberration (CHL cell line) and *in vitro* sister chromatid exchange (CHL/IU cell line) assays.
Levofloxacin caused no impairment of fertility or reproduction in rats at oral doses as high as 360 mg/kg/day, corresponding to 3,150 times the highest recommended human ophthalmic dose.

Pregnancy: Teratogenic Effects. Pregnancy Category C:
Levofloxacin at oral doses of 810 mg/kg/day in rats, which corresponds to approximately 7,000 times the highest recommended human ophthalmic dose, caused decreased fetal body weight and increased fetal mortality.
No teratogenic effect was observed when rabbits were dosed orally as high as 50 mg/kg/day, which corresponds to approximately 400 times the highest recommended maximum human ophthalmic dose, or when dosed intravenously as high as 25 mg/kg/day, corresponding to approximately 200 times the highest recommended human ophthalmic dose.
There are, however, no adequate and well-controlled studies in pregnant women. Levofloxacin should be used during pregnancy only if the potential benefit justifies the potential risk to the fetus.

Nursing Mothers:
Levofloxacin has not been measured in human milk. Based upon data from ofloxacin, it can be presumed that levofloxacin is excreted in human milk. Caution should be exercised when QUIXIN® is administered to a nursing mother.

Pediatric Use:
Safety and effectiveness in infants below the age of one year have not been established. Oral administration of quinolones has been shown to cause arthropathy in immature animals. There is no evidence that the ophthalmic administration of levofloxacin has any effect on weight bearing joints.

Geriatric Use:
No overall differences in safety or effectiveness have been observed between elderly and other adult patients.

Adverse Reactions: The most frequently reported adverse events in the overall study population were transient decreased vision, fever, foreign body sensation, headache, transient ocular burning, ocular pain or discomfort, pharyngitis and photophobia. These events occurred in approximately 1-3% of patients. Other reported reactions occurring in less than 1% of patients included allergic reactions, lid edema, ocular dryness, and ocular itching.

Dosage and Administration:
Days 1 and 2:
Instill one to two drops in the affected eye(s) every 2 hours while awake, up to 8 times per day.
Days 3 through 7:
Instill one to two drops in the affected eye(s) every 4 hours while awake, up to 4 times per day.
How Supplied: QUIXIN® (levofloxacin ophthalmic solution) 0.5% is supplied in a white, low density polyethylene bottle with a controlled dropper tip and a tan, high density polyethylene cap in the following size:

5 mL fill in 5 cc container - NDC 68669-135-05
Storage:
Store at 15° – 25°C (59° – 77°F).
Rx Only.
Manufactured by:
Santen Oy, P.O. Box 33, FIN-33721 Tampere, Finland
Santen†
Marketed by:
VISTAKON® Pharmaceuticals, LLC
Jacksonville, FL 32256 USA
Licensed from:
Daiichi Pharmaceutical Co., Ltd., Tokyo, Japan

U.S. PAT. NO. 5,053,407
Vistakon Pharmaceuticals, LLC
March 2004 Version
Shown in Product Identification Guide, page 106

Wyeth Pharmaceuticals
Division of Wyeth
P.O. BOX 8299
PHILADELPHIA, PA 19101

PHOSPHOLINE IODIDE® ℞
(echothiophate iodide for ophthalmic solution)

SECTION 8

INTRAOCULAR PRODUCT INFORMATION

The information concerning each product in this section has been prepared by the manufacturer, and edited and approved by the manufacturer's medical department, medical director, or medical counsel.

For those products that have official package circulars, the descriptions in *Physicians' Desk Reference For Ophthalmic Medicines* must be in full compliance with Food and Drug Administration regulations. For more information, please turn to the Foreword. In presenting the following material, the publisher is not necessarily advocating the use of any product listed.

Bausch & Lomb, Incorporated
**180 EAST VIA VERDE
SAN DIMAS, CA 91773**

Direct Inquiries to:
Customer Services (800) 338-2020

Bausch & Lomb, Incorporated, manufactures a complete line of ophthalmic products, including refractive surgery systems, foldable and PMMA intraocular lenses, phacoemulsification and vitreoretinal microsurgical equipment, handheld ophthalmic surgical instruments, and viscoelastics.

Bausch & Lomb, Incorporated, manufactures and distributes refractive surgery products including microkeratomes, excimer laser systems and disposable blades. Intraocular lens products include silicone one-piece foldable IOLs, which can be inserted through incisions of less than 3mm incision.

Bausch & Lomb, Incorporated, also offers the Joffort System®, a line of three-piece foldable lenses, plate haptic lenses with single-handed Passport® lens inserters, and the Hydroview® and Meridian Composite Hydrogel Foldable UV-Absorbing IOL. Bausch & Lomb, Incorporated also distributes Amvisc® and Amvisc® Plus sodium hyaluronate, Ocucoat® methylcellulose along with the Millennium™ Microsurgical Phacoemulsification system.

Bausch & Lomb, Incorporated, provides a wide selection of pre-market approved lenses available for posterior and anterior chamber. IOLs are available in many styles, including one-piece designs and special high and low diopter powers. Bausch & Lomb, Incorporated offers Vitrasert® Sterile intravitreal implant with Cytovene (ganciclovir 4.5 mg) for the treatment of CMV retinitis.

For information on refractive surgery systems or intraocular lenses or any other products, please contact your Bausch & Lomb, Incorporated sales representative at 800-338-2020.

AMVISC® PLUS ℞
(sodium hyaluronate)

Description: AMVISC® PLUS is a sterile nonpyrogenic solution of sodium hyaluronate. AMVISC® PLUS contains 16 mg/mL of sodium hyaluronate dissolved in a physiological sodium chloride phosphate buffer solution (pH 6.8 – 7.6). In the limit of zero shear rate (1), the viscosity is 132,000 cP (132 Pa s) at 25°C and the osmolality is approximately 340 milliosmoles.

Characteristics: Sodium hyaluronate is a high molecular weight polysaccharide composed of sodium glucuronate and N-acetylglucosamine. Sodium hyaluronate is ubiquitously distributed throughout the tissues of the body and is present in high concentrations in such tissues as vitreous humor, synovial fluid, umbilical cord and the dermis of rooster combs. Sodium hyaluronate functions as a tissue lubricant (1,2) and it is thought to play an important role in modulating the interactions between adjacent tissues. It can also act as a viscoelastic support maintaining a separation between tissues. Sodium hyaluronate prepared from different materials may have different molecular weights but is thought to have the same chemical structure. Sodium hyaluronate is also elaborated by certain bacteria as a protective substance. Those bacteria may be cultured by fermentation process to yield sodium hyaluronate. The sodium hyaluronate in AMVISC® PLUS is prepared from the dermis of rooster combs (2). It has a molecular weight greater than 1,000,000, is reported to be nonantigenic (3,4), does not cause foreign body reactions, is nonpyrogenic and is well tolerated in human eyes (5). AMVISC® PLUS does not interfere with normal wound healing processes.

Indications: AMVISC® PLUS is indicated for use as a surgical aid in ophthalmic anterior (6) and posterior (5) segment procedures including • extraction of a cataract • implantation of an intraocular lens (IOL) • corneal transplantation surgery • glaucoma filtering surgery • surgical procedures to reattach the retina.

Because of its lubricating and viscoelastic properties, transparency and ability to protect corneal endothelial cells (7), AMVISC® PLUS helps maintain anterior chamber depth and visibility, minimizes interaction between tissues, and acts as a tamponade and vitreous substitute during retina reattachment surgery. AMVISC® PLUS also preserves tissue integrity and good visibility when used to fill the anterior and posterior segments of the eye following open sky procedures.

Contraindications: At the present time there are no contraindications to the use of AMVISC® PLUS when used as a surgical aid in ophthalmic surgical procedures.

Applications:
1. Cataract surgery and IOL implantation—The required amount of AMVISC® PLUS is slowly infused through a needle or cannula into the anterior chamber. The protective effect of AMVISC® PLUS as an aid is optimized when the injection is performed prior to cataract extraction and insertion of the IOL and is effective for both intra- and extracapsular cataract procedures. AMVISC® PLUS may be applied to the IOL prior to insertion. Additional AMVISC® PLUS can be injected as required to facilitate surgical procedures (SEE PRECAUTIONS).
2. Corneal transplant surgery—The corneal button is removed and the anterior chamber filled with AMVISC® PLUS until it is level with the surface of the cornea. The donor graft is then placed on top of the AMVISC® PLUS and sutured into place. Additional AMVISC® PLUS can be used as required to aid in surgical procedures (SEE PRECAUTIONS).
3. Glaucoma filtration surgery—AMVISC® PLUS is injected through a corneal paracentesis to restore and maintain anterior chamber volume during the performance of the trabeculectomy. Additional AMVISC® PLUS can be used as required to aid in the surgical procedures (SEE PRECAUTIONS).
4. Intraocular injection in conjunction with scleral buckling procedures for retina reattachment—After release of subretinal fluid and development of buckling by tying the mattress sutures, air is injected into the vitreous cavity and then exchanged with AMVISC® PLUS injected through a needle (22 to 30 gauge) passed via the pars plana epithelium. The volume of AMVISC® PLUS injected (2–4 mL) will vary with the volume of the subretinal fluid released and the space occupied by the buckle.

Precautions: Those precautions normally considered during anterior segment and retina reattachment procedures are recommended. There may be increased intraocular pressure following surgery (8) caused by preexisting glaucoma or by the surgery itself. For these reasons the following precautions should be considered.
• An excess quantity of AMVISC® PLUS should not be used. • AMVISC® PLUS should be removed from the anterior chamber at the end of surgery to prevent or minimize post-operative intraocular pressure increases (spikes). • If the postoperative intraocular pressure increases above expected values, correcting therapy should be administered. • AMVISC® PLUS is prepared from a biological source and the physician should be aware of the possible effects of using any biological materials. • Reuse of cannula should be avoided. Even after cleaning and rinsing, resterilized cannula could release particulate matter as AMVISC®

Continued on next page

Amvisc Plus—Cont.

PLUS is injected. It is recommended that disposable cannula be used when administering AMVISC® PLUS. • There have been isolated reports of diffuse particulates or haziness appearing after injection of AMVISC® PLUS into the eye. While such reports are infrequent and seldom associated with any effects on ocular tissues, the physician should be aware of this occurrence. If observed, the particulate matter should be removed by irrigation and/or aspiration.

Adverse Reactions: Sodium hyaluronate is a natural component of the tissues of the body and is extremely well tolerated in human eyes. Transient postoperative inflammatory reactions were reported in clinical trials (5) and oral and topical steroid preparations were administered. AMVISC® PLUS is tested in animals to determine that each batch is essentially noninflammatory. Since sodium hyaluronate molecules are noninflammatory, any phlogistic response is considered to be caused by the surgical procedures. The best index of the degree of phlogistic response is the postoperative clarity of the vitreous cavity. As outlined above transient postoperative increase in intraocular pressure has been observed following the use of sodium hyaluronate in anterior segment surgery. On rare occasions postoperative reactions including inflammation, corneal edema and corneal decompensation have been reported. The relationship to the use of AMVISC® PLUS has not been established.

Adverse Reaction Reporting: Adverse reactions and/or potentially sight-threatening complications that may be reasonably regarded as AMVISC® PLUS related and that were not previously expected in nature, severity or degree of incidence should be reported to Bausch & Lomb Surgical at 800-338-2020 or 909-624-2020. Outside the USA call your customer service affiliate.

How Supplied: AMVISC® PLUS is a sterile viscoelastic preparation supplied in a disposable glass syringe delivering either 0.5 mL or 0.8 mL of sodium hyaluronate dissolved in physiological sodium chloride phosphate buffer solution. Each mL of AMVISC® PLUS contains 16 mg of sodium hyaluronate. Sodium hydroxide and/or hydrochloric acid are added to adjust pH (if necessary). AMVISC® PLUS is sterile filtered and aseptically transferred to syringes. The filled syringes are sealed and final package sterilized (R). Contents of unopened and undamaged pouches are sterile. Refrigerated AMVISC® PLUS should be allowed to reach room temperature (approximately 20 to 45 minutes, depending on volume) prior to use.

For Intraocular Use: Store at 2–8°C. Protect from freezing.

Caution: Federal U.S. law restricts this device to sale by or on the order of a physician.

References:
1. Arshinoff, Steve A., MD: "Dispersive and Cohesive Viscoelastic Materials in Phacoemulsification;" Ophthalmic Practice; 13:3, 1995.
2. Swann DA. Studies of Hyaluronic Acid. I. The preparation and properties of rooster comb hyaluronic acid. Biochim Biophys Acta 1968; 156:17.
3. Richter W. Non-immunogenicity of purified hyaluronic acid preparations tested by passive cutaneous anaphylaxis. Int Arch Allergy 1974; 47:211.
4. Richter, W, Ryde EM, Zetterstrom EO. Non-immunogenicity of a purified sodium hyaluronate preparation in man. Int Arch Appl Immunol 1979; 59:45.
5. Pruett RC, Schepens CL, Swann DA. Hyaluronic acid vitreous substitute. A six year clinical evaluation. Arch Ophthalmol 1979; 97:2325.
6. Pape LG, Balazs EA. The use of sodium hyaluronate (Healon®) in human anterior segment surgery. Ophthalmol 1980; 87:699.
7. Miller D, Stegmann R. Use of Na-hyaluronate in anterior segment eye surgery. AM Intra-Ocular Implant Soc J 1980; 6:13.
8. Miller D, Stegmann R. The use of Healon® in intraocular lens implantation. Int Ophthalmol Clinics 1982; 22:177.

Size	Reorder #
0.5 mL	60051
0.8 mL	60081

Manufacturer:
Bausch & Lomb Incorporated
Rochester, NY 14609 U.S.A.
EU Authorised Representative: Bausch & Lomb Incorporated
Regent Park • Kingston Road
Leatherhead KT22, 7PQ UK
®/™ Trademarks of Bausch & Lomb Incorporated
© 2003 Copyright of Bausch & Lomb, Incorporated. All rights reserved.
PO11-602-01   PIN 555-200   Rev. 12/96

AMVISC® ℞

Information listed for AMVISC® Plus also applies to AMVISC® with the following exceptions.
- AMVISC® contains 12 mg/mL sodium hyaluronate adjusted to yield approximately 40,000cs dissolved in physiological saline.
- AMVISC® is a sterile viscoelastic preparation supplied in a disposable glass syringe delivering either 0.5 mL or 0.8 mL sodium hyaluronate dissolved in physiological saline. Each mL of AMVISC® contains 12 mg sodium hyaluronate adjusted to yield approximately 40,000cs, 9 mg of Sodium Chloride and q.s. Sterile Water for Injection USP.

For more information regarding AMVISC® Plus or AMVISC® viscoelastics contact: Bausch & Lomb (800) 338-2020 180 East Via Verde San Dimas, CA 91773
®/™ Trademarks of Bausch & Lomb Incorporated

MILLENNIUM™ MICROSURGICAL SYSTEM

The Millennium™ Microsurgical System is a modular designed unit allowing for expanded ophthalmic surgical capability and integration of future technology. It offers anterior and/or posterior segment functionality with unlimited surgeon programming and software upgrades via a CD-ROM. The Millennium™, with Advanced Flow and venturi modules, is the only dual aspiration pump system for ophthalmic surgery, providing both flow and vacuum-based response. Additional features include Dual Linear™ control, surgeon-controlled parameter and mode adjustment, voice confirmation. Functions include ultrasound, bipolar, vitrectomy, illumination, air/fluid, automated scissors, viscous fluid module, LIGHTNING™ high speed vitrectomy cutter, cart with automated IV pole.

Contact your local representative or Bausch & Lomb, Incorporated at 1-800-338-2020.

OCUCOAT® ℞
(2% hydroxypropylmethylcellulose)

Description: OCUCOAT® is a sterile, isotonic, nonpyrogenic viscoelastic solution of highly purified, noninflammatory, 2% hydroxypropylmethylcellulose with a molecular weight greater than 80,000 daltons. OCUCOAT® is supplied in 1 mL syringes. Each mL provides 20 mg/mL of hydroxypropylmethylcellulose dissolved in a physiological balanced salt solution containing 0.49% sodium chloride, 0.075% potassium chloride, 0.048% calcium chloride, 0.03% magnesium chloride, 0.39% sodium acetate, 0.17% sodium citrate and water for injection. The osmolarity of OCUCOAT® is 285 ± 32 mOsM, the viscosity is 4000 ± 1500 cst, and the pH is 7.2±0.4.

Characteristics: OCUCOAT® is an ophthalmic surgical aid for use in anterior segment surgery.
OCUCOAT®:
1. Is a space occupying, tissue protective substance
2. Exhibits excellent flow properties
3. Is completely transparent
4. Is nonantigenic
5. Is easily removed from the anterior chamber
6. Contains no proteins which may cause inflammation or foreign body reactions
7. Requires no refrigeration or restrictive storage conditions
8. Does not interfere with normal wound healing process
9. Clears the trabecular meshwork in 24 hours (98% clearance rate)

Indications: OCUCOAT® is indicated for use as an ophthalmic surgical aid in anterior segment surgical procedures, including cataract extraction and intraocular lens implantation. OCUCOAT® maintains the anterior chamber during cataract surgery and thereby allows for more efficient manipulation with less trauma to the corneal endothelium and other ocular tissues.

Contraindications: At present, there are no known contraindications to the use of OCUCOAT® when used as recommended.

Precautions: Precautions are limited to those normally associated with the ophthalmic surgical procedure being performed.
There may be transient increased intraocular pressure following surgery because of pre-existing glaucoma or due to the surgery itself. For these reasons, the following precautions should be considered:
- OCUCOAT® should be removed from the anterior chamber at the end of surgery.
- If the postoperative intraocular pressure increases above expected values, appropriate therapy should be administered.

Adverse Reactions: Clinical testing of OCUCOAT® showed it to be extremely well tolerated after injection into the human eye.
A transient rise in intraocular pressure postoperatively has been reported in some cases.
Rarely, postoperative inflammatory reactions (iritis, hypopyon), as well as incidents of corneal edema and corneal decompensation, have been reported with viscoelastic agents. Their relationship to OCUCOAT® has not been established.

Clinical Applications: In anterior segment surgery, OCUCOAT® should be carefully introduced into the anterior chamber using a 20 gauge or smaller cannula. OCUCOAT® may be injected into the chamber prior to or following delivery of the crystalline lens. Injection of OCUCOAT® prior to lens delivery will provide additional protection to the corneal endothelium and other ocular tissues. Injection of the material at this point is significant in that a coating of OCUCOAT® may protect the corneal endothelium from possible damage arising from surgical instrumentation during the cataract extraction surgery.

OCUCOAT® may also be used to coat an intraocular lens as well as tips of surgical instruments prior to implantation surgery. Additional OCUCOAT® may be injected during anterior segment surgery to fully maintain the chamber or to replace fluid lost during the surgical procedure. OCUCOAT® should be removed from the anterior chamber at the end of surgery. Rather than aspirate OCUCOAT® from the eye with the OCUCOAT® syringe, it is recommended that OCUCOAT® be aspirated using an automated I/A device, or irrigated using an irrigation syringe or a BSS squeeze bottle.

How Supplied: OCUCOAT® is a sterile, nonpyrogenic, viscoelastic preparation supplied in a 1 mL single use glass syringe with a Luer tip and a Luer lock cannula. OCUCOAT® syringes are aseptically packaged and terminally sterilized. The sterility expiration date is on the outer package.

Store at room temperature; avoid excessive heat (60° C). Protect from light. For intraocular use.

Warning: Manufactured with CFC-12, a substance which harms public health and environment by destroying ozone in the upper atmosphere.

Caution: Federal (USA) law restricts this device to sale by or on the order of a physician.

For intraocular use only. Discard unused contents of OCUCOAT® syringe after each use. Do not resterilize.

Contact your local representative or Bausch & Lomb directly at (800) 338-2020.

KEY TO CONTROLLED SUBSTANCES CATEGORIES

Products listed with the symbols shown below are subject to the Controlled Substances Act of 1970. These drugs are categorized according to their potential for abuse. The greater the potential, the more severe the limitations on their prescription.

CATEGORY	INTERPRETATION
ℂ_II	**HIGH POTENTIAL FOR ABUSE.** Use may lead to severe physical or psychological dependence. Prescriptions must be written in ink, or typewritten and signed by the practitioner. Verbal prescriptions must be confirmed in writing within 72 hours, and may be given only in a genuine emergency. No renewals are permitted.
ℂ_III	**SOME POTENTIAL FOR ABUSE.** Use may lead to low-to-moderate physical dependence or high psychological dependence. Prescriptions may be oral or written. Up to 5 renewals are permitted within 6 months.
ℂ_IV	**LOW POTENTIAL FOR ABUSE.** Use may lead to limited physical or psychological dependence. Prescriptions may be oral or written. Up to 5 renewals are permitted within 6 months.
ℂ_V	**SUBJECT TO STATE AND LOCAL REGULATION.** Abuse potential is low; a prescription may not be required.

KEY TO FDA USE-IN-PREGNANCY RATINGS

The U.S. Food and Drug Administration's use-in-pregnancy rating system weighs the degree to which available information has ruled out risk to the fetus against the drug's potential benefit to the patient. The ratings, and their interpretation, are as follows:

CATEGORY	INTERPRETATION
A	**CONTROLLED STUDIES SHOW NO RISK.** Adequate, well-controlled studies in pregnant women have failed to demonstrate a risk to the fetus in any trimester of pregnancy.
B	**NO EVIDENCE OF RISK IN HUMANS.** Adequate, well-controlled studies in pregnant women have not shown increased risk of fetal abnormalities despite adverse findings in animals, or, in the absence of adequate human studies, animal studies show no fetal risk. The chance of fetal harm is remote, but remains a possibility.
C	**RISK CANNOT BE RULED OUT.** Adequate, well-controlled human studies are lacking, and animal studies have shown a risk to the fetus or are lacking as well. There is a chance of fetal harm if the drug is administered during pregnancy; but the potential benefits may outweigh the potential risk.
D	**POSITIVE EVIDENCE OF RISK.** Studies in humans, or investigational or post-marketing data, have demonstrated fetal risk. Nevertheless, potential benefits from the use of the drug may outweigh the potential risk. For example, the drug may be acceptable if needed in a life-threatening situation or serious disease for which safer drugs cannot be used or are ineffective.
X	**CONTRAINDICATED IN PREGNANCY.** Studies in animals or humans, or investigational or post-marketing reports, have demonstrated positive evidence of fetal abnormalities or risk which clearly outweighs any possible benefit to the patient.

YOUR TRUSTED DRUG INFORMATION SOURCE...

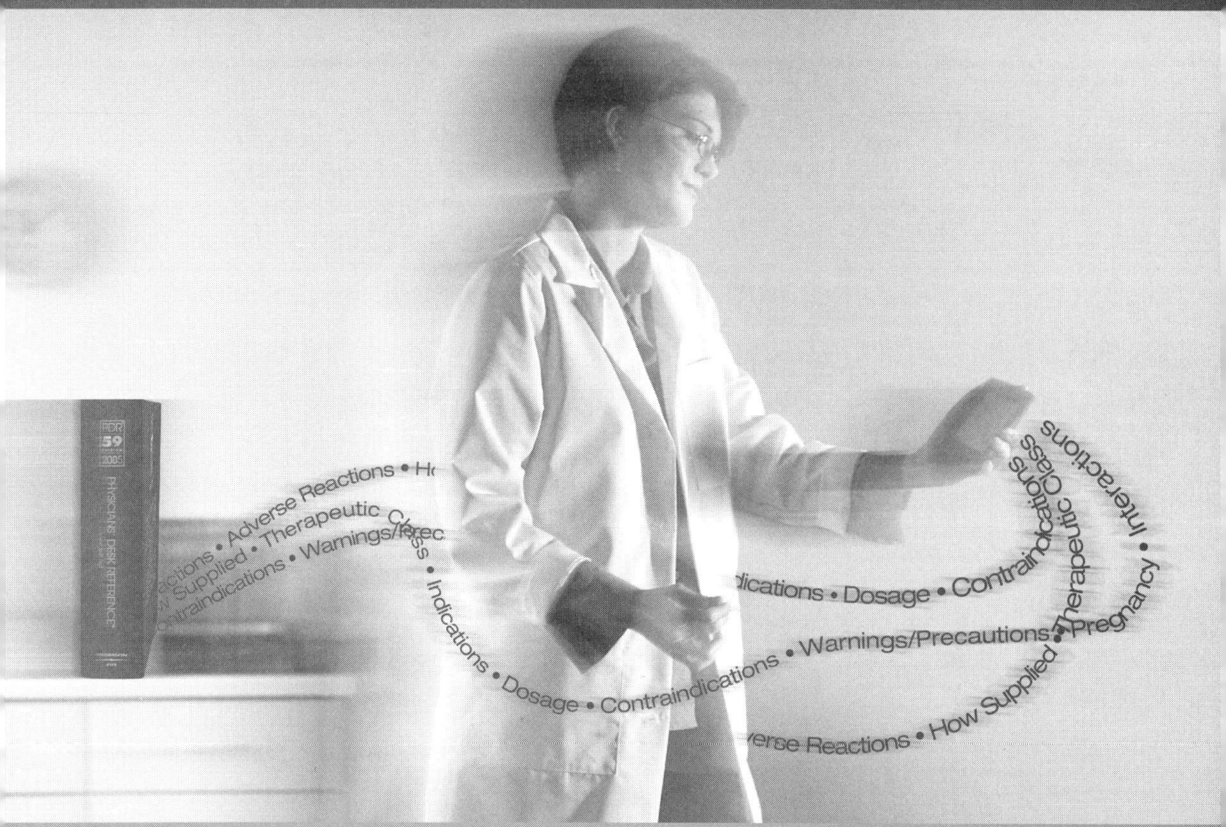

...NOW IN AN INSTANT!

mobilePDR®

With all of the drug information programs available, why not use the one from the company synonymous with drug information? mobilePDR is our *FREE** handheld download available for either your Palm® OS or Pocket PC device.

mobilePDR *offers key drug reference such as:*

- Drug look-up by brand or generic name, therapeutic class or indication
- Drug interaction search between 2 and 32 drugs
- Critical drug updates and information in our "What's New" feature
- Current drug information you trust from PDR updated nightly

And...

- *FREE* – entire program & technical support have no hidden costs
- Downloads quick and easily at **www.PDR.net**
- Uses about 3MB memory on device
- Downloads without interference from your existing desktop or ISP firewall
- Allows you to update content and software whenever you sync – no more installing and uninstalling to get new features

mobilePDR *... Consider the source.*

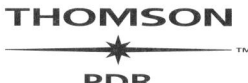

*The download of mobilePDR is free to U.S.-based MDs, DOs, NPs, and PAs in full-time patient practice, and to U.S. medical students and residents.

QUICK. EASY. CONCISE.
THE PERFECT MONTHLY PORTABLE PDR!

SPECIAL PRICE! $49

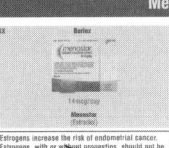

Helpful Drug Comparison Section

Over 1,200 Abbreviated Drug Monographs
270 pages including Dosage, How Supplied, Interactions and Adverse Reactions

Recent Approvals
Monthly comprehensive drug profiles of newly approved products

---

A 12-month subscription to the PDR Monthly Prescribing Guide is yours for the **special offer price of $49!** Get abbreviated FDA-approved drug information on over 2,000 products across all therapeutic classes.

Call us at **800-432-4570** or visit **www.PDRbookstore.com** to place your order today!

THOMSON PDR

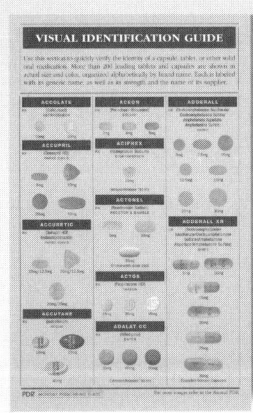

EXCLUSIVE PDR 5-COLOR PILL IMAGES SECTION

16 Page Insert of the Top 600 Oral Medications Every Month!

Mention Keycode: OPH05ES